Essentials *of* PEDIATRIC CARDIOLOGY

Essentials of PEDIATRIC CARDIOLOGY

SECOND EDITION

Anita Khalil
MBBS MD FIAP FIMSA
Consultant Pediatrician and Pediatric Cardiologist
The Heart Centre
Lajpat Nagar, New Delhi, India

Former Director Professor Pediatrics
Maulana Azad Medical College
New Delhi, India

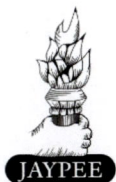

JAYPEE BROTHERS MEDICAL PUBLISHERS
The Health Sciences Publisher
New Delhi | London

Jaypee Brothers Medical Publishers (P) Ltd.

Headquarters

EMCA House
23/23-B, Ansari Road, Daryaganj
New Delhi 110 002, India
Landline: +91-11-23272143,
+91-11-23272703+91-11-23282021,
+91-11-23245672
E-mail: jaypee@jaypeebrothers.com

Overseas Office

JP Medical Ltd.
83, Victoria Street, London
SW1H 0HW (UK)
Phone: +44-20 3170 8910
E-mail: info@jpmedpub.com

Corporate Office

Jaypee Brothers Medical Publishers (P) Ltd.
4838/24, Ansari Road, Daryaganj
New Delhi 110 002, India
Phone: +91-11-43574357
Fax: +91-11-43574314
E-mail: jaypee@jaypeebrothers.com

EU GPSR Authorised Representative
Logos Europe, 9 rue Nicolas Poussin
17000, La Rochelle, France
Phone: +33 (0) 6 67 93 73 78
E-mail: Contact@logoseurope.eu

Website: www.jaypeebrothers.com
Website: www.jaypeedigital.com

© 2011 Jaypee Brothers Medical Publishers

The views and opinions expressed in this book are solely those of the original contributor(s)/author(s) and do not necessarily represent those of editor(s) of the book.

All rights reserved. No part of this publication may be reproduced, stored or transmitted in any form or by any means, electronic, mechanical, photocopying, recording or otherwise, without the prior permission in writing of the publishers.

All brand names and product names used in this book are trade names, service marks, trademarks or registered trademarks of their respective owners. The publisher is not associated with any product or vendor mentioned in this book.

Medical knowledge and practice change constantly. This book is designed to provide accurate, authoritative information about the subject matter in question. However, readers are advised to check the most current information available on procedures included and check information from the manufacturer of each product to be administered, to verify the recommended dose, formula, method and duration of administration, adverse effects and contraindications. It is the responsibility of the practitioner to take all appropriate safety precautions. Neither the publisher nor the author(s)/editor(s) assume any liability for any injury and/or damage to persons or property arising from or related to use of material in this book.

This book is sold on the understanding that the publisher is not engaged in providing professional medical services. If such advice or services are required, the services of a competent medical professional should be sought.

Every effort has been made where necessary to contact holders of copyright to obtain permission to reproduce copyright material. If any have been inadvertently overlooked, the publisher will be pleased to make the necessary arrangements at the first opportunity. The **CD/DVD-ROM** (if any) provided in the sealed envelope with this book is complimentary and free of cost. **Not meant for sale**.

Inquiries for bulk sales may be solicited at: jaypee@jaypeebrothers.com

Essentials of Pediatric Cardiology

First Edition: 2003
Second Edition: 2011, **Reprint: 2025**

ISBN 978-81-8448-993-4
Typeset at JPBMP typesetting unit

Printed at: Samrat Offset Pvt. Ltd.

Foreword

The field of cardiology is generally viewed as difficult by the practical pediatricians. Understandably, there is some disinclination towards adopting this specialty as an area of particular interest. Also, often, there is a tendency to refer the pediatric cardiology cases directly to a "specialist". This trend can result in suboptimal management and care for some of the cardiac patients during the most demanding period of their lives—infancy and childhood.

The essential of the subject for pediatric practice can be presented and taught in a simplified manner. The author in her publication has endeavored to present state-of-art information on the important aspect of pediatric cardiology in a lucid and simplified manner. The topics chosen are of direct relevance to the practicing pediatricians and the residents. This book will act as a source of inspiration to the practicing pediatricians and infuse interest in residents and younger colleagues.

I would like to congratulate Dr Anita Khalil for carrying on the hard work on the superspecialty of pediatric cardiology even after relinquishing the charge of the subspecialty chapter on pediatric cardiology. This second edition of the first monograph which was released in 2003, is a testimony of her unstinted dedication to the subject.

Panna Choudhury
National President
Indian Academy of Pediatrics, 2009

Preface to the Second Edition

Since the publication of 1st edition of "Essentials of Pediatric Cardiology" in 2003, important advances have been made not only in the diagnosis but also in the medical and surgical management of children with congenital and acquired heart diseases. These advances make it necessary to update the book. Extensive updating and revisions have been made to the level that is appropriate for primary care physicians, residents, postgraduates and medical students. Despite extensive revision, the book maintains the original goal of providing non-cardiologists with fundamental and practical information for the management of children with cardiac problems. Thus, the general layout of the book has been preserved to serve as a small reference book, avoiding excessive theoretical details and surgical techniques found in superspecialty textbooks.

Pediatric cardiology is now recognized as a distinct superspecialty, and dedicated fellowship programs are being conducted in some selected superspecialty centers. Quality of pediatric cardiac care has also improved significantly since the last few years, and this has been made possible by the new superspecialty hospitals that are opening all over and they are offering specialized treatment in pediatric cardiology and other specialties, for the needy children who do not have the ability to go overseas for treatment. This is just the beginning, the existing number of centers is not enough to take care of all the affected children. Many more centers have to be opened and many more pediatricians and pediatric cardiologists have to be trained.

Topics (like) congestive heart failure, hypertension, arrhythmias, congenital heart disease and rheumatic heart disease, rheumatic fever, myocardial diseases, cardiac imaging, perinatal cardiology, etc. are some of the chapters in the book that have been dealt with in a simplified manner and recent advances concerning the topics have also been incorporated to make the reading comprehensive.

I wish to acknowledge the assistance extended towards me in getting the manuscript ready. Mr PN Shukla has always been of immense help to me for the last 25 years and now his grandson Shashank Mishra was most helpful with his untiring efforts to get the manuscript ready in a record period of time. M/s Jaypee Brothers Medical Publishers (P) Ltd., New Delhi, India, have been generous enough to come forward to publish the book for me, it is always the last minute dash which is the story of most of the projects. Lastly, I would like to thank a large number of well wishers, all the members of my family especially my husband and my two daughters who have always been a huge source of encouragement and a tower of strength for any venture that I have embarked upon.

Anita Khalil

Preface to the First Edition

Cardiovascular problems make up a significant proportion of the medical and surgical emergencies which arise in the neonatal period and early infancy. Despite the existence of highly specialized forms of investigations (echocardiography, angiocardiography, cardiac catheterization) which enable a precise diagnosis to be made of all congenital cardiopathies, the task of the pediatricians first and later on the pediatric cardiologists—is not as simple in the first few months of life as it is later on in older children with cardiac lesions. Since early diagnosis of congenital heart disease is the rule, it is the responsibility of the professionals to decide which patient would need domiciliary care and who should be referred to an advanced center for specialized care.

Since I started teaching pediatric cardiology, I felt that there was a need for a book that was written primarily for non-cardiologists, such as medical students, residents and practitioners. Although many excellent pediatric cardiology textbooks are available, they are not very helpful to the non-cardiologists, since they are filled with many details that are beyond the comprehension of the practitioners. This book is intended to meet the need of non-cardiologist practitioners for improving their skills in arriving at a clinical diagnosis of cardiac problems, using basic tools available in their place of work. Although areas of clinical diagnosis, e.g. History taking, physical examination and routine investigations like X-ray chest and electrocardiography have not been dealt with, this book serves as a quick reference to pediatric cardiology, e.g. there are updated chapters on congestive cardiac failure, hypertension, arrythmias with special mention on pacemakers, etc. An attempt has been made to update the knowledge of the practising pediatricians and postgraduates on the subject of pediatric cardiology, so that judicious referral and detailed investigations are carried out in deserving patients. I hope the readers would find the contents stimulating.

Anita Khalil

Contents

1. Congestive Cardiac Failure — 1
2. Hypertension in Children — 22
3. Arrhythmias — 42
4. Pacemakers in Children — 73
5. Cardiac Imaging — 77
6. Congenital Heart Disease: General Aspects — 101
7. Congenital Heart Disease: Specific Lesions Diagnostic Approach to Congenital Heart Disease — 122
8. Perinatal Cardiology — 214
9. Rheumatic Fever: Recent Advances — 263
10. Rheumatic Heart Disease: Valvular Defects — 283
11. Myocardial Disorders — 304
12. Cardiac Infections — 357
13. Primary Prevention of Atherosclerotic Cardiovascular Disease Beginning in Childhood — 389

Index — *411*

CHAPTER 1

Congestive Cardiac Failure

Congestive cardiac failure (CCF) is defined as the inability of the heart to maintain an output required to sustain the metabolic needs of the body at rest or during stress (systolic failure) without evoking certain compensatory mechanisms.[1] In addition, inability of the heart to receive blood into ventricular cavities at low pressure during diastole (diastolic failure).[2] Presence of myocardial failure distinguishes CCF from peripheral circulatory congestion resulting from mechanical obstruction as in constrictive pericarditis.

Congestive cardiac failure by itself is not a diagnosis. It is a manifestation of an underlying anatomical or pathological cause affecting the heart.

HEART FAILURE SYNDROMES

Clinically, heart failure syndromes are of 3 types:
1. *Shock:* This is a situation of acute circulatory collapse (low output state) which has to be treated immediately. The etiological factors include septicemia, gastroenteritis, hypoplastic left heart syndrome, aortic atresia, cardiomyopathies, etc.
2. *Acute heart failure:* This is an emergency when there is acute decompensation of left ventricle due to fluid overload, hypertensive crisis, rupture of papillary muscle, severe mitral stenosis, etc.
3. *Chronic heart failure:* This is that situation when there is stable balance between diminished systemic flow and activation of compensatory hemodynamic and neurohormonal responses.

ETIOPATHOGENESIS

Though diastolic failure was not recognized earlier, systolic failure however is much more common. The causes of systolic cardiac failure can be divided into two groups according to age (Table 1.1). The commonest cause of CCF in infants is congenital heart disease, whereas in older children, it is rheumatic fever and rheumatic heart disease.

Table 1.1: Causes of CCF at different ages

1. Fetus
   a. Severe anemia -hydrops fetalis
   b. Supraventricular tachycardia
   c. Complete heart block
2. Neonate
   a. Birth to 1 week
      - Hypoplastic left heart syndrome
      - Birth asphyxia-hypoxic cardiomyopathy
      - Transposition of great arteries (TGA)
      - Coarctation of aorta-systemic A-V fistula
   b. 1 week to 1 month
      - Coarctation of aorta
      - TGA
      - Endocardial fibroelastosis
      - Large shunts (VSD, PDA)
      - Viral myocarditis
      - Cor pulmonale
      - Fluid overload
3. Infant
   a. 1-3 months
      - TGA
      - Endocardial fibroelastosis
      - Total anomalous pulmonary venous connection (TAPVC)
      - Coarctation of aorta
   b. 3-6 months
      - Endocardial fibroelastosis
      - Supraventricular tachycardia
      - Large VSD, PDA
      - TGA
   c. 6-12 months
      - Large VSD, PDA
      - Endocardial fibroelastosis
      - Pulmonary venous anomaly
4. Toddler
   - Supraventricular tachycardia
   - Large VSD, PDA
   - AV malformation

Contd...

Contd...
- Acute hypertensive crisis
- Anomalous origin of left coronary artery (LCA)
5. Older child and adolescent
   - Rheumatic carditis
   - Infective endocarditis
   - Acute glomerulonephritis
   - Viral myocarditis
   - Dilated cardiomyopathy
   - Thyrotoxicosis
   - Constrictive pericarditis
   - Drugs, e.g. Adriamycin
   - Hemosiderosis

Congenital Heart Disease (CHD)

Infants with CHD have a relatively healthy myocardium and if they do not manifest with CCF in the first year of life, they are not likely to do so in the next 10 years unless complicated by anemia, infection, arrhythmias or bacterial endocarditis. Congenital heart disease with volume or pressure overload is the most common cause of CCF in the pediatric age group. Lesions with volume overload such as ventricular septal defect (VSD), patent ductus arteriosus (PDA) and endocardial cushion defect (ECD) are the commonest cause of CCF in the first 6 months of life. Infants with left to right shunt tend to develop CCF around 6-8 weeks of life. At birth, the pulmonary vascular resistance is high but there is a gradual fall during the first few weeks of life. Patients with transposition of great arteries (TGA) with intact ventricular septum and total anomalous pulmonary venous connection (obstructed) manifest with CCF within the first week of life, otherwise TGA with ventricular septal defect or unobstructed anomalous pulmonary venous connection, the CCF develops by the age of 6-8 weeks following physiological fall in pulmonary vascular resistance.

Acquired Heart Diseases

1. *Myocardial disease:* Viral myocarditis usually occurs in children more than 1 year of age. The commonest cause of myocarditis is Coxsackie B virus infection leading on to dilated cardiomyopathy. There are other viral infections, e.g. adenoviruses, cytomegaloviruses, etc. which also give rise to myocarditis.[3] The primary myocardial disease causing CCF include glycogen storage disease, endocardial fibroelastosis, medial necrosis of coronary arteries and anomalous origin of left coronary artery.
2. *Metabolic abnormalities:* Severe hypoxia and acidosis, as well as hypoglycemia and hypocalcemia can cause CCF in newborns.

Arrhythmias

Three fourths of patients with arrhythmias leading on to CCF are below 4 months of age. Heart rates above 180 per minute tend to precipitate CCF and if the tachycardia persists for 24 hours, 20% of patients develop CCF and after 48 hours, 50% go into CCF. There is a tendency for the recurrence of arrhythmias if the onset is after 4 months of age.

Anemia

In children with normal hearts, protracted decrease of hemoglobin levels of around 5 gm/dl can result in CCF, whereas higher hemoglobin level (7-8 gm%) can precipitate CCF in children with diseased cardiac status. Infants are more prone to CCF because of prolonged anemia.

Rheumatic Fever and Rheumatic Heart Disease

Rheumatic carditis and valvular involvement of rheumatic etiology are the commonest cause of CCF in older children.[4]

Hypertension

Systemic hypertension due to acute glomerulonephritis and aorto-arteritis are the next common causes leading on to CCF in older children and adolescents.

PATHOPHYSIOLOGY

The manifestations of CCF are caused largely by the physiological compensations called into play to combat the inadequate oxygen delivery. The oxygen delivery is dependent on the oxygen content of blood and the cardiac output, while the cardiac output in turn is determined by the preload, afterload, myocardial contractility and the heart rate (Flow chart 1.1).

a. **Preload**—Filling volume of the heart. It is basically a function of venous return and compliance of ventricles.
b. **Afterload**—The resistance the ventricles face on ejection of blood. It can be described as the intra-venous wall stress that develops during ejection and is determined by ventricular pressure, diameter and wall thickness. The simplest approximation of afterload can be obtained by the magnitude of aortic pressure.
c. **Myocardial contractility**—Signifies the efficiency and vigour of the contraction of the myocardium. A decrease in the contractility, the reserve of the ventricles as a pump becomes insufficient to meet body requirement and therefore CCF is the systemic manifestation of inadequate pump function of heart. The fall in cardiac output leads to activation of several neurohormonal

Flow chart 1.1: Neurohormonal and compensatory mechanisms in heart failure[5]

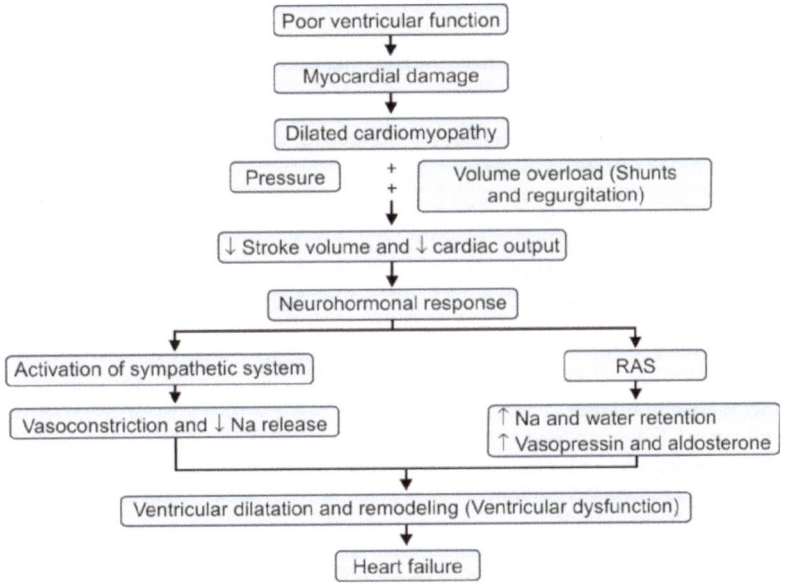

compensatory mechanisms aimed at improving the mechanical environment of the heart. Activation of sympathetic system tries to maintain cardiac output with an increase in heart rate increased myocardial contractility and peripheral vasoconstriction. Similarly stimulation of renin - angiotensin system (RAS) also helps to improve the cardiac output and maintain perfusion of vital organs with retention of salt and water which sometimes unfortunately overreacts and this results in further deterioration of cardiac contractility, establishing a vicious cycle of failure begetting failure.[6]

d. **Heart rate** is directly related to the cardiac output and is used as a compensatory mechanism by the body to maintain optimal cardiac output by increasing or decreasing the heart rate. The cardiac output is the net product of heart rate and the stroke volume per beat. If the stroke volume falls, the heart rate increases in response to increased catecholamine secretion to compensate for the fall in cardiac output.

CLASSIFICATION

The classification of heart failure as per NYHA and Ross is given in Tables 1.2 and 1.3 respectively.

Table 1.2: Heart failure-functional classification (NYHA)

Class I	Asymptomatic
	No limitation to ordinary physical activity-no fatigue, dyspnea or palpitation.
Class II	Mild-limitation of physical activity
	Unable to climb stairs.
Class III	Moderate-Marked limitation
	Shortness of breath on walking on flat surface.
Class IV	Severe-Orthopnea-breathless even at rest
	No physical activity is possible

Table 1.3: Ross classification

	Heart failure in infants
Mild	• Intake < 3.5 ounces/feed
	• Respiratory rate > 50/min.
	• Abnormal respiratory pattern
	• Diastolic filling sounds
	• Hepatomegaly
Moderate	• Intake < 3 ozs/feed or time taken/feed > 40mins
	• Diastolic filling sounds
	• Respiratory rate > 60/min
	• Moderate hepatomegaly
Severe	• Heart rate > 170/min
	• Decreased perfusion - mottling of hands and feet
	• Severe hepatomegaly

CLINICAL FEATURES

Neonates

1. In newborn infants, CCF manifests with respiratory distress and feeding difficulty.
2. Early onset of poor perfusion—seen as pale, sallow or cyanotic grey complexion.
3. Tachycardia and rhythm disturbances due to hypoxia.
4. Four limb BP measurements—help in confirming or ruling out aortic obstructive lesions, e.g. coarctation of aorta.

5. Critical coarctation or other ductus dependent lesions present between 3-10 days of life as the ductus begins to close, leading on to poor peripheral perfusion.
6. Hyperactive precordium, abnormal heart sounds and murmurs indicate an underlying large shunt leading on to CCF.

Infants

1. Poor feeding with easy fatiguability leading on to failure to thrive, respiratory distress, baseline tachypnea and diaphoresis—features of increased pulmonary flow.
2. Cyanosis, hypotonia and shock—are late manifestations.
3. Slow weight gain—manifesting as facial puffiness, pedal edema.
4. Ventricular septal defect (large)—most common acyanotic heart disease to present in this age group. The two most common models of presentation are:
   a. Progressive CCF in early infancy.
   b. Recurrent episodes of chest infection.
5. Relatively uncommon causes in later infancy, e.g. TAPVR (unobstructed) and anomalous origins of coronary artery from pulmonary artery—lead onto myocardial dysfunction and ventricular dilatation manifesting with features of CCF.

Children and Adolescents

1. Classical manifestations include—progressive exertional dyspnea, anorexia, easy fatigability, abdominal pain, anasarca and pedal edema.
2. Physical examination—tachycardia, gallop rhythm, tachypnea, elevated JVP, enlarged tender liver, pulsatile precordium, cardiomegaly and presence of basal crepitations in the lungs.

MANAGEMENT

The general aims of management are to achieve increase in cardiac performance, augment peripheral perfusion and decrease pulmonary and systematic venous congestion. The initial therapy is aimed at stabilizing the infant's condition for diagnostic purposes, e.g. echocardiography and possibly an angiocardiography also, because in all situations, the decision to intervene surgically or to continue with medical management requires a definitive anatomical diagnosis.

Before starting treatment, a few investigations have to be carried out, which include:

X-ray chest: Cardiomegaly—usual cardiac status of children with CCF (Figs 1.1A and B).

Electrocardiogram: Helpful in diagnosis of underlying heart disease by revealing selective chamber enlargement or hypertrophy.

Echocardiogram: Assessing ventricular function and diagnosing underlying heart defects.

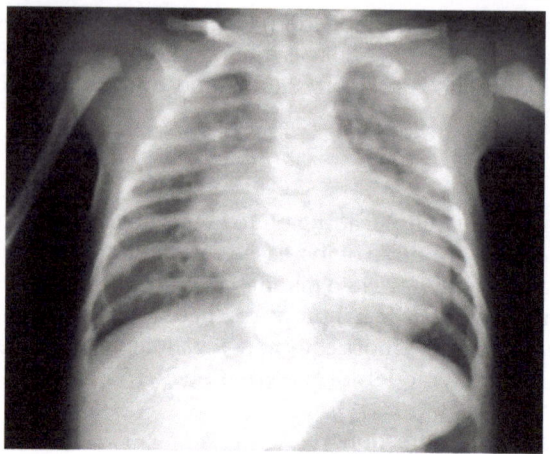

Fig. 1.1A: Chest radiographs of patients with congestive cardiac failure with cardiomegaly

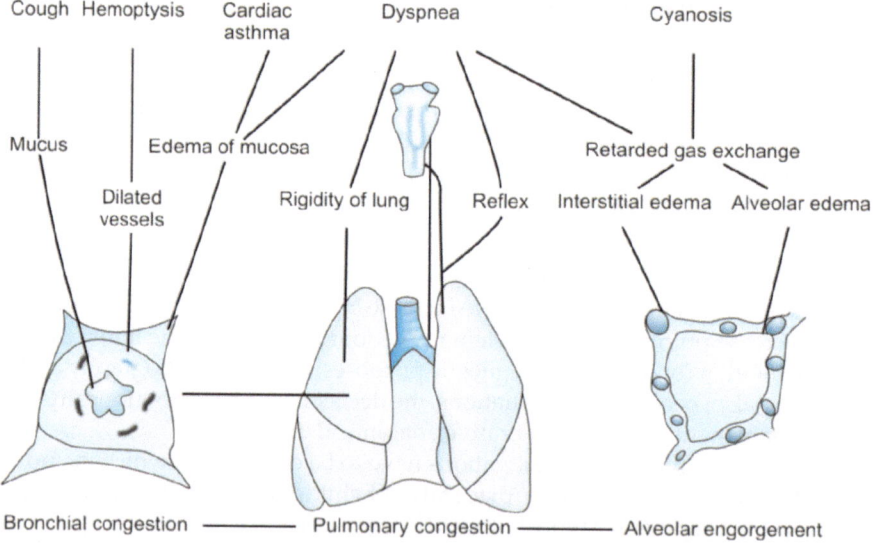

Fig. 1.1B: Clinicopathological correlation of congestive cardiac failure

Serum electrolytes/ABG: May be altered in critically ill patients. The serum sodium may be low, however total body sodium and water are increased.

Cardiac catheterization: Preoperative assessment of complex and complicated cardiac lesions.

MRI: Accurate assessment in complex congenital heart disease.

Myocardial biopsy: It helps in clinching diagnosis in myocarditis.

TREATMENT

Treatment of chronic heart failure includes:
1. Medical
2. Devices
3. Surgical

Medical Therapy—Aims:
1. To reduce morbidity and hospitalization.
2. Improve quality of life, enhance exercise capacity and improved long term survival.
3. To maintain normal growth.
4. To decrease neurohormonal activation and halt or delay the progression of heart failure.

Medical Therapy
1. Non-pharmacological and pharmacological.

Non-Pharmacological-General Therapy
1. *Counselling*—Making parents and patients understand the disease and principles of treatment.
2. *Fluid*—Fluid intake to be restricted in severe cases of CCF.
3. *Salt*—High salt content to be avoided, e.g. pickle, chips, papad, etc.
4. All immunizations should be given.
5. *Regular exercises*—Physiotherapy should be encouraged.
6. *Nutrition*—Diet
   Nutrition has to be emphasized upon, because in chronic CCF failure to thrive and finally growth failure ultimately result because of prolonged undernutrition.

Calorie and Protein Requirement
   Caloric requirement is greater than a normal child—120-160 Kcal/Kg/day.

Caloric density has to be increased to 24-36 Kcal/ounce. This can be achieved by adding corn oil and sugar to the milk or formula in phases. If the patient is not able to accept feeds, then nasogastric feeding may have to be resorted to. Because of its long half life, serum pre-albumin is a more reliable parameter of nutritional status compared to albumin. The children should be advised to avoid the use of extra salt and high sodium containing foods.

Precipitating and aggravating factors in CCF include anemia, hypertension, infective endocarditis, myocarditis, thyrotoxicosis, drug toxicity, fever, infections, arrhythmias and pulmonary embolism. If the patient is not responding well, the aggravating factors should be looked for and managed.

There is some evidence that immunosuppressive therapy may be useful in patients with active myocarditis.

Pharmacological Therapy

Myocardial performance begins to decrease when approximately 20% of the contractile units of the heart are impaired. With further destruction, decompensation sets in rapidly. Renal blood flow is decreased in direct proportion to the reduction in cardiac output. Reduction in renal flow causes increased tubular reabsorption of sodium and water causing an increase in blood volume which results in increased venous pressure (preload) and edema formation. There is an increase in intracellular and extracellular sodium content. The reduced cardiac output is associated with increased ventricular diastolic pressures, the atrial pressure and the systemic vascular resistance, which is related to increased vascular stiffness. The management of CCF consists of a "four pronged attack" for the correction of inadequate cardiac output.
1. Augment myocardial contractility.
2. Improve myocardial performance by reducing the heart size.
3. Reduce cardiac work and thus improve cardiac function.
4. Correct the underlying cause.

Augmenting Myocardial Contractility

Inotropic Drugs

Inotropic drugs improve the myocardial contractility in an acute crisis by the use of dopamine or dobutamine.[7] In a chronic situation using digoxin is an important component of CCF management. The use of inotropic agents has often been disputed using the argument that stimulating the failing myocardium may further damage it and that the heart is already exposed to potent inotropic agents in CCF.[6] On the other hand, an increase in myocardial contractility decreases the preload and reflexly the afterload with consequent diminished oxygen consumption which is beneficial for the failing heart. Digitalis has been demonstrated to be superior to captopril in improving the quality of life.[8] Some of the other non-digitalis ionotropic agents and diuretics are described in Table 1.4.

Digitalis

The digitalis group of drugs act by the inhibition of Na-K ATPase which in turn leads to an increase in intracellular sodium which is exchanged for Ca by the sarcolemmal membrane resulting in better excitation-contraction coupling. Digoxin augments myocardial contractility, reduces preload,

Congestive Cardiac Failure

Table 1.4: Non-digitalis inotropic agents and diuretics

Agent administration	Route of	Dose
Intropic agents		
1. Isoproterenol	IV	0.05-0.5 mcg/kg/min infusion
2. Dopamine	IV	0.05-20.0 mcg/kg/min infusion (maximum dose 50 mcg/kg/min)
3. Dobutamine	IV	5.0-10.0 mcg/kg/min infusion (maximum dose 40 mcg/kg/min)
4. Amrinone	IV	0.75 mg/kg bolus over 2 min then 5-10 mcg/kg/min infusion (maximum dose 10 mg/kg/day)
5. Milrinone	IV	0.25-1 µg/kg

afterload and also myocardial O_2 consumption. It is useful in controlling heart rate in paroxysmal atrial tachycardia and atrial fibrillation. Digoxin has half-life of 36 hours and the initial effect is after 30 minutes and a peak percent is excreted unchanged in the urine. Therapeutic levels of the drug should be maintained between 0.08-0.16 microgram/dl (Table 1.5).

Though rapid digitalization is considered safe in children, slow digitalization may be considered in a less sick child whereby 7 to 10 days would be required to achieve the desired levels by daily maintenance dosing. Special care needs to be taken when administering digoxin with diuretics as hypokalemia induced by loop diuretics precipitates digitalis toxicity. Anorexia, nausea and vomiting are amongst the earliest signs of digitalis intoxication. The most frequent arrhythmia caused by digitalis is premature ventricular beats. First-degree heart block in the form of prolongation of P-R interval necessitates withdrawal of the drug. Any new arrhythmias developing on the drug should be considered to be digoxin related, until proved otherwise. When tachyarrythmias develop from digitalis intoxication, withdrawal of the drug and treatment with oral potassium, phenytoin and

Table 1.5: Recommended doses of digoxin in children

Age	Total digitalizing dose (mcg/kg)	Daily maintenance dose (mcg/kg)
Premature infant	21 IV	5 IV
Full term neonate (up to 3 months)	30 IV	8-10 IV or PO q 12 hr
Infants <2 yr		40-60 PO 10-12 POq 12 hr
Children > 2 yr	30-40 PO	8-IO PO q 12 hr
Higher doses may be used in supraventricular tachycardia		

lidocaine are indicated. Potassium is preferably given orally and must not be given in the presence of hyperkalemia.

Sympathomimetic Agents

Dopamine and dobutamine are the most effective of the sympathomimetic amines used in the management of CCF especially with a view to tide over an acute crisis in patients with compromised peripheral perfusion. Dopamine is a naturally occurring precursor of norepinephrine with actions on dopaminergic and adrenergic receptors. At doses of 1 to 2 µg/kg/min it dilates the renal and mesenteric blood vessels causing an increase in renal blood flow and sodium excretion. At doses of 10 µg/kg/min, it has an inotropic effect on the heart whereas at doses of 10 to 20 µg/kg/min peripheral vasoconstrictive action dominates raising the blood pressure. Higher doses cause generalized vasoconstriction and hence are not useful. A major problem with all sympathomimetics is that of progressive loss of responsiveness which may become evident within 8 hours of continuous infusion. Dobutamine is a synthetic catecholamine with a potent inotropic but poor vasoconstrictive action. It is given in continuous infusions of 2.5 to 10 µg/kg/min and is considered especially useful in cardiogenic shock as it causes no increase in the afterload. These drugs combine inotropic effect with peripheral vasodilatation.[7]

Phosphodiesterase Inhibitors

These drugs combine inotropism with peripheral vasodilatation—reduce afterload and decrease myocardial oxygen demand. They also increase cardiac output, reduce ventricular pressure, enhance ventricular emptying without altering heart rate.

Amrinone is a bipyridine with both positive inotropic effect with peripheral vasodilatation thus reducing afterload. They act by selectively inhibiting a specific phosphodiesterase. They increase the cardiac output, reduce ventricular filling pressure and enhance the ventricular emptying without a change in heart rate and blood pressure. Thus the myocardial oxygen demand is decreased. The drug is administered in dosage of 0.075 mg/kg intravenously initially and then by an infusion of 5-10 µg/kg/min. Side effects include hypotension and reversible thrombocytopenia. It is useful only to tide over an acute situation.

Milrinone is an analog which has been tried orally for prolonged use. It increases exercise capacity and cardiac output. However some studies have shown an increase in long-term mortality precluding its routine use. It is said to be 30-50 times more potent than amrinone and useful in treating those patients who are refractory to standard therapy.

Levosimendan—Most useful drug but is under research trial—will probably replace inotropes in future.

Reducing the Heart Size

Diuretics

The drugs to achieve this objective are diuretics (Table 1.6). By reducing the circulating blood volume, the venous return is decreased causing a reduction in the preload and the ventricular end-diastolic volume. Following the reduction in heart size, myocardial function improves and the cardiac output tends to increase. By reducing the sodium and water content of the arterial wall, its stiffness is reduced. Moreover, loss of sodium and water results in decrease in blood pressure and thus the afterload. It must be kept in mind, however, that the decrease in blood volume by diuretics leads to decreased renal perfusion. If this is achieved vigorously it may result in hypotension and increase in blood urea nitrogen.

The commonest diuretics being used are:

Loop diuretics
- *Furosemide (Lasix):* It does not reduce renal flow. It can be used alone or in combination with a potassium sparing diuretic like spironolactone or amiloride.
- *Side effects*—hyponatremia, hypokalemia and hypochloremic alkalosis.
- *Bumetanide*—an analogue of furosemide.

Table 1.6: Diuretics

Agents	Class	Action	Dose	Side effects
Loop diuretics	Loop	Inhibit Na^+ $2Cl^-$ K^+ Cotransport	PO 4 mg/kg/dose	hyponatremia
			I/V 1-2 mg/kg/dose Up to 6 mg	hypokalemia hypochloremic alkalosis
Bumetanide Ethacrynic acid, torsemide			0.015-0.1 mg/kg/dose	
Thiazide/Thiazide like diuretics Chlorothiazide		Inhibit Na^+Cl^- Cotransport	10-20 mg/kg/dose	hyponatremic alkalosis
Hydrochlorothiazide		Distal tubule	1-2 mg/kg/dose	↑ glucose
Metolazone		-do-		
Indapamide		-do-	0.2-0.4 mg/kg/24 hrs	↑ uric acid
Aldosterone Receptor Antagonists (K^+ Sparing) Spironolactone	collecting duct	↑ Na, ↑ Cl	1-4 mg/kg/day	Gynecomastia
Eplerenone	-do-	↓ K		

- *Torsemide*—Loop diuretic with anti-aldosterone properties. It is better tolerated than furosemide and has comparatively less hypokalemic effect.

In infants, diuretics cause an increase in plasma renin levels in those with a large left to right shunt. To get better results, a thiazide diuretic may be added to an already administered loop diuretic. The thiazide diuretic metolazone, administered in conjunction with a loop diuretic (Furosemide/Torsemide) can be uniquely successful in effecting a diuresis in edematous or diuretic resistant patients.

Although spironolactone and eplerenone are potassium sparing diuretics, their beneficial effects in heart failure are probably less related to their diuretic effects than other effects. Though spironolactone is a drug well established in pediatric practice, eplerenone is a drug in research studies in adults and has not yet been used in children.

Reducing Cardiac Work and Improving Working Environment

With the pump dysfuction, compensatory neurohumoral mechanisms initiate a vicious cycle. Peripheral arteriolar constriction leads to increased wall stress (afterload) whereas venoconstriction results in increased venous return (preload) and high ventricular filling pressure. The normal heart can easily cooperate with increased pre and afterloads, but the failing myocardium working on the lower segment of the Starling's law curve is unable to do so. The rationale for using vasodilators is to improve the working environment of the heart (Table 1.7). Vasodilators make the pump function more efficiently by reducing the workload and ventricular filling pressures without augmenting the contractility and thus the oxygen requirements. The sites of action and doses of various vasodilators are given in Table 1.8.

Table 1.7: Classification of vasodilators

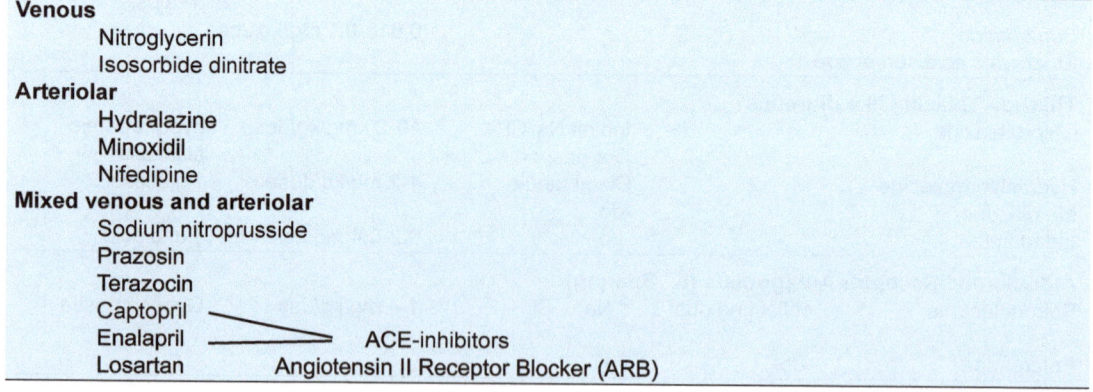

Table 1.8: Doses and mode of administration of vasodilators

Agent	Site of action	Dose	Tolerance
Nitroglycerine	Venous	0.05-20 mcg/kg/min IV infusion	Common
Iso-sorbide dinitrate	Venous	0.01 mg/kg q 6 hr PO (maxi. Dose 2 mg/kg/day)	Common
Nitroprusside	Venous + arteriolar	0.05-1.0 mg/kg/IV q 6 hr	Rare
Hydralazine	Arterial	0.05-1.0 mg/kg/IV q 6 hr 1.7 mg/kg/dose PO	Occasional
Prazosin	Venous + arterial	5.25 mcg/kg/dosePO q 6 hr	Common
Nifedipine	Venous + arterial	0.3 mg/kg/dose q 6 hr PO	Rare
Captopril	Venous + arterial	Neonate: 0.4-1.6 mg/kg/day PO/Infants: 0.5-6.0 mg/kg/day in 3 div doses PO Children: 12.5 mg q 12 hr PO	
Enalapril	Venous + arterial	0.1-0.5 mg kg/day in two div doses, PO	
Losartan	Venous + arterial	0.5-6 mg/kg/day once daily PO	
Minoxidil	Arterial	0.2 mg/kg/day initial dose increase slowly up to 1.0 mg/kg/day PO	Occasional

The drugs (nitroglycerin) acting on veins-increases venous capacitance,[10] thereby reducing venous return, ultimately relieving pulmonary and systemic venous congestion. Arterial dilators (hydralazine) reduce systemic impedance (afterload), thereby increasing cardiac output.

Vascular smooth muscle has certain unique properties. Intracellular calcium ion concentration is increased predominantly by the receptor operated channels and minimally by the potential dependent channels, as most blood vessels resist depolarization. The intracellular calcium regulates the contractile process probably by myosin light chain kinase via calmodulin to phosphorylate myosin light chain.

Despite different mechanisms of action, all vasodilators favorably alter the short term hemodynamic response. Long term trials of some of these drugs have shown continued benefits. Captopril and isosorbide dinitrate improve symptomatic status and exercise capacity. Hydralazine and prazosin, however, were not found consistently more effective than placebo during long term use. There is a higher incidence of tolerance with the use of latter drugs because they ultimately stimulated vasoconstrictor mechanisms that offset the acute vasodilatory response. The long term efficacy of isosorbide dinitrate persists due to its venodilator effect on pulmonary vasculature even though tolerance develops to the arteriolar vasodilation. Angiotensin converting enzyme inhibitors execute multi-pronged action like preventing the degradation of bradykinin and stimulating prostaglandin production thus providing the long term efficacy.[9]

Angiotensin Converting Enzyme Inhibitors (ACE-inhibitors)

The vasodilators also redistribute the blood flow to regional beds. Reduced hospitalization and mortality has been shown with ACE-1 as vasodilator therapy. ACE inhibitors produce their effects through at least three mechanism; inhibition of the angiotension-converting enzyme, inhibition of norepinephrine release from sympathetic nerve endings. ACE-1 are at present considered to be the first line of therapy in mild, moderate, severe or very severe CCF and can be used in monotherapy in mild congestive heart failure. In pediatric practice, patients of CCF showing adequate response with diuretics and digoxin should receive ACE-l as the third drug.[11] Uncommonly, dry irritating cough can be a significant and troublesome side effect of ACE-1 therapy. Since ACE-1 or Losartan cause potassium retention, supplements of potassium and potassium sparing diuretics like triamterene or amiloride should not be given at the same time. The safer diuretic would be furosemide combined with metolazone in a small dose. Combining two agents acting at different vascular beds with variable mechanisms like isosorbide dinitrate and hydralazine has been found to provide additive benefit.[12] ACE-inhibitors are contraindicated in renal vascular disorders, e.g. renal artery stenosis, coarctation of aorta and aorto-arteritis.

Angiotensin II Receptor Blockers (ARB)

Losartan Potassium-non peptide selective at 1 receptor antagonist, has hemodynamically same effects as ACE-inhibitors. They are more beneficial in elderly patients because, they lack brady kinin potentiating activity—so there is no cough as a side effect. In salt depleted patients, it can cause hypotension.

Calcium Channel Blockers

Nifedipine and diltiazem have also been used in CCF. The trials have shown hemodynamic benefits although less favorable as compared to other vasodilators. Nifedipine cannot be recommended as the initial vasodilator agent except when additional indications like systemic hypertension coexists. Its predominant effect is on the resistance of vessels and hence needs to be combined with diuretics and venodilators. It's use should be avoided with other negative inotropic agents in patients with left ventricular failure and also with relatively low blood pressure. However, most studies do not favor use of calcium channel blockers in CCF since they do not improve short term or long term exercise capacity. Nifedipine, diltiazem and verapamil have been shown to have a negative inotropic effect which can lead to clinical or hemodynamic deterioration. In long term use, calcium channel blockers activate sympathetic and renin angiotensin system thus adversely affecting CCF and have been found to increase mortality in CCF due to systolic dysfunction.

Beta Adrenergic Antagonists

These drugs are carvedilol, bisoprolol, metoprolol XL and they are reserved for those patients who are clinically stable on ACE inhibitors, diuretic and digitalis. These drugs reduce afterload, and also reduce adrenergic drive.

It is widely recognized that myocardial cell loss irrespective of the basic cause precipitates in a vicious cycle where excessive sympathetic activity causes myocardial beta receptor "down regulation" in addition to the peripheral vasoconstriction. The prognosis of patients with CCF is inversely related to the circulating catecholamine levels. If catecholamines indeed contribute to pathogenesis of CCF, it will be worth while trying a beta blocker. The improvement in ventricular function occurs slowly over a period of months. Other studies lend support to this concept, including one where cardiac transplantation for end-stage CCF could be avoided with the use of beta blockers.

Correcting the Underlying Cause

It is outside the scope of this review to cover this aspect of management of CCF except to emphasize that CCF is a manifestation of an underlying disease and the primary aim should be to identify and correct the pathological basis of CCF.

Device Therapy

Two major advances in treatment of heart failure and prevention of sudden cardiac death in adults is to use devices in adults. Experience with use of cardiac re-synchronization therapy in children with systemic ventricular dysfunction and heart failure is small but increasing.

1. *Mechanical device used in heart failure include:*
   a. *Intra-aortic balloon pump*—this is the most commonly used device to improve cardiac function and maintain circulation, especially in the preoperative stage before valve replacement or cardiac transplantation (Figs 1.2A and B).
   b. *Ventricular assist device*—this device is under investigation as an alternate to cardiac transplantation (Fig. 1.3).
2. *Cardiac resynchronization*-Biventricular Pacing—this is an emerging mode of therapy in resistant chronic CCF. The installed pacemaker synchronizes left ventricular contraction, which leads to increase in left ventricular ejection fraction and cardiac index. This ultimately leads on to improved quality of life.
3. *Implantable cardiac defibrillator*—Treatment of choice in those who have survived sudden cardiac arrest. This is programmed when the heart rate goes beyond a certain rate. Other investigational devices are in an experimental state.

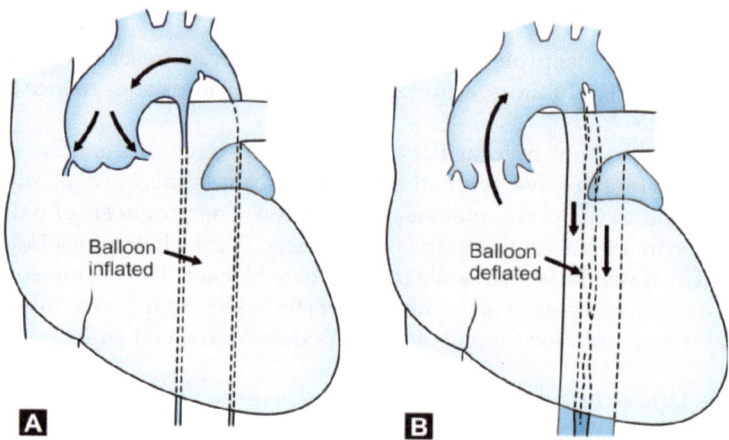

Figs 1.2A and B: Intra-aortic balloon pump. The balloon inflated during cardiac diastole increases coronary artery infusion. (A) Left ventricular afterload is decreased as the balloon is deflated during cardiac systole (B)

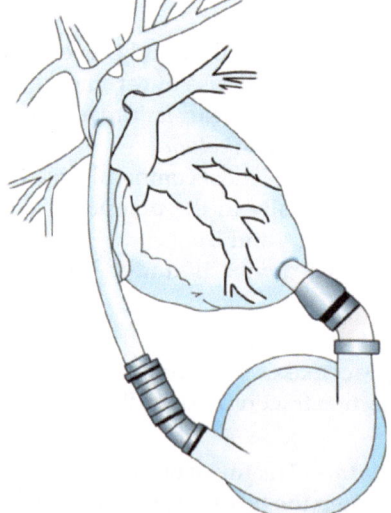

Fig. 1.3: Ventricular assist device

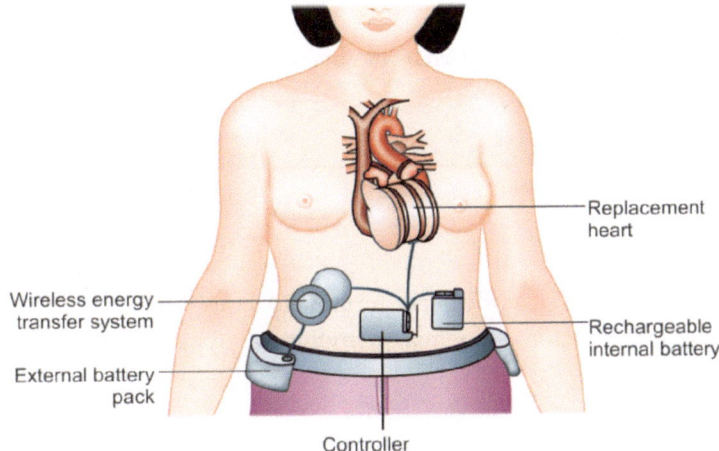

Fig. 1.4: External pneumatic counter pulsation—an electric motor driven artificial heart. (*Courtesy:* Colucci WS, Braunwald E–Atlas of heart failure (cardiac function and dysfunction 4th Ed.)

4. *External pneumatic counter pulsation* prevents ventricular remodeling therapy and preventing further ventricular dilatation. This is an electric motor driven artificial heart which can be implanted in the thoracic cage with all its attachments (Fig. 1.4).

Surgical Therapy

1. *Mitral valve reconstruction:* This surgery is indicated in patients with gross mitral regurgitation with left ventricular dysfunction where medical therapy is unable to correct remodeling.
2. *Ventricular reduction surgery-Batista procedure:* Surgical removal of 20-40 % akinetic wall of left ventricle to reshape LV. But this has not given good results and later LV assist devices will be required.
3. *Coronary artery bypass grafting (CABG)*—indicated in young patients with established coronary artery disease and also in those children with anomalous origin of coronary artery from pulmonary artery (ALCAPA). This surgery gives favorable results in those with severe left ventricular dysfunction (LVEF < 30%).
4. *Cardiac transplantation:* Ideal for late stage heart disease but the biggest limitation is lack of donors.
   Indications
   - End stage heart failure
   - Dilated cardiomyopathy, restrictive cardiomyopathy, hypoplastic left heart syndrome.

Contraindications
- Malignancy,
- Systemic medical disorders—Hypertension, diabetes mellitus, bleeding disorders, etc.
- Active infection—HIV, HBB, HBC.

GUIDELINES FOR MANAGEMENT OF CCF

- Bed rest—Propped up position
- Humified oxygen
- Diet-Salt restricted
- Infants—Nasogastric feeding, calorie dense formula (0.8 cal/ml)
- Control of precipitating factors—Anemia, arrhythmias, hypertension, infective endocarditis, electrolyte disturbance.
- Pharmacological
  - Digoxin-Inotropic drug
  - Diuretics
  - Furosemide, spironolactone,
  - Vasodilators - hydralazine
  - ACE inhibitors - captopril, enalapril
  - Angiotensin receptor antagonists - losartan
  - Beta blockers - atenolol, carvedilol
- Devices and surgery
  - IABP, pacemaker/defibrillator,
  - Ventricular assist devices

    Valve replacement

    Heart transplantation

REFERENCES

1. Behram RE. The cardiovascular system. In: Textbook of pediatrics (16th Edn) Behram RE, Kleighmen RM, Nelson WE, Vaughan VC. Philadelphia. WB Saunders Company, 2000 pp.
2. Francis GS. Neurohormonal Mechanisms involved in congestive heart failure. Am J Cardiol 1985;55:15A-21A.
3. Perloff WH. Physiology of Heart and Circulation. In : Cardiovascular problems in Pediatric Critical Care. Eds. Swedlow DB, Raphaely Rc. New York. Churchill Livingstone 1986;1-85.

4. Martin P O', Laughlin MD. Congestive heart failure in children. Pediatric Clin of N America 1999;46(2):263-73.
5. Eugene Braunwald. Heart Failure. In: Harrison's Principles of Internal Medicine. (13th Edn). Isselbacher KJ. Braunwald E, Wilson ill Martin JB Fauci AS Kasper DL. WB SaundersCompany 1994:998-1009.
6. Lejemtel TH, Sonnenblick EH. Should the failing myocardium be stimulated? N Engl J Med 1984;310: 1384-86.
7. Unverferth DE, Megorein RD, Levis RP. Long term benefit of dobutamine in patient with congestive cardiomyopathy. Amer Heart J 1980;100:622-25.
8. Young B, et al. Prospective randomized study of ventricular failure and efficacy of digoxin. J Am Coil Cardio 1992;19:259A-262A.
9. Packer M, et al. Comparison of Vasodilatation and ACE inhibition (Enalapril) on exercise capacity and quality of life in chronic CHF. N Eng J Med 1987;317:799- 801.
10. Vaksmann G, Khayat P, Godart F, et al. Effects of transdermal Nitroglycerine in children with congestive heart failure: A Doppler Echo-cardiography study. Pediatr Cardiol 2001-02;22:11-13.
11. Tripathi KD. Plasma Kinins, Angiotensins and ACE Inhibitors in Essentials of Medical Pharmacology (3rd edn) 1994;176-85.
12. Nasser A, Dietz JR, Siddique M, et al. Effects of Kaliuretic peptide on sodium and Water Excretion in persons with Congestive Heart Failure. Am J Cardiol 2001;88:23-29.

CHAPTER 2

Hypertension in Children

Hypertension in infancy and childhood is rare, may be undiagnosed, though it is now a recognized concept that the roots of "essential" hypertension extend back into childhood[1] with persistence of rank order with age, a concept known as "Tracking".[2] Till about a decade ago, most occurrences of hypertension in childhood were believed to be due to secondary hypertension and "primary" or "essential" hypertension was believed to be exceedingly rare. But now recent studies have inferred that because of more frequent routine blood pressure recordings in children, mild essential or primary or essential hypertension is being increasingly diagnosed and is stated to be the commonest cause of high blood pressure in children.[3] Blood pressure elevation is established as an important risk factor for the development of cardiovascular disease in adults. In the Framingham study, elevated blood pressure is associated with increased incidence of myocardial infarction, cerebrovascular heart disease, left ventricular hypertrophy and congestive heart failure.[4] A 10 mm increase in systolic blood pressure is associated with a 20% increased risk of cardiovascular events in adults in the age group of 35-64 years.[5]

Definition

Blood pressure is the lateral pressure exerted on the vessel wall by the blood contained there in. It is a function of two major factors, cardiac output and peripheral resistance. The definitions of pediatric hypertension are based on cross-sectional studies in children, which have shown continuous rise in level of blood pressure from infancy through adolescence.

Hypertension has been defined on the basis of the age and sex of the child as the finding at 3 different blood pressure readings:
1. Above 90th percentile rank of age and sex.
2. Above 95th percentile of normal value for age and sex (Task force Report 1977).
3. Above 95th percentile for age and sex with values between 90th and 95th percentile classified as high normal blood pressure (Task force Report 1987).[1]

Prevalence of Primary and Secondary Hypertension

Discovery of blood was an epoch making event brought about by William Harvey in 1628. Although the definition of hypertension is somewhat arbitrary, the prevalence of hypertension in childhood and adolescents is estimated between 1-3%, and more recent estimates have placed the prevalence at approximately 5%.[6] Majority of these children have only a mild increase in blood pressure (primary) but there is a small group of children with much higher blood pressures (secondary hypertension). The prevalence of persistent secondary hypertension is about 0.1%,[7] and renal disease predominates (80%) in this group. Mild hypertension rarely causes any lasting effect but severe sustained hypertension in children carries a high risk of morbidity and mortality. Essential hypertension is being diagnosed in children because of routine recording of blood pressure in children. A prevalence of hypertension in Indian children has been reported to be 1.8% (4-16 years of age)[8] and amongst the hospitalized children with hypertension, 72% are of renal origin. Coarctation of aorta is relatively rare though aorto-arteritis is more common.[9] Neonatal hypertension is rare though it is being recognized more frequently as a sequelae to umbilical artery characterization.

Target Organ Effects

Hypertension is clearly associated with increased risk for cardiovascular disease in adults and treatment of hypertension results in decreased risk over time. Elevated blood pressure is also a component of metabolic syndrome, which is associated with increased risk of cardiovascular disease in adults.

The Bogalusa study has shown that blood pressure elevation is related to the presence of fatty streaks and fibrous plaques in aorta, coronary arteries which show that systemic blood pressure elevation plays an important role in early stages of atherosclerosis.

Blood pressure elevation has also been associated with increased left ventricular mass in children and adolescents. This is important because left ventricular hypertrophy has been identified as an independent risk factor for cardiovascular disease in adults. Some studies have found an association between blood pressure elevation and increased carotid IMT (intima media thickness) whereas others have not. This area requires further study.[14]

Newborn

The normal systolic blood pressure in a full term newborn on
1st day   –   70 mm
1 month   –   85 mm

In preterms-the systolic and diastolic blood pressures are independent of birth weight and gestational age and tend to correlate with low Apgar scores.

A newborn is hypertensive when:
Full term - systolic blood -> 90 mm Hg
- diastolic BP -> 60 mm Hg
Preterm - systolic BP -> 80 mm Hg
- diastolic BP -> 50 mm Hg

Definition of Hypertension by Age Group (2nd Task force 1987)[1]

Age group	Blood pressure
Newborn 1-7 days	systolic 96 mm Hg
8-30 days	112/74 "
3 months-5 years	116/76 "
6 years-9 years	122/78 "
10-12 years	126/82 "
13-15 years	136/86 "

Blood Pressure Correlation with Height and Weight

Body weight or body mass index is the strongest determinant of blood pressure in children and abnormal weight gain and obesity are the pivotal factors in blood pressure elevation in children and adolescents.

Larger (heavier and or taller) children have higher blood pressure than small children of same age.[10] The correlation of higher blood pressure range associated with height and obesity has been given importance particularly for patients with high normal pressure (borderline 90th-95th percentile), which will be considered normal if the child is taller or has higher lean body mass or obesity. Barker has proposed that infants born with low birth weight owing to fetal undernutrition, with decreased renal mass and changes in vascular structure and function would be predisposed to future hypertension.[10]

Classification of Hypertension

Classification of hypertension in children and adolescents is given in Table 2.1. Clinically, it depends on the severity of hypertension (2nd Task Force 1987)

Borderline or mild - Systolic and/or diastolic B.P. repeatedly between 90th-95th percentile for age and sex.

Moderate - Blood pressure level repeatedly exceeding 95th percentile by 15 mm or less and without any target organ involvement. This is usually the precursor of essential hypertension.

Table 2.1: Classification of hypertension in children and adolescents

	SBP or DBP percentile[a]	Frequency of BP measurement
Normal	< 90th percentile	Recheck at next scheduled physical examination.
Prehypertension	90th to <95th or BP exceeds 120/80 mm Hg even if below 90th percentile upto <95th percentile[b]	Recheck in 6 months
Stage 1 hypertension	95th-99th percentile plus 5 mm Hg	Recheck in 1-2 weeks or sooner if the patient is symptomatic. If persistently elevated on two additional occasions evaluate or refer to source of care within 1 month.
Stage 2 hypertension	> 99th percentile plus 5 mm Hg	Evaluate or refer to source of care within 1 week or immediately if the patient is symptomatic

SBP, systolic blood pressure; DSP, dystolic blood pressure.
a. For sex, age, and height measured on at least three separate occasions, if systolic and diastolic categories are different, categorize by the higher value.
b. This occurs typically at 12 years old for SBP and for DBP.

Severe - Blood pressure levels repeatedly exceeding 95th percentile by 15 mm or more with target organ involvement

There are a few terms associated with hypertension:

Accelerated hypertension—when there is recent increase over previous hypertensive level associated with evidence of vascular changes in fundus but no papilloedema.

Malignant hypertension—with elevated BP, there is papilloedema and retinal hemorrhage and exudates may also be present.

Measurement of Blood Pressure in Children

The 2nd Task force (1987) gives the following recommendations:
1. All children-3 years and above should have routine measurement of blood pressure.
2. Mercury sphygmomanometer is preferred to aneroid manometer.
3. Three cuff sizes are necessary for different age groups. The cuff size refers to the inner inflatable bladder and the cuff should be long enough to completely encircle the circumference of the arm and wide enough to cover approximately 45-55% of the right upper arm between the acromion

and the olecranon. The length of bladder should be between 80-100% of the circumference of arm and the ratio between two should be 1:2.
4. The child should be in a comfortable sitting position (infant many be supine) in congenial surroundings with right arm fully exposed and resting on supportive surface at the heart level, and the diaphragm of the stethoscope should be placed on the exposed brachial artery.
5. Systolic blood pressure is determined by the onset of the "tapping" korotkoff sound. Whereas the muffling of the korotkoff sounds (fourth korotkoff sounds) was previously thought as the diastolic pressure. American Heart Association has recently established the disappearance of sounds (fifth korotkoff sound) as the diastolic pressure in children of all ages including adolescents.
6. Increased blood pressure is clearly associated with obesity and height, the association with weight is believed to be a causal one, and body mass index (BMI) gives an accurate measure of obesity.

$$BMI = \frac{Weight\ (kg)}{Height\ (m^2)}$$

$$BMI > 30 \text{ - obese}$$
$$25\text{-}30 \text{ - overweight}$$
$$< 25 \text{ - normal}$$

7. *In newborns and infants:* The optimum method for measurement of blood pressure is the indwelling arterial umbilical artery or renal artery catheter which is often in place. An alternative method is the oscillometric monitor, which correlates reasonably well with intra-arterial recording.

Etiology (Tables 2.2A and B)

Pathophysiology

1. *Genetic predisposition:* A familial influence on blood pressure can be identified early in life. Children from families with hypertension tend to have higher blood pressure than do children from normotensive families. A heterogeneous group of factors contribute to the risk for essential hypertension aside from genetic predisposition. These include reactivity of vascular smooth muscles and the kidney and the interaction of the renin angiotensin system, cardiac index, obesity, hormonal and environmental factors. In the last 5 years, there have been important revelations in the genetic predisposition towards hypertension, which include "candidate genes" which highlight the role of renin angiotensin system. Other genetic aspects include "lithium counter transport machinery", the association with insulin resistance, sodium sensitivity and gene influenced body mass index.[11]
2. *Environmental factors:* Dietary sodium, potassium and calcium intake.

Table 2.2A: Hypertension can be etiologically classified into those leading on to transient and sustained hypertension

Transient	Acute glomerulonephritis
	Henoch Schonlein purpura, hemolytic uremic syndrome
	Guillain Barre syndrome, acute poliomyelitis
	Burns-salt and water retention, lead poisoning
	Drugs - Atropine
	Sympathomimetic drugs
	Steroid therapy
Sustained	1. Renal
	• Diseases of renal parenchyma
	– Chronic glomerulonephritis
	– Reflux nephropathy
	– Obstructive uropathy
	– Renal dysplasia
	– Polycystic kidney disease
	– Chronic renal failure
	– Renovasular disease
	• Renal artery stenosis
	– Fibromuscular dysplasia
	– Neurofibromatosis
	• Renal artery anomalies
	– Aneurysm, thrombosis, A-V fistula. Aorto-arteritis
	– Renal tumors
	– Wilm's tumor
	– Hamartoma
	2. Coarctation of aorta
	• Thoracic
	• Abdominal
	3. Endocrinal
	• Catecholamine excess
	– Pheochromocytoma
	– Neuroblastoma
	– Corticoid excess
	– Congenital adrenal hyperplasia
	– Conn's syndrome
	– Cushings syndrome
	– Low renin states (mineralocorticoid excess)
	4. Primary (Essential) hypertension

Table 2.2B:[1] Hypertension-agewise classification (Taskforce 1987)

Newborn	-	Infancy-Renal artery thrombosis Renal artery stenosis Coarctation of aorta Bronchopulmonary dysplasia Elevated intracranial pressure.
Infancy-6 years	-	Acute glomerulonephritis Acute pyelonephritis Polycystic disease Renal artery stenosis Coarctation of aorta
6-10 years	-	Renal artery stenosis Aorto-arteritis Chronic renal failure Essential hypertension
Adolescence	-	Essential hypertension Chronic renal failure

Sodium Intake

In adults with established hypertension, decrease in dietary sodium intake may lower the blood pressure, but in infants and adolescents, it is less clear. The blood pressure response to sodium restriction in obese adolescents was effective in lowering BP in females but not in male adolescents. This response is correlated to higher fasting plasma insulin concentration, higher aldosterone level and increased activity of the sympathetic nervous system. In reviewing the literature, it emerges that sodium sensitivity in the young seems to be linked to race, family history and obesity and though little effect is seen with restricted sodium intake over a few weeks, a sustained reduction in sodium intake over years may have an effect on blood pressure, in the adolescents.

Potassium[19]

Potassium plays a role in the regulation of the blood pressure by its natriuresis and suppression of renin production and release. Potassium intake has been shown to have an inverse relationship with both systolic and diastolic blood pressure in children, and dietary potassium and the ratio of potassium to sodium may be more important than dietary sodium alone in its relationship to systolic blood pressure.

Calcium[20]

Preliminary data support an inverse correlation of dietary calcium to blood pressure in children, presumably secondary to increased intracellular calcium levels, which in turn, increase smooth muscle tone and vascular resistance of arterioles.

Diagnostic Evaluation of Hypertensive Children (Flow chart 2.1)

Many children with mild hypertension are asymptomatic and hypertension is diagnosed as a result of routine BP measurement. Whenever a young child is found to be hypertensive, renovascular disease should be strongly suspected.

Clinical Picture

1. General-headache, dizziness, nausea, vomiting, irritability and personality changes.
2. Specific-stroke, congestive cardiac failure, renal failure, convulsions, encephalopathy.

History—Past and Present

1. Neonatal - history of umbilical artery catheterization, bronchopulmonary dysplasia.
2. Cardiovascular - history of diagnosis of coarctation of aorta
   - history of palpitation, headache, excessive sweating (excessive catecholamine levels)
3. Renal - h/o obstructive uropathy urinary tract infection, renal surgery, oliguria, hematuria, enuresis, nocturia.
4. Endocrinal - Weakness, muscle cramps (hypokalemia, hyperaldosteronism), age of menarche, sexual development.
5. Medications - Corticosteroids, amphetamines-antiasthmatic drugs, nephrotoxic, antibiotics-aminoglycoside.
6. Habits - Smoking, narcotic drugs-cocaine
7. Family history - Essential hypertension, obesity, stroke, renal disease, etc.

Physical Examination

General

- Accurate measurement of BP—average of at least 3 readings in the sitting and standing positions to be taken
- Presence of edema (facial and periorbital)-renal disease

Flow chart 2.1: Evaluation and management of children and adolescents with hypertension[16]

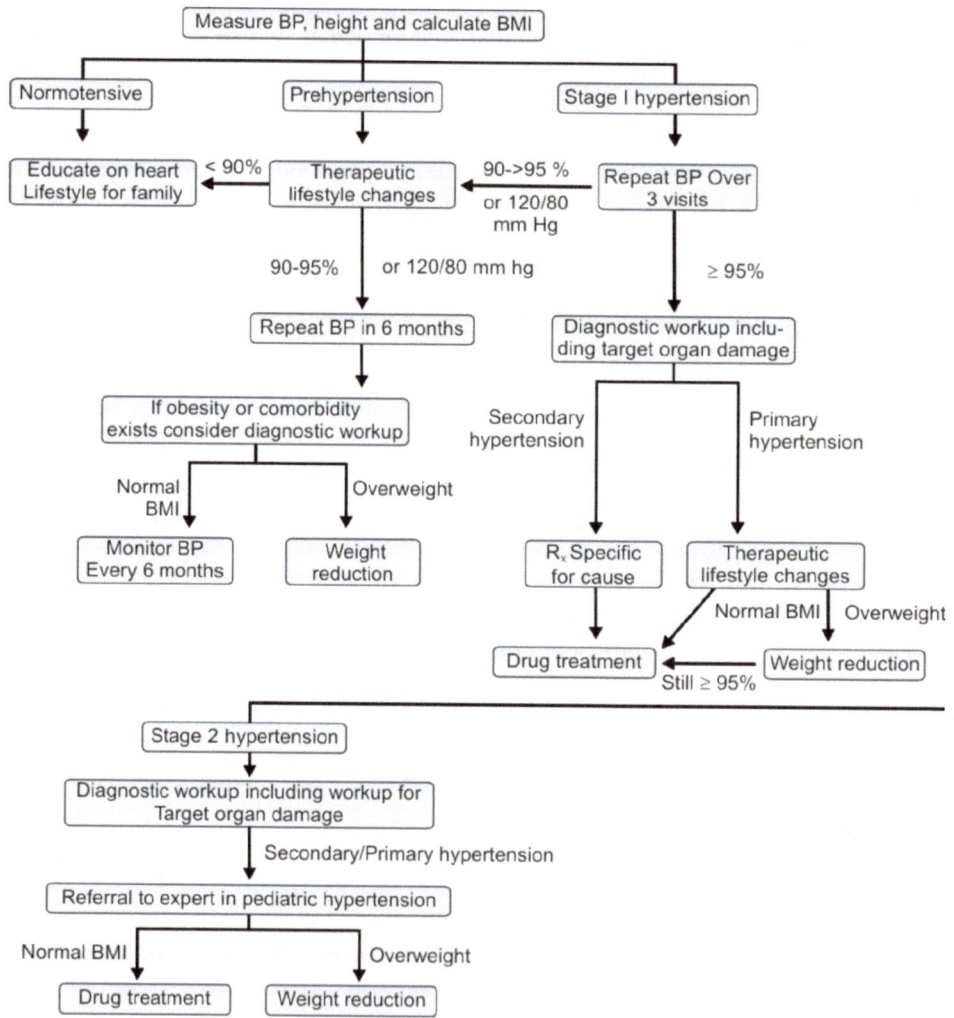

- Ear, nose, throat-Adenotonsillar hypertrophy
  - Snoring
  - Sleep apnea
- Height, weight
  - Growth retardation, Truncal obesity } Chronic renal failure, Cushings syndrome, Insulin resistance syndrome, SLE
- Skin
  - Episodic pallor
    Flushing, diaphoresis } Phenochromocytoma
    Acne, hirsutism, striae } Cushing syndrome
    Acanthosis nigricans } Type 2 diabetes, SLE
- Genitalia
  - Ambiguous Virilization } Adrenal hyperplasia
- Moonface, obesity, abdominal striae, buffalo hump
  - Cushings syndrome
- CVS–tachycardia, absent or delayed peripheral pulses-coarctation of aorta; aorto-arteritis.
- Abdomen
  - Epigastric bruit-coarctation of aorta
  - Lumps in renal angle Wilm's tumor, polycystic kidney.
- Fundus–for vascular changes and papilloedema
- CNS–presence of neurologic deficit in stroke

Staging/Phasing of Evaluation of Hypertensive Patient

As primary hypertension is diagnosed more frequently in children-a stepped phase evaluation is recommended.

Phase I: Broad screening

- Complete hemogram
- Urinalysis with urine culture and sensitivity, blood urea, serum creatinine, uric acid, serum electrolytes, calcium

- X-ray chest and ECG
- Echocardiogram-essential before starting medication for the basal assessment of LV mass and determining target organ damage (if primary hypertension is suspected)
- Lipid profile (if primary hypertension suspected)
- Intravenous pyelogram
- Renal ultrasound-(indicated in secondary hypertension).

Phase II: Specific screening (non-invasive diagnostic procedure)
- Renal scan-with angiotensin converting enzyme inhibitor
- Micturating cystourethrogram (if reflux suspected)
- 24 hours urine
  - VMA and catecholamines
  - 17 keto and 17 hydroxysteroids
- Plasma renin and cortisol and serum aldosterone
- CT scan for kidneys and adrenals

Phase III: Invasive
When no organic cause has been found in phase I and II
- Renal artery imaging-aortography
- Venography for renal vein renin levels
- Digital subtraction angiography

Phase IV
- Renal biopsy

Treatment of Hypertension

The goal of treatment of hypertension in children is to achieve a reduction of blood pressure below the 90-95th percentile for age, gender and height and prevention of the long term effects of persistent hypertension. Available means of treatment include non-pharmacological and pharmacological methods.[12]

Non-Pharmacologic Therapy of Hypertension

In general initial, approach to treatment includes therapeutic changes in lifestyle.

Lifestyle Modifications

If patients are overweight, then aggressive weight control management should be brought about. The modification of lifestyle is focused on changing diet and physical activity which can have beneficial effect on control of blood pressure.

Diet

In children and adolescents, much of the observed primary hypertension is at least in part related to being overweight. With the increasing prevalence and severity of childhood obesity, weight management is an increasing aspect of non-pharmacologic management of hypertension. Weight management ultimately brings about gradual reduction in blood pressure readings and also improvement in main component of metabolic syndrome.

Salt

High salt, low potassium and obesity are the principal associations with hypertension.[13] Even though there is an association between dietary intake of salt and hypertension, moderate short term restriction of dietary salt does not reduce blood pressure in adolescents, it gets reduced by weight reduction. Infancy may be an important period in relation to dietary sodium. Those on low sodium diet had significantly lower blood pressure than normal sodium group.[18]

Potassium

In pre-adolescent girls and boys, BMI and heart rate and not sodium and potassium are the major determinants of blood pressure level. A family history of hypertension appears to be a stronger predictor of enhanced cardiovascular reactivity than race. So there is not enough evidence to show that potassium supplementation brings down blood pressure.[19]

Calcium

In a study conducted on adolescent African American children, calcium supplementation brought down the diastolic blood pressure, but in another biracial adolescent study, calcium supplementation brought about a decrease in systolic blood pressure.[20] The treatment effect largely disappeared after 6 weeks.

Obesity[15]

Body mass is the strongest predictor of blood pressure and moreover obesity is considered a cause of hypertension. Strategies aimed at reducing BMI in childhood, if these changes track into adulthood, may reduce the probability of cardiovascular disease in adulthood. Programs of behavior modification and parental involvement may lead to significant weight losses in obese children, which if sustained could have an important effect on adult risk for hypertension and coronary heart disease.[16] In children, where 8-10 % reduction in BMI is obtained, reduction in blood pressure ranges between 8-16 mm Hg. Since treatment of obesity and maintenance of weight loss are difficult, it is important to focus on prevention of abnormal weight gain in childhood.[21]

Physical Activity

The recommendation that exercise (aerobic exercises) be included in a program to reduce weight and also blood pressure level, generally is predicted on the interactive effects of weight loss and exercise. Strategies that incorporate multiple lifestyle interventions have been successful in reducing blood pressure levels in children. Exercise is indicated in young athletes who have elevated blood pressure and they should be encouraged to follow a diet and continue to exercise which will help them to achieve the ideal body weight. Regular physical activity is a useful component of therapeutic lifestyle changes to treat hypertension in children.

Pharmacological Treatment of Hypertension (Tables 2.3 and 2.4)

The therapeutic goal for children and adolescents with hypertension is to lower the blood pressure below the 95th percentile for age, sex and height. However, for those children with diabetes or chronic renal disease, a more aggressive goal is appropriate to bring the blood pressure below 90th percentile to prevent cardiovascular diseases in future.

The approach to treatment in children and adolescents includes starting a low dose of the initial medication. Blood pressure should be monitored and dose increased till the ideal blood pressure is achieved, or side effects appear. If the first choice of medication is not as effective as desired, medication from another class may be started in a low dose and titrate upwards till the ideal BP is achieved. Sometimes, it is necessary to add a second drug from another class for desired blood pressure lowering. In addition to longitudinal follow up of blood pressure, it is important to look out for side effects and also look for target organ damage (Flow chart 2.2).

Table 2.3:[16] Indications for treatment with antihypertensive medications

- Symptomatic hypertension
- Secondary hypertension
- Stage 2 hypertension
- Hypertension (stage 1 or 2) with established target organ damage
- Hypertension (stage 1 or 2) with the presence of other risk factors for cardiovascular disease
- Persistent hypertension (stage 1 or 2) despite implementation of therapeutic lifestyle changes

Table 2.4:[17] Antihypertensive drug therapy for chronic hypertension in children

Class	Drug	Dose	Dose interval	Comments
1. Angiotensin Converting enzyme (ACE) inhibitor	Captopril	0.3-0.5 mg/kg/dose Maximum 6 mg/day	TDS	1. All ACE-inhibitors are contraindicated in pregnancy 2. Check serum potassium and creatinine to monitor hyperkalemia and azotemia. 3. Cough and angioedema are less common with newer members than captopril. 4. FDA approval for ACE-inhibitors with pediatric labeling is limited to children > 6 yrs of age and to creatinine clearance > 30 ml/min/1.73 m^2
	Enalapril	0.08-5 mg/kg/day Maximum-0.6 mg/kg/day up to 40 mg/day	BD	
	Lisinopril	0.07 mg/kg/day up to 5 mg/day Maximum-0.6 mg/kg/day up to 40 mg/day	QID	
2. Angiotensin-receptor Blocker (ARB)	Irbesartan	6-12 yrs-75-150 mg/day > 13 yrs-150-300 mg/day	QID	Same as ACE–Inhibitors.
	Losartan	0.7 mg/kg/day up to 50 mg/day. Max. 1.4 mg/kg/Day. Up to 100 mg/day	QID	
3. Adrenergic blocking Agents. a. α and β blocker	Labetalol	1-3 mg/kg/day Max. 10-12 mg/kg/day up to 1200 mg/day	BD	• Contraindicated in asthma and overt heart failure. • Not to be used in insulin dependent diabetics.
α blocker	Prazocin	0.5-0.1mg/kg/day	TDS	• Postural hypotension
β blocker	Atenolol	0.5-1 mg/kg/day Max-2 mg/kg/day up to 100 mg/day	QID	• Drug of choice for mild to moderate hypertension
	Metoprolol	1-2 mg/kg/day Max – 6 mg/kg/day up to 600 mg/day	BD	• Should not be used in insulin dependent diabetics.

Contd...

Contd...

	Propranolol	1-2 mg/kg/day Max. 4 mg/kg/day up to 600 mg/day	BD-TDS	Contraindicated in asthma and heart failure
4. Calcium channel blocker	Nifedipine	0.25-3 mg/kg/day	BD	Drug of choice in severe hypertension, given sublingually, may cause tachycardia
	Amlodipine	6-17 years 2.5-5 mg once daily	-	
5. α-Agonist	Clonidine	> 12 years 0.2 mg/day Max. 2.4 mg/day	BD	May cause dry mouth and sedation can cause rebound hypertension
6. Diuretics	Hydrochloro Thiazide	1 mg/kg/day Max. 3 mg/kg/day Up to 50 mg	QID	Patients on diuretics should have electrolytes monitoring
	Furosemide	0.5-2.0 mg/kg/dose Max. 6 mg/kg/day	BD-QID	Useful drug in resistant hypertension in renal diseases
	Spironolactone	1 mg/kg/day Max. 3.3 mg/kg/day up to 100 mg/day	BD-QID	Tachycardia and fluid retention can occur.
	Triamterene	1-2 mg/kg/day Max. 3-4 mg/kg/day, up to 300 mg/day	BD	Potassium sparing. May cause hyperkalemia if given with ACE-inhibitors and ARBS.
	Amiloride	0.4-0.625 mg/kg/day Max. 20 mg/kg/day	QID	Tachycardia and fluid retention can occur
7. Vasodilator	Hydralazine	0.75 mg/kg/day Max. 7.5 mg/kg/day	QID	Hydralazine can cause a lupus like syndrome
	Minoxidil	Children < 12 years 0.2 mg/kg/day Max. 50 mg/day Children >12 years 5 mg/kg/day Max. 100 mg/day	TDS-QID	Minoxidil is for patients who are resistant to other drugs. Can cause hypertrichosis
	Diazoxide	2.5 mg/kg/day Max. 10 mg/day		Can cause hyperglycemia, hyperurecemia 2nd line drug for hypertensive emergency

Flow chart 2.2: Treatment of childhood hypertension-stepped care approach[21]

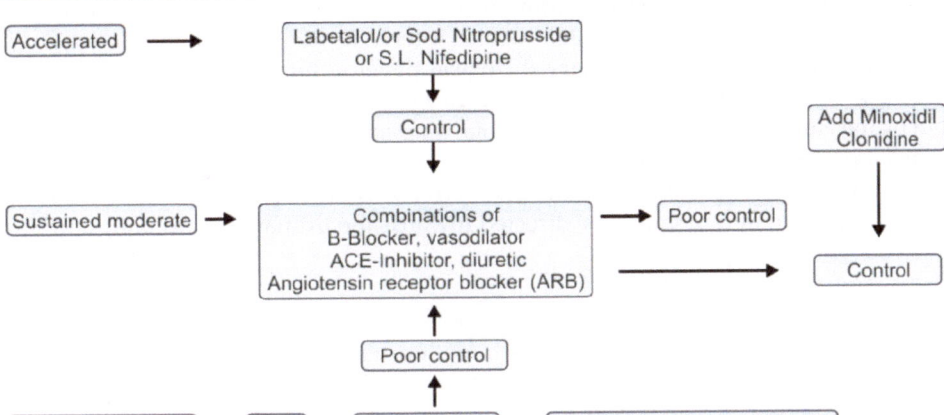

Severe sustained hypertension in childhood should be treated, because the incidence of morbidity and mortality is higher without treatment. The therapeutic options available must be chosen on the individual merits of a particular case. Complications of untreated hypertension are hypertensive encephalopathy, visual impairment, cerebral hemorrhage, left ventricular failure and acute renal failure.

Neonatal Hypertension (Table 2.5)

In the first week of life, systolic blood pressure rises 1-2 mm Hg per day, thereafter rising 1-2 mm Hg per week for the first 6 weeks. In healthy term infants, the 95th percentile of systolic blood pressure is 95 mm Hg at 4 days of age and 113 mm Hg at 6 weeks of life.[22]

Table 2.5:[12] Conditions for which neonates and infants should have measurement of blood pressure

1. Prematurity-Neonatal complications.
2. Congenital heart disease.
3. Renal parenchymal disease or urologic malformation.
4. Evidence of elevated intracranial pressure.
5. Treatment with drugs that raise blood pressure.

The causes of hypertension in the neonate are renovascular, renal parenchymal, neoplastic, cardiovascular, endocrinal, etc. The most common cause is renovascular disease following umbilical artery catheterization, thrombosis of patent ductus arteriosus or dehydration.[23]

Many infants with bronchopulmonary dysplasia develop hypertension, probably because of prolonged use of bronchodilators, diuretics and oxygen therapy. Coarctation of aorta should be ruled out by measuring BP in all 4 limbs and cranial ultrasound should be done to rule out increased intracranial tension.

Severe renovascular hypertension in the newborn responds to ACE-inhibitors.[24] Treatment for other causes e.g., coarctation, should be directed towards the primary abnormality.

Treatment of Severe Hypertension

Severe hypertension may occur in children and adolescents when the blood pressure goes beyond 99th percentile for age, sex and height. This situation needs prompt evaluation and treatment (Table 2.6).[25]

Table 2.6:[6] Antihypertensive drugs for management of severe hypertension in children

Drug	Class	Recommended dose	Route	Comments
		Most useful		
Esmolol	β-blocker	100-500 µg/kg/min	IV infusion	Very short-acting; constant infusion preferred. May cause profound bradycardia. Produced modest reductions in BP in a pediatric clinical trial.
Hydralazine	Vasodilator	0.2-0.6 mg/kg/dose	IV, IM	Should be given every 4 hrs when given IV bolus.
Labetalol	α and β	Bolus: 0.2-1.0 mg/kg	IV bolus or infusion.	Asthma and overt heart failure are relative contraindications.
Nifedipine	Calcium channel blocker	1-3 µg/kg/min	IV infusion	May cause reflex tachycardia
Sodium Nitroprusside	Vasodilator	0.53-10 µg/kg/min	IV infusion	Monitor cyanide levels with prolonged (>72h) use or in renal failure; or coadminister with sodium thiosulfate.

IV = intravenous; BP = blood pressure; IM = intramuscular.

Hypertensive Emergencies

Hypertensive crisis require antihypertensive therapy to lower blood pressure quickly and expeditiously. The speed with which BP is lowered depends on level of hypertension and presence of cerebral edema, left ventricular failure and/or renal failure. Lowering blood pressure too rapidly, however incurs the risk of underperfusion of the vital organs.

Antihypertensive agents used in such situations are relativity safe and predictable. The commonly used agents are, sublingual nifedipine, intravenous labetalol (α and β blocker), rapidly acting angiotensin converting enzyme inhibitors and I/V nitroprusside in intensive care setting only for short periods because of its side effects. It is recommended that the blood pressure be lowered by < 25% in first 8 hours with normalization in 24-48 hour period. Doses are listed in (Tables 2.7 and 2.8).

SUMMARY

Hypertension is an important clinical entity in children and adolescents that may be associated with early atherosclerosis and other target organ diseases. Recognition of hypertension requires blood pressure measurement on regular basis on children 3 years and above. Hypertension is often accompanied with obesity and other cardiovascular risk factors. Treatment of hypertension

Table 2.7:[25] Parental drug therapy in hypertension emergencies

	Drug of choice	Alternative	Avoid
1. Encephalopathy	Np.Lp,Dz	Hz	-
2. Acute pulmonary edema	Np. Hz Dz	-	Lp
3. Acute renal failure	Lp. Hz. Dz.	-	Np
4. Subarachnoid hemorrhage	Np. Lp-Dz.	Hz	-
5. Malignant hypertension	Np. Lp, Dz	Hz	-

Np-Nitroprusside   Lp-Labetalol   Dz-diazoxide   Hz-Hydralazine

Table 2.8:[25] Antihypertensive drug therapy for hypertensive emergencies

1. Nifedipine	-	0.25-0.5 mg/kg sublingually-repeated twice if no response.
2. Sodium nitroprusside	-	0.5-/µg/kg/min I/v initially may be increased to 8 µg/kg/min-max.
3. Labetalol	-	0.2-mg/kg-increased incrementally to 1 mg/kgl dose Maintenance-0.25-2 mg/kg/hour
4. Diazoxide	-	1-5 mg/kg/dose I.V.bolus up to max of 150 µg/dose

requires a stepwise approach, usually starting with therapeutic lifestyle changes and progressing to pharmacologic treatment. For most patients, the goal should be to lower blood pressure below 95th percentile for age, sex and height.

REFERENCES

1. Update on 1987 Task Force Report on High Blood Pressure in children and Adolescent: a working group report from the National High Blood Pressure Education Program working group on Hypertension Control in Children and Adolescent. Pediatrics 1996;98:649-58.
2. Bao W, Threefoot SA, Srinivasan SR, et al. Essential hypertension predicted by tracking of elevated blood pressure from childhood adulthood: the Bogalusa Heart study. Am J Hypertens 1995;8:657-65.
3. Kaplan NM, Devereux RB, Miller HS. Task force 4: Systemic hypertension. J Am Col Cardiol 1994;24: 885-88.
4. Mac Mahon S, Peto R, Cutler J, et al. Blood pressure, Stroke and coronary heart disease. Part 1, Prolonged differences in blood pressure-prospective observational studies corrected for regression dilution bias. Lancet 1990;335:765-74.
5. Kannel WB. Hypertension: Epidemiological appraisal. In: Robinson K ed. Preventive Cardiology: A guide for clinical practice. Armonk, NY: Futura publishing 1998;1-14.
6. Sorof G, Lai D, Turner J, et al. Overweight ethnicity and the prevalence of hypertension in school aged children. Pediatrics 2004;113:475-82.
7. Berenson GS, Srinivasan SR, Rao W, et al. Association between multiple cardiovascular risk factors and atherosclerosis in children and young adults: the Bogalusa Heart study. N Engl J Med 1998;338:1650-56.
8. Sachdev Y. Normal blood pressure and hypertension in Indian children. Indian Pediatr I984;21:41-45.
9. Shrivastava S, Srivastava RN, Tandon R. Idiopathic obstructive aorta-arteritis in children. Indian Pediatr 1986;23:403-405.
10. Barker D. The fetal origins of hypertension. J Hypertens Supplement 1996;14:117s-120s.
11. Nwankwo MU, Lorenz JM, Gardiner JC. A standard protocol for blood pressure measurement in the newborn. Pediatrics 1997;99:E-10.
12. Hypertension in Moss and Admom's Heart Disease in Infants, Children and Adolescents including the fetus and young adults. Eds. Allen HD; Driscoll DJ, Driscoll DJ, Shadar RE, Felter TF. (7th ed), Lippincott, Wilkins and Wilkins 2008.
13. Hegyi T, Carbone MT, Anwar M, et al. Blood pressure ranges in premature infants I: the first hours of life J Pediatr 1994;124:627-33.
14. Lauer RM, Clarke WR, Beaglehole R. Level, trend and variability of blood pressure during childhood: The Muscatine study. Circulation 1984;69:242-49.
15. Donahue RP, Prineas RJ. Gomez O, et al. Tracking of elevated systolic blood pressure among low and overweight adolescents: the Minneapolis children's blood pressure study. J Hypertension 1994;12:303-08.
16. Bartosh SM, Aronson AJ. Childhood hypertension: An update on Etiology, Diagnosis and Treatment. PCNA 1999;46(2):562-68.

17. Sachieken RM. Systemic hypertension in Heart Disease in Infants, children and adolescents. Moss AJ, Adams JH, Emmanouilides GC Eds, Published by Williams and Wilkins, Baltimore USA, 2001;7:1400-12.
18. Dyer A, Elliott P, Chee D, et al. Urinary biochemical markers of dietary intake in the INTER SALT study. Am J Clin Nutr 1997;16:1246s-1253s.
19. Sorof JM, Fennan A, Cole N, et al. Potassium intake and cardiovascular reactivity in children with risk factors for essential hypertension. J Pediatr 1997;131:87-94.
20. Dwyer JH, Dwyer KM, Scribner RA, et al. Dietary calcium, supplementation and blood pressure in African American adolescents. Am J Clin Nutr 1998;68:648-55.
21. Brownell KD, Kelman JH, Stunkard J. Treatment of obese children with and without their mothers: Change in weight and blood pressure. Pediatrics 1983;71:515-23.
22. Blowey DL, Warady BL, Alon V. Hypertension in the neonatal period. Child Nephrol Urol 1992;12:113-18.
23. Alagappan A, Malloy MH. Systemic hypertension in very low birth weight infants with brouchopulmonary dysplasia: Incidence and risk factors. Am J Perinatol 1998;15:3-8.
24. Schilder JL, Van den Anker JN. Use of enalapril in neonatal hypertension. Acta Paediatr 1995;84:1426-28.
25. Calhun DA, Opan PS. Treatment of hypertension crisis. N Engl J Med 1990;323:1177-83.

CHAPTER 3

Arrhythmias

DISORDERS OF CARDIAC RHYTHM AND CONDUCTION

Cardiac Arrhythmias

Cardiac arrhythmias are relatively infrequent in infants and children compared to adults and most of them are benign and do not signify underlying heart disease. Cardiac arrhythmias are rhythm disturbances which result from abnormal impulse generation such as automaticity or triggered depolarization, abnormal impulse conduction such as conduction block or delay, functional or fixed re-entry circuits and abnormalities in autonomic influence.[1]

Arrhythmias in children are being diagnosed with increasing frequency primarily because of awareness amongst pediatricians and pediatric cardiologists along with advances in investigative technologies, e.g. 24 hours ambulatory electrocardiography, echocardiography in all its advanced forms, e.g. transoesophageal and 3-dimensional, etc, which help in evaluating and managing the arrhythmias on an urgent basis. Otherwise these arrhythmias complicate fast and go into either low output state or near fatal dysrhythmias like ventricular tachycardia or fibrillation. Moreover since complex cardiac surgeries are being done, there is an increase in rhythm disorders in the post operative period, about which the intensivist has to anticipate and be prepared to manage.

Anatomy and Physiology of Conduction System (Fig. 3.1)

The specialized conducting tissues in the heart comprise of the sinoatrial (SA) node, internodal tracts connecting the SA node to the atrioventricular (AV) node, Bundle of His and the Purkinje fibers. The sinoatrial node is the pacemaker which is a cluster of automatic cells near the junction of SVC and right atrium. This tissue exhibits automaticity, which is the ability to spontaneously generate impulses. The rate of impulse generation is fastest in the SA node which normally dictates the rate and rhythm of heart beat. The SA node is influenced by the vagus (cardio-inhibiting) and sympathetic (cardio-stimulating) nerves. The impulse generated in the SA node spreads throughout both atria and to the AV node from where it passes via the Bundle of His to supply both ventricles

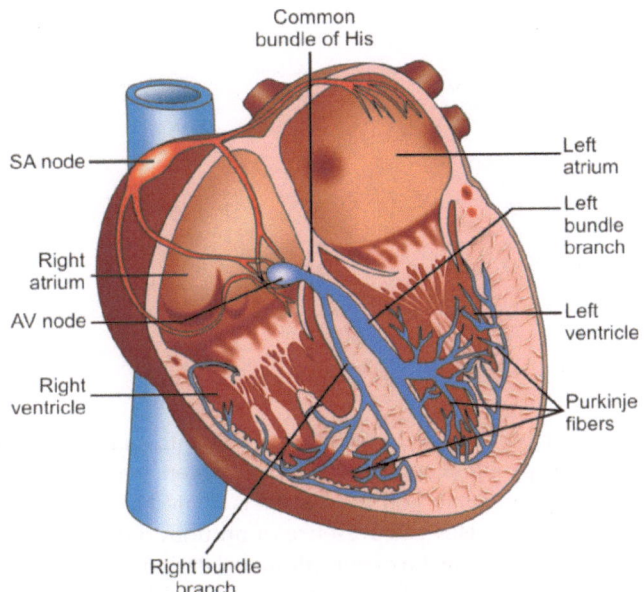

Fig. 3.1:[1] The normal conduction pathway. The electrical impulse begins in the SA node and is transmitted to the AV node, bundle of His, bundle branches and Purkinje fiber network. (From Grauer K: A practical guide to ECG implementation, St Louis, 1992, Mosby)

through the Purkinje fibers. The atrioventricular node (AV node) is situated in the anteromedial portion of RA anterior to coronary sinus. The cardiac fibers are excitable and certain specialized cells in the conduction system (SA node and AV node) depolarize spontaneously and this ability is called "automaticity". The rate at which automatic cells fire is controlled primarily by the automatic nervous system and secondarily by changes in the local environment which include potassium concentration, pH, PO_2 and extracellular calcium concentration.

If the SA node ceases to function, the intrinsic rhythmicity of the AV node takes over at a slower rate (50-60/min in older children and 100/min in infants). If the AV node and Bundle of His also cease to conduct impulses, the ventricles produce their own idioventricular rate (30-40/min). Anomalous development or injury to any segment results in an abnormal situation or propagation of electrical activity resulting in arrhythmias.

The major risks of cardiac disorders are:

Bradycardia brings about hemodynamic alterations which results in decrease in cardiac output and slow and irregular rhythm may result in syncope or cardiac arrest.

The younger the child, faster the heart rate. Tachycardia is defined as a heart rate beyond the upper limit of normal for the patient's age and bradycardia is defined as a heart rate slower than the lower limit of normal. Normal resting heart rates by age are presented in Table 3.1.[4]

Table 3.1: Heart rate[4]

The normal heart rates varies with age:

Age	Resting HR/bpm	Average
1-30 days	110-165	125
1-6 months	105-145	120
6-12 months	90-125	110
1-3 years	90-110	100
3-8 years	65-110	90
8-12 years	55-110	80
12-16 years	50-90	70

Features of Presentation

History

Although, the only definitive way to diagnose arrhythmias is to record an ECG, information from patient's history may be helpful in diagnosing the problem and assessment of urgency in reaching the diagnosis. The pattern of presentation of arrhythmias in young patients is related to the age of the patient, the duration and heart rate and in many cases the presence of an underlying defect. Infants cannot verbally communicate a sensation of tachycardia or symptoms related to arrhythmia. A careful history often shows that the infant may have been fussy, lethargic, irritable and sleepy and feed poorly for sometime before recognition of arrhythmias. Diaphoresis, coughing, pallor and cyanosis are directly related to the duration of arrhythmias and degree of circulatory congestion secondary to the arrhythmias. Infants with supraventricuiar tachycardia do not manifest with congestive cardiac failure in the first 24 hours. If SVT lasts for 24 to 36 hours, then CCF manifests in 19% of the 50% of those with SVT for at least 48 hours (Nadas).[2]

Signs and symptoms of arrhythmias at the time of presentation in the patients over 5 years of age differ dramatically from those in infancy, palpitations and irregular pulse being one of the more common complaints.

Rapid, abrupt onset of palpitations with equally abrupt spontaneous termination suggests paroxysmal supraventricular tachycardia and not sinus tachycardia. Parents or patients can be taught to count the pulse during such episodes. They can usually tell whether the fast rhythm is regular (SVT and ventricular tachycardia) or irregular (Atrial fibrillation or atrial flutter with block).

Symptoms associated with palpitation give a clue to the severity of the problem. Syncopal attacks occur as the result of hemodynamic compromise caused by the arrhythmia (rapid supraventricular tachycardia, atrioventricular block) and are ominous because they are associated with sudden death. Sensation of palpitation in the neck may result in regurgitation of blood into systemic venous system.

Patients, who point to specific area on the chest wall, indicating the location of chest pain, rarely have a pathologic tachyarrhythmia. Termination by valsalva maneuvers, gagging or facial immersion in cold water suggests re-entrant SVT. A review of past medical history, associated structural cardiac disease, non-cardiac cause of palpitation especially hyperthyroidism should also be considered. Sudden infant death syndrome remains the commonest cause of death in infants outside the neonatal period. Despite the well documented drop in incidence, it still affects approximately 2/1000 infants.

Physical Examination

Careful inspection and auscultation aid in diagnosing underlying cardiac defect. Arrhythmias are often associated with congenital heart disease, both before and after corrective or palliative surgery. During the episodes, the rate, rhythm, BP, and arterial and venous (cannon waves in jugular veins) pulsations should be noted.

Electrocardiographic Monitoring

The electrocardiographic diagnosis of arrhythmia's mechanism is vital for determining the best treatment, especially when anti-arrhythmic medications are contemplated. Failure to document the tachycardia/bradycardia can lead to inappropriate treatment. Resting 12 lead ECG should be obtained. For reference a standard cardiac cycle as noted on ECG is shown in Figure 3.2.

The P wave represents atrial depolarization, QRS represents ventricular depolarizations, whilst the PR interval represents the time for signal to travel from sinus node to the A-V node, etc.

Sinus Rhythm (Fig. 3.3)

Implies normal sequence of conduction originating in the sinus node proceeding to ventricles via A-V node and bundle of His to the Purkinje system. P wave precedes each QRS complex with regular P-R interval.

An initial determination is made as to whether the QRS duration and morphology during tachycardia are normal or increased. The narrow QRS (usually under 80 milliseconds) are caused by supraventricular tachycardia, whilst the wide QRS may be caused by ventricular tachycardia or SVT with sustained aberrant conduction of bundle branch block. In children, most wide complex tachycardias are of ventricular origin. Next, the relationship between P waves and QRS complexes is determined, and if possible this relationship is often diagnostic. For example a narrow QRS tachycardia with AV dissociation and an atrial rate lower than ventricular rate may be diagnosed as functional ectopic tachycardias. For rhythms with 1 : 1 relation between P wave and QRS complexes, the relative timings of the respective waves is often helpful, e.g. wave close to preceding QRS, close

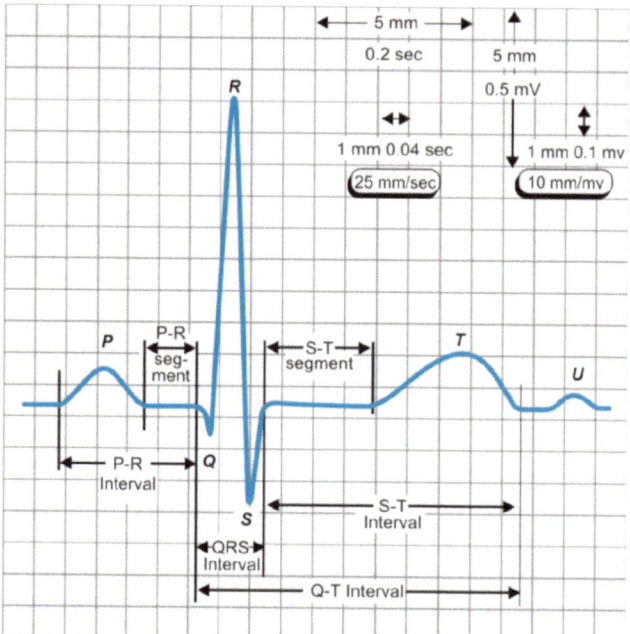

Fig. 3.2: Normal electrocardiogram

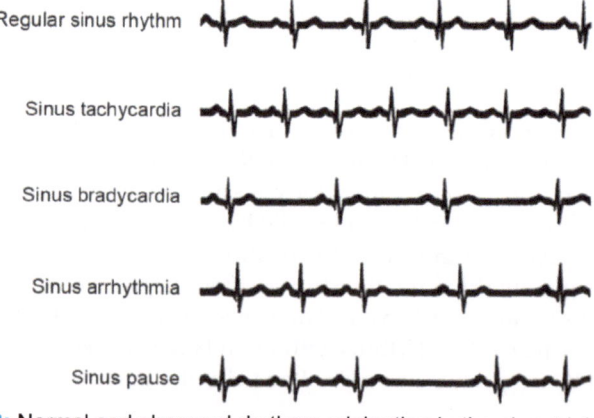

Fig. 3.3: Normal and abnormal rhythms originating in the sinoatrial node[3]

to following QRS or on top of QRS. These characteristics help to differentiate between accessory pathway tachycardia, atrial tachycardia and atrioventricular nodal re-entry.

Clinical classification of arrhythmias (Fig. 3.4 and Table 3.2):
1. Is the R-R interval regular? If regular (< 0.8 second variation), the answers to further questions will categorize the rhythm.

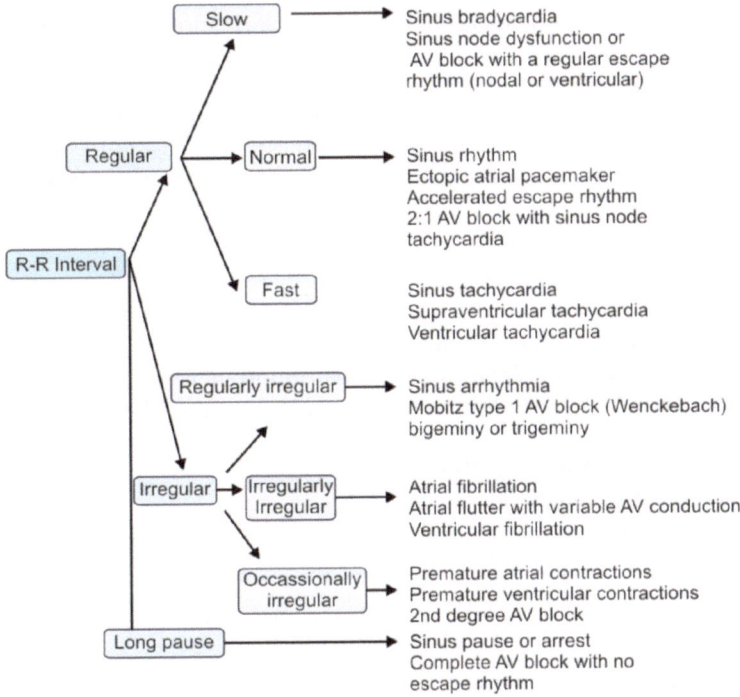

Fig. 3.4: Algorithm for identification of cardiac rhythm[5]

Table 3.2: Clinical classification of arrhythmias[4]

1. Heart rate	-	increased/decreased.
2. Heart rhythm	-	regular/irregular.
3. Site of origin	-	supraventricular/ventricular.
4. ECG complexes	-	narrow/broad

2. Whether the ventricular rate is normal, decreased or increased for the patients age and clinical condition.
3. Whether the QRS duration is normal or prolonged (normally under 0.08 seconds). If the QRS duration is prolonged, the specific morphology must be determined.
4. Atrial activity: Whether there are P waves, flutter or fibrillation waves (best seen in leads II and V_1). If P waves are visible, the P wave axis must be determined. Normal sinus P waves have an axis of + 40° to + 90°. Finally, the relation of atrial depolarization to the QRS complexes must be determined.
5. If the RR intervals are irregular, then it has to be determined whether they are regularly or irregularly irregular or there is a basic regular RR interval into which an irregular RR interval is introduced.

Using this method of analysis most of the arrhythmias can be broadly classified into
1. Tachyarryhthmias
2. Bradyarryhthmias

Tachyarrhythmias

All the rhythms that originate in the sino-atrial node (sinus rhythm) and are faster than normal are tachyarrhythmias. They also represent a variety of fast abnormal rhythms originating either in atria or ventricles of the heart. Tachyarrhythmias may be further classified into:
1. Sinus tachycardia.
2. Premature ventricular contractions (PVCs).
3. Supraventricular tachycardia (SVT).
4. Ventricular tachycardia.
5. Atrial fibrillation.
6. Atrial flutter.
7. Ventricular fibrillation.

Recognition of Tachyarrhythmias

Tachyarrhythmias may cause non specific signs and symptoms that differ according to age of patient. Clinical findings may include palpitations, light headedness, dizziness, fatigue and syncope. In infants, the tachyarrhythmia may be undetected for long periods until cardiac output is significantly impaired and infant develops signs of congestive heart failure such as poor feeding, rapid breathing and irritability. Other symptoms associated with tachyarryhthmias are:

1. Respiratory distress/failure often due to pulmonary edema.
2. Shock with hypotension or poor end organ perfusion.
3. Altered consciousness.
4. Sudden collapse with rapid detectable pulses.
   If the rhythm is unstable, it causes signs and symptoms of poor tissue perfusion.

Sinus Tachycardia

The sinus tachycardia(ST) is defined when heart rate is more than 160/minute in an infant, more than 140/min but less than 200/min in children (Fig. 3.5). The children may manifest with fever, anxiety and may present either in a state of shock or may be with manifestations of congestive heart failure. The underlying cause has to be treated which includes fever, fluid loss, metabolic stress, injury pain, anxiety, anemia or drugs.

ECG characteristics:
- Heart rate is increased.
- P waves are normal.
- P-R interval is constant.
- R-R interval varies with heart rate.
- QRS complex is narrow.

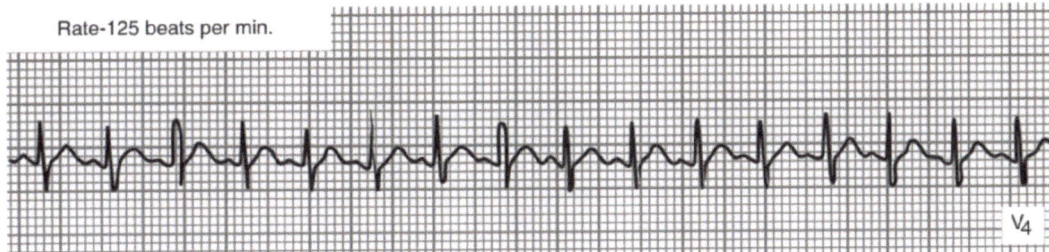

Fig. 3.5: Sinus tachycardia (heart rate 180/min) in a febrile 10 month old infant

Sinus Arrhythmia

Sinus arrhythmia is a phasic variation in heart rate. The heart rate increases during inspiration and decreases during expiration. The arrhythmia occurs with maintenance of characteristics of sinus rhythm. No treatment is indicated.

Supraventricular Tachycardia (SVT)-Atrioventricular Re-entrant Tachycardia

Pre-excitation Syndromes (Fig. 3.6)

Supraventricular tachycardia (SVT) is an abnormally fast rhythm originating above the ventricles. It is most commonly caused by a re-entry mechanism that involves an accessory pathway or the A-V conduction system. SVT is the most common significant arrhythmia in children.[6]

SVT tends to be sustained. Most SVTs in the young have a narrow QRS complex, under 80 millisecond in duration. After conversion to sinus rhythm, the QRS morphology should be the same as during SVT. However some young patients with SVT may manifest a wide QRS morphology. Thus, wide QRS tachycardias in infants (and not in older children) may be aberrant forms of SVT.

SVT is caused by one of the following mechanisms (Figs 3.7A and B):
1. Accessory pathway re-entry (AVRT) tachycardia.
2. AV Nodal re-entry tachycardia (AVNRT)
3. Ectopic atrial focus-primary atrial tachycardia
4. Junctional ectopic tachycardia (JET)

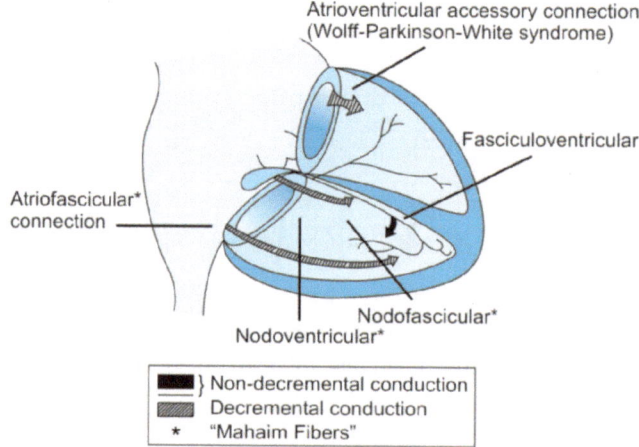

Fig. 3.6: Types of ventricular pre-excitation. Typical accessory AV connections display nondecremental (all or one) conduction. Various patterns of pre-excitation with decremental antegrade conduction have been included under the designation Mahaim fibers. Catheter and surgical ablation results have indicated atriofascicular conditions

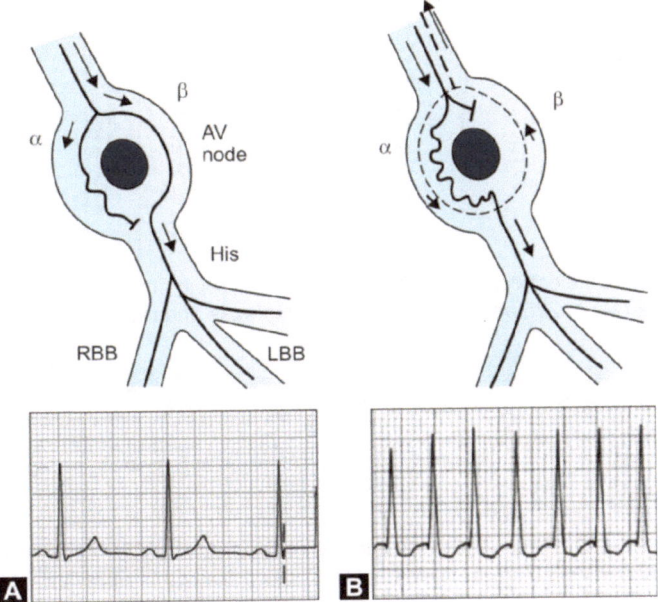

Figs 3.7A and B:[2] Schematic diagram of dual pathways of atrioventricular (AV) node. (A) Normal conduction, resulting in normal sinus rhythm. (B) Re-entrant circuit, resulting in AV nodal re-entrant SVT. RBB = Right bundle branch; LBB = left bundle branch

In general, the rate of SVT in patients under 1 year of age is faster than older patients. Rates from SVT range from 220-280 beats/minute in younger patients compared to 180-240 beats/minute in an older child (Fig. 3.8). The characteristic features include abrupt onset and termination, fixed cycle length, normal QRS complexes and usually an absence of clearly discernible P waves. In pediatric patients, two tachycardia mechanisms, atrioventricular re-entry tachycardia (AVRT) and AV nodal re-entry tachycardia (AVNRT) predominate in an age dependent manner.

Accessory pathway re-entry (AVRT) tachycardia: Most commonly involves an abnormal rhythm circuit that allows a wave of depolarization to travel in a circle, between atria and ventricles. It includes either a re-entry mechanism within the AV node or it involves the AV node as an accessory pathway. A re-entrant circuit is established as a wave of depolarization is conducted to the ventricle through the AV node and then back to the atrium using an accessory pathway. Accessory pathway

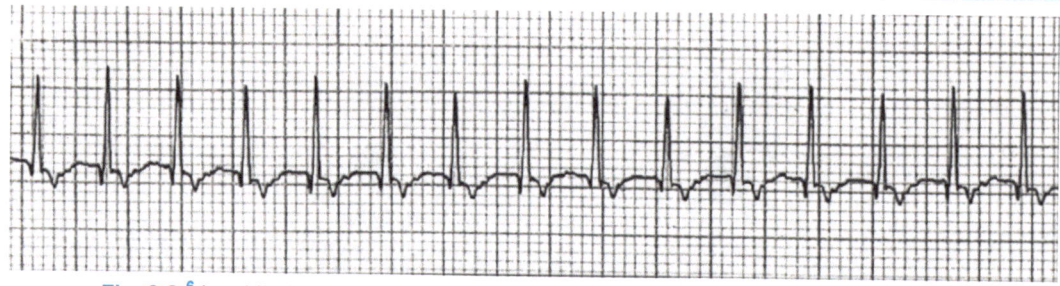

Fig. 3.8:[6] Lead II electrocardiograph rhythm strip showing supraventricular tachycardia at a rate of 225 beats, narrow QRS complexes and retrograde inverted

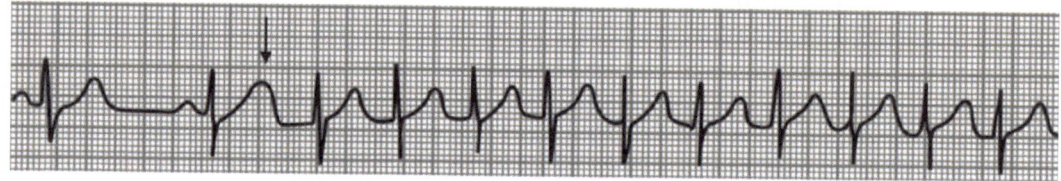

Fig. 3.9: V1 Electrocardiographic rhythm strip showing AV nodal re-entry tachycardia (AVNRT) with narrow QRS complex and absent P wave

SVT is the most common cause of non sinus tachycardia in children. A common example of a condition that produces SVT via an accessory pathway is Wolff-Parkinson White (WPW) syndrome in which ventricular pre-excitation (producing a "delta" wave) on ECG is visible during sinus rhythm.

AV nodal re-entry (AVNRT) tachycardia: It is the commonest cause of the SVT in adulthood. SVT may also result from re-entry using dual pathways (fast and slow) within the AV node. It is commonly associated in congenital heart disease (e.g., Ebstein anomaly, single ventricle and following cardiac surgery). This decreases cardiac output leading on to congestive cardiac failure (Fig. 3.9).

Clinical presentation:

Infants - Poor feeding, rapid breathing, irritability, unusual sleepiness, pallor, vomiting

Older children - Palpitation, shortness of breath, chest pain, discomfort, dizziness, lightheadedness and fainting

SVT is well tolerated in most infants and older children. It can however lead to congestive heart failure and clinical evidence of shock, particularly when there is underlying congenital heart disease or myocarditis and left ventricular function is impaired.

ECG Characteristic of SVT

Heart rate — Infants — >220/minute.
Children - >180/minute.
P wave — absent or abnormal.
R-R interval — Often constant
QRS Complex usually narrow in 90% of children.

Pre-excitation syndrome: It represent a group of electrophysiologic abnormalities in which atrial impulses are conducted partly or completely prematurely to the ventricles via a mechanism other than the normal AV node.

Wolff-Parkinson-White syndrome (WPW syndrome) (Fig. 3.10): WPW syndrome is the most common form of cardiac pre-excitation syndrome. Although commonly seen in normal hearts, there is an increased prevalence among patients with congenital heart disease, hypertrophic cardiomyopathy and cardiac rhabdomyomas. Overall incidence in healthy subject is up to 2/1000. The presence of multiple accessory connections is increased in presence of congenital heart disease especially Ebstein's anomaly where abnormal development of valve annulus is fundamental to both the electrical and anatomic anomalies.

WPW syndrome is characterized by tachycardia (240 + 40/min) with short P-R interval due to rapid anterograde (atria to ventricle) conduction and a broad slurring of QRS complex producing delta waves caused by premature activation of ventricle through the accessory pathway (bundle of Kent) followed by depolarization of ventricles through the AV node and bundle of His.

Narrow QRS duration in orthodromic reciprocating tachycardia whereas wide QRS in antidromic reciprocating tachycardia.

Clinically complaints of palpitation, exertional dyspnea with occasional cardiovascular collapse may be there. Ambulatory electrocardiographic monitoring (Holter monitoring) is used to capture any abnormality on ECG when symptoms occur.

ECG-Short P-R interval with abnormal P wave axis and slurring of QRS complex producing delta waves.

Echocardiography-used to diagnose structural lesions (Ebstein's anomaly, rhabdomyoma, endocarditis, etc.) associated with arrhythmias.

Management of SVT (Fig. 3.11)

1. Vagal stimulatory maneuvers-carotid sinus massage, pressure on eyeball, gagging-effective in older children but rarely in infants. Placing an icebag on face is more effective in infants. A glove filled with ice placed on infants face for 20 seconds or pelting it with water is useful.

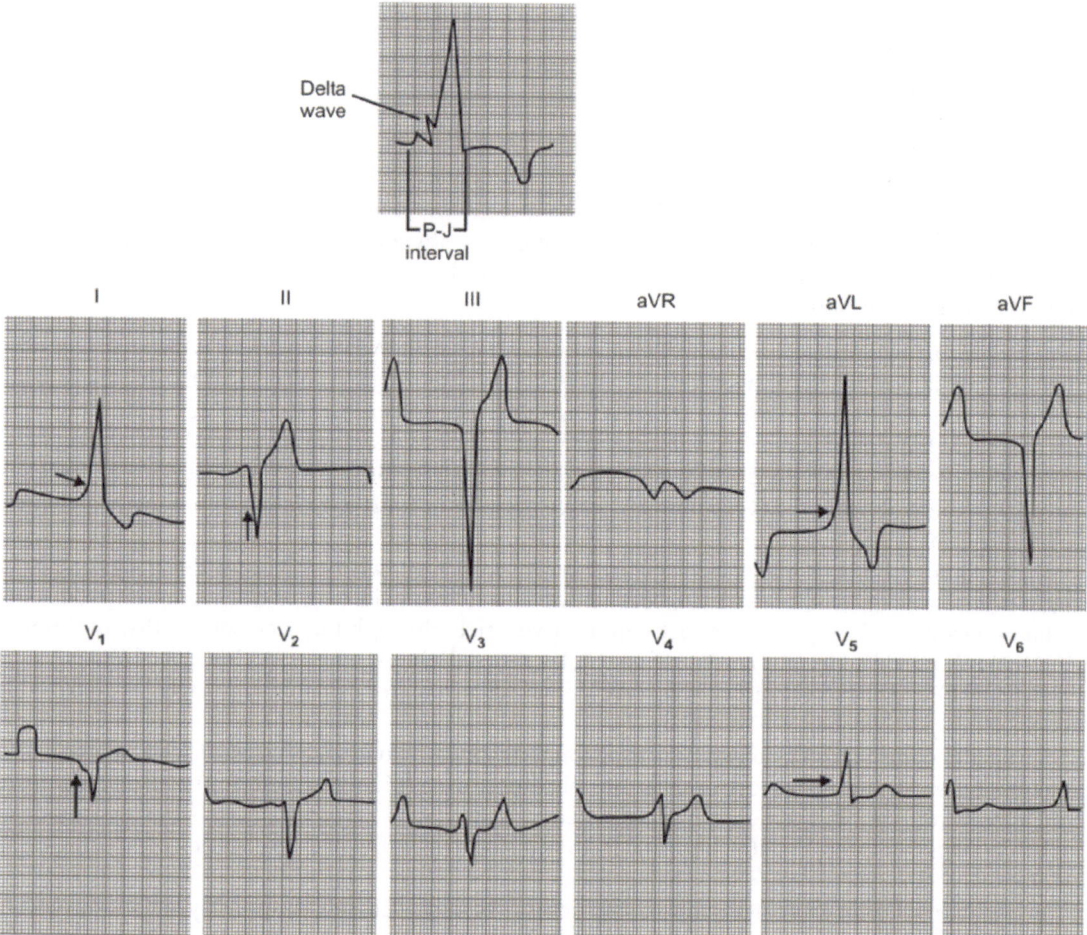

Fig. 3.10: Monitor recording from a patient with intermittent Wolff-Parkinson-White syndrome. The second and third beats display short PR intervals with delta wave with no change in the atrial rhythm

Arrhythmias

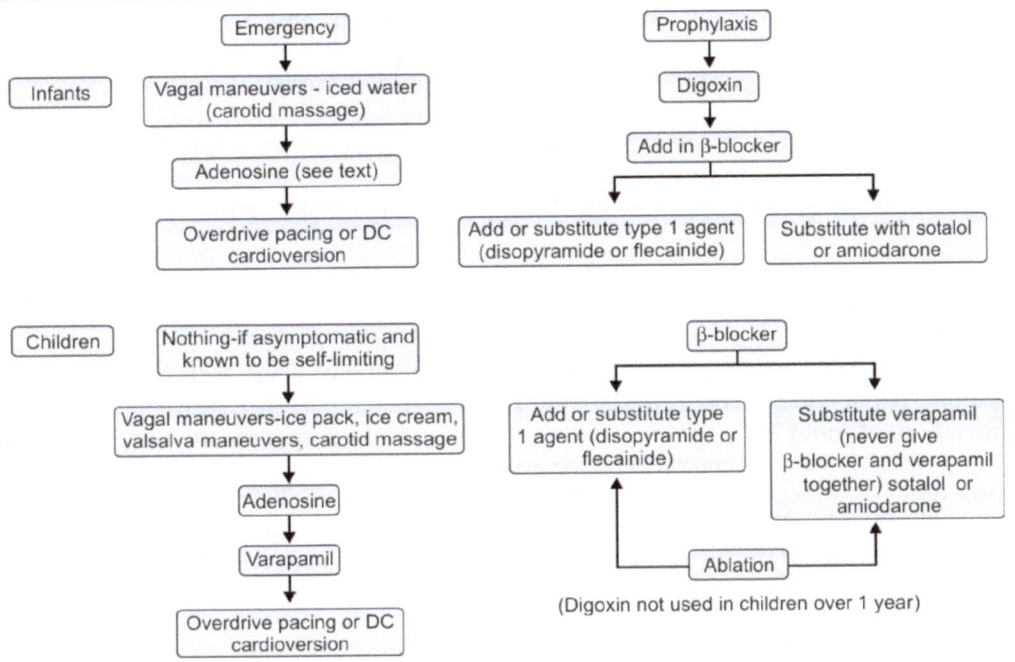

Fig. 3.11:[5] Algorithm for management of SVT in infants and children

2. Adenosine-drug of choice in SVTs with re-entry circuits, but not effective in irregular tachycardias like atrial flutter, fibrillation or ventricular tachycardia.
   Mode of action-Transiently blocks AV node conduction and sinus node pacemaking activity.
   - Usual effective dose 0.1 mg/kg (maximum dose-6 mg/kg) given in instalments of rapid saline flush.
   - Side effect-Severe bronchospasm reported in known asthmatic patients.
3. If adenosine is not available-DC cardioversion in infants with CCF-0.5 joule/kg-2 joule/kg. This should be followed by digitalization for 3-6 months to prevent recurrence.
4. In older children, intravenous propranolol or verapamil may be tried-but they are not drugs of choice and require careful monitoring.

5. In patients with postoperative atrial tachycardia-intravenous amiodarone administration has given excellent results.
6. Overdrive transoesophageal pacing or atrial pacing in those resistant cases that have already undergone digitalization.
7. Finally intracardiac radiofrequency ablation techniques are now available for life threatening arrhythmias which give permanent cure.
8. Radiofrequency ablation or surgical interruption of accessory pathways-in case medical management fails.

Atrial Flutter

Atrial flutter is an uncommon narrow complex tachyarrhythmia in children. The pacemaker lies in single re-entry circuit and "circus movement" in right atrial tissue which is the mechanism of this arrhythmia. Atrial flutter is characterized by a strictly regular atrial rate (F wave with "saw tooth" configuration) of about 300 beats/min, followed by ventricular response with varying degrees of block (e.g., 2:1, 3:1, 4:1) and a normal QRS complex (Fig. 3.12).

Atrial flutter may suggest a significant cardiac pathology and possible causes are structural heart disease with dilated atria, myocarditis, and previous surgery involving atria (Mustard procedure, Fontan operation, or ASD repair), rheumatic heart disease and digitalis toxicity. The ventricular rate determines eventual cardiac output.

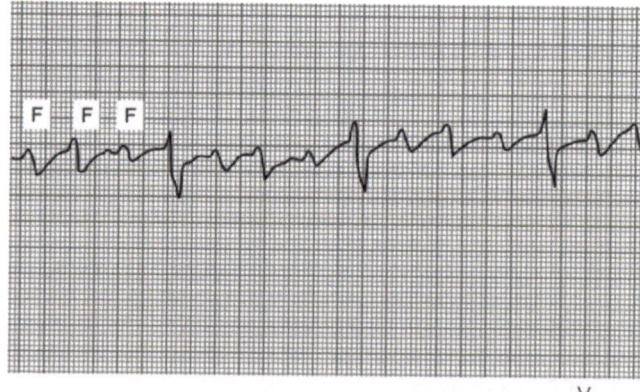

Fig. 3.12: Atrial flutter with characteristic "saw tooth" undulating P waves

Management

1. Digitalization-once digitalis toxicity is ruled out.
2. Propranolol-1-4 mg/kg/day in 3 divided doses.
3. Amiodarone-still in experimental stage in children.
4. Synchronized DC cardioversion-treatment of choice if drug treatment fails.
5. Quinidine and procainamide (class I)-required for maintenance.

Atrial Fibrillation (AF) (Fig. 3.13)

There are multiple small migratory re-entry circuits in the right atrium leading to absence of co-ordinated atrial contraction. It is characterized by fast atrial rate (f wave at a rate of 350-600 beats/min) and an irregular ventricular response with normal QRS complexes. It is associated with structural heart diseases like dilated atria, myocarditis, digitalis toxicity or previous atrial surgery. The rapid ventricular rate with loss of co-ordinated contraction of the atria and the ventricles, decreases the cardiac output, similar to atrial flutter.

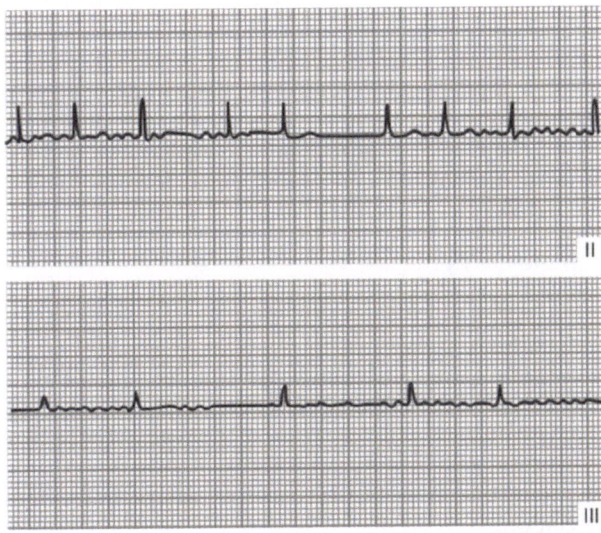

Fig. 3.13:[9] Lead II recording of atrial fibrillation displaying a course baseline and an irregular ventricular rhythm

Atrial fibrillation also suggests a significant cardiac pathology which include congenital or rheumatic heart disease involving mitral or aortic valve and dilated atria, myocarditis or cardiomyopathy and digitalis toxicity.

Ventricular Arrhythmia (Fig. 3.14)

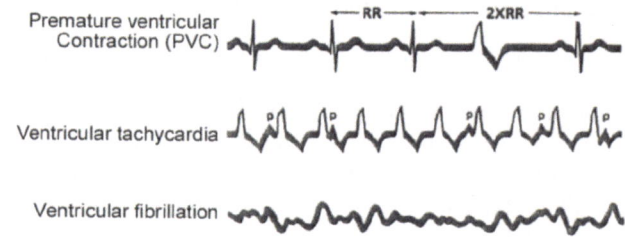

Fig. 3.14: Ventricular arrhythmias. (From Park MK, Guntheroth WG: How to Read Pediatric ECGs, 3rd ed. St. Louis, Mosby, 1992)

Premature Ventricular Contraction (PVC)

A bizarre wide QRS complex appears earlier than anticipated and T wave points in the opposite direction. A full compensatory pause usually appears which indicates that the sinus node is not prematurely discharged by the PVC. PVCs that are asymptomatic and have no hemodynamic consequences do not require treatment. Occasional PVCs may be treated with beta blockers, atenolol 1-2 mg/kg in a single daily dose.

Ventricular Tachycardia (VT)

VT is a series of 3 or more repetitive beats originating from the ventricle distal to the bifurcation of Bundle of His. It is also defined by a rate faster than 120 beats/min in children. On the surface electrocardiogram each QRS complex is different from the underlying sinus rhythm and normally shows ventricular atrial dissociation (Figs 3.15A and B). This is the most important consideration because the QRS complex may not be absolutely wide for the age of the patient. Also if the child has tachycardia with a bundle branch block morphology, the chances are greater than 90% that it is of ventricular origin. Other points that favor the diagnosis of ventricular tachycardia are:
1. Atrioventricular dissociation,
2. Intermittent fusion or sinus capture beats.
3. Morphology of ventricular tachycardia similar to single PVC's.

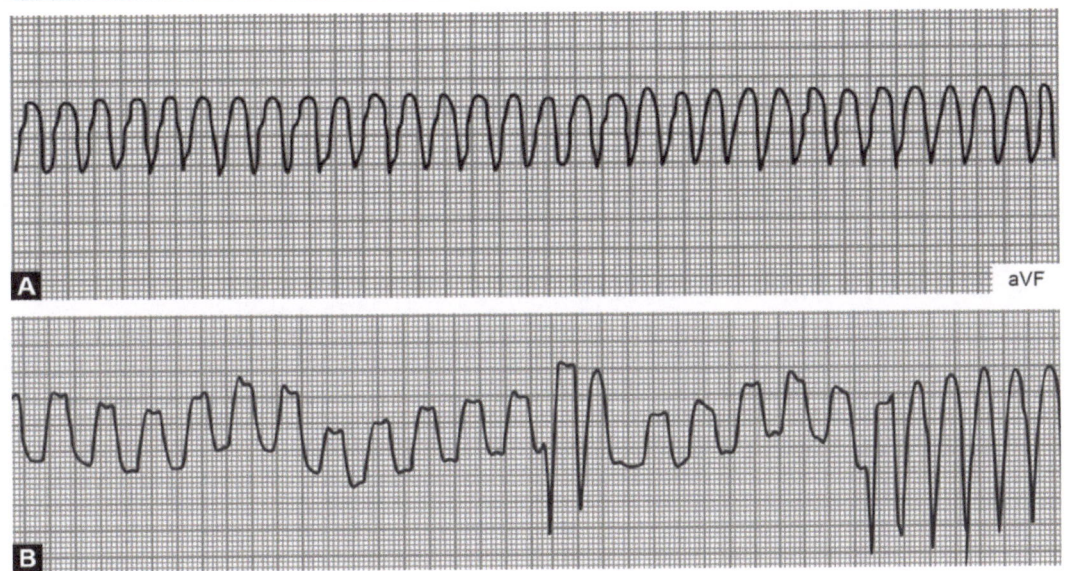

Figs 3.15A and B: Ventricular tachycardia. (A) Monomorphic; (B) Polymorphic (torsades de pointes)

Clinically, the child may be asymptomatic or present with syncope. Rapid ventricular rate may often compromise stroke volume and cardiac output and may deteriorate into ventricular fibrillation. Most children who develop VT have underlying heart disease, prolonged QT syndrome, myocarditis/cardiomyopathy, electrolyte imbalance, hyperkalemia, hypocalemia, etc. Almost all types of ventricular arrhythmias should be treated in patients who are otherwise seriously ill and have acute onset of arrhythmia. Multiparous PVCs, couplets and ventricular tachycardia should be treated immediately.

Management: Ventricular tachycardia signifies a serious myocardial pathology or dysfunction. Immediate treatment with sustained symptomatic tachycardia starts with an assessment of patient's hemodynamic status.

1. VT is promptly treated with synchronized direct current cardioversion in patients with low cardiac output (0.5-1 joule/kg).
2. If the patient is conscious, intravenous bolus of lidocaine (1mg/kg/dose over 1-2 min) followed by intravenous drip of lidocaine (20-50 µg/kg/min).
3. If cardioversion fails, the patient may become hypoxic, acidotic or hypocalcemic.

4. In postoperative VT resistant to other drugs, amiodarone has shown good results.
5. If antiarryhthmic control is inadequate, invasive electrophysiological studies should be considered.

Pulseless VT may be monomorphic or polymorphic (QRS complexes vary in appearance). Torsades de pointes is an arrhythmia in which the QRS gradually changes from one morphology to another. The ventricular rate can vary from 150-250/mt. It can be seen in conditions associated with a markedly prolonged baseline QT intervals or other conditions e.g. drug toxicity. This tends to, recur and to resolve spontaneously but may deteriorate into ventricular fibrillation. Tosades de pointes is treated with magnesium sulphate.

Long QT Interval Syndrome (LQTS)

Long QT Interval syndromes are rare congenital disorders associated with serious ventricular arrhythmias. Torsade de pointes is the characteristic ventricular tachyarrhythmia which is almost pathognomonic of long QT syndromes. The first symptomatic episode is usually in childhood. The clinical history is almost diagnostic, with repeated episodes of syncope associated with emotional stress, sudden fight or physical stress.

Ventricular Fibrillation

On the surface electrocardiogram, ventricular fibrillation is a series of low amplitude, rapid, irregular depolarizations without identifiable QRS complexes. It is an arrhythmia which is of malignant magnitude and mostly terminates fatally. The depolarizations are disorganized and resemble electrical interference in electrode contact with patient. Trans-oesophageal cardiac recording and stimulations are well recognized (Fig. 3.16).[7] This technique is useful in diagnosing the atrial/ventricular relationship in patients with small P wave or when P waves are buried in QRS complexes or T waves.

Management of Ventricular Fibrillation (Flow chart 3.1)

If ventricular fibrillation either does not respond to first attempt at defibrillation, bretylium tosylate may be tried. It is important to note that the onset of action of bretylium takes 3 to 6 minutes and the 1/2 life is quite long, therefore the line of administration of bretylium should be noted carefully and successive defibrillation planned. Multiple doses of bretylium are probably not necessary.

Management after restoring sinus rhythm is directed at finding the underlying abnormality. Ventricular fibrillation is the rarest cardiac arrhythmia found in children and also most dangerous. The majority of children who have ventricular fibrillation have either a structurally normal heart or a prolonged QT interval/WPW syndrome. Ventricular fibrillation with WPW syndrome is an absolute indication for surgery. Thus children with ventricular fibrillation should be extensively evaluated for detection of congenital or acquired heart disease.

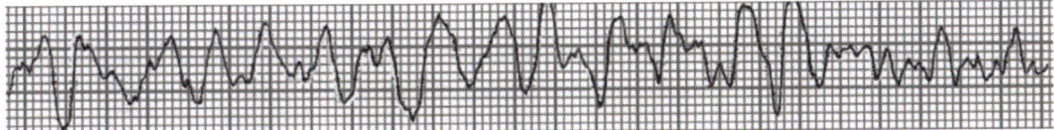

Fig. 3.16: Holter recording showing ventricular fibrillation

Flow chart 3.1: Treatment of ventricular fibrillation/pulseless ventricular tachycardia in accordance with Resuscitation Council, UK Guidelines 1997.

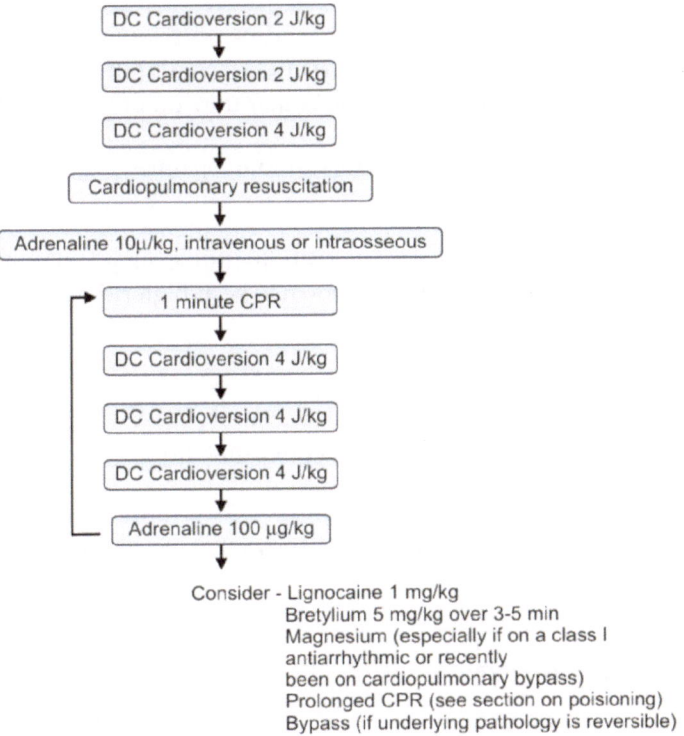

Consider - Lignocaine 1 mg/kg
Bretylium 5 mg/kg over 3-5 min
Magnesium (especially if on a class I antiarrhythmic or recently been on cardiopulmonary bypass)
Prolonged CPR (see section on poisioning)
Bypass (if underlying pathology is reversible)

Overdrive ventricular pacing may be used by pacing at a rate 30-50 beats minute faster than the tachycardia, for 5 to 10 minutes and then stop pacing. However, with this method one should be prepared to use immediate cardioversion or defibrillation.

Chronic Treatment[9,10]

Cardiac arrhythmia suppression trial (CAST) include certain drugs for further treating already established patients with arrhythmias. These drugs are classified into 3 major groups:

Class IA: Quinidine, Procainamide

These are essential for ventricular arrhythmia only after other drugs have failed and should not be used in patients with long QT interval and should be used continuously in patients with depressed left ventricular function and sinus node dysfunction.

Class IB: Phenytoin/Mexiletine

Major indication for postoperative congenital heart disease especially those with abnormal hemodynamics, also in LQTs and MVP. Their value is that they do not depress left ventricular function when given orally.

β-blockers are of major use in children with LQTs, cardiomyopathies.

Class III: Amiodarone/Sotalol

The major indication for amiodarone is in patients with life threatening arrhythmias who have paroxysmal symptoms such as syncope and those known to be at high risk for sudden death.

Bradyarrhythmias
Approach to identification of cardiac rhythm
- Slow ventricular rate is when
  - impulse formation in SA node is blocked.
  - Intrinsic rhythmicity of A-V block node takes over (50-60/min)
  - Commonest condition in newborn
  - Blocked atrial contractions
- When SA and AV node are both blocked-idioventricular rhythm (30-50/min) which is generated in the ventricles.

Bradyarrhythmias

Bradyarrhythmias may be classified into:
1. Sinus bradycardia.
2. Sinus node dysfunction.
3. Atrioventricular conduction disturbances.
    a. First degree A-V block.
    b. Second degree A-V block.

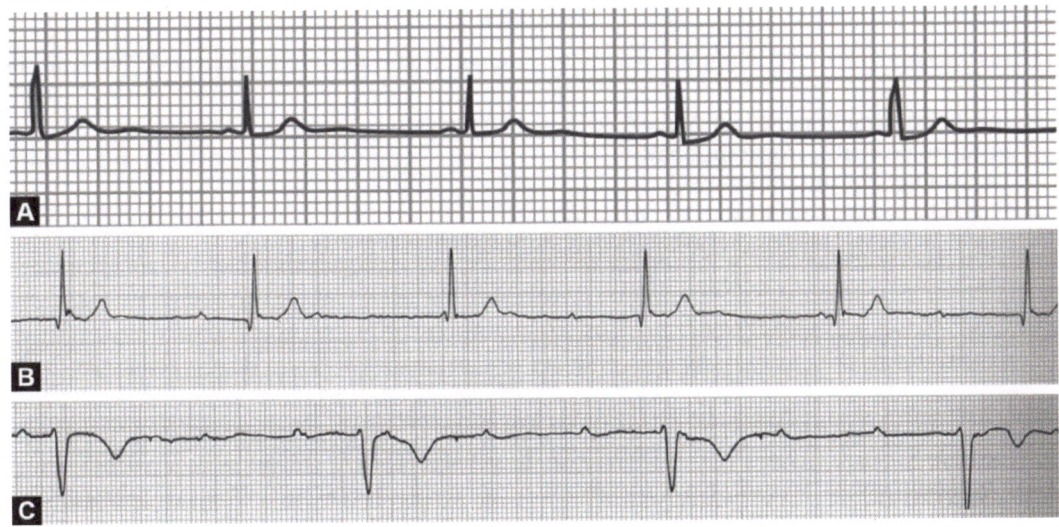

Figs 3.17A to C: Bradycardia. (A) Sinus bradycardia. (B) Junctional escape rhythm. (C) Idioventricular escape rhythm

   c. Third degree (complete) A-V block.
   d. Bundle branch blocks.

Sinus Bradycardia

- Characteristics of sinus rhythm but rate is lower than the normal for that age.
- The heart rate is slow normally also when the vagal stimulation is high
- Especially in athletes, hypothermia, hypothyroidism, hyperkalemia, obstructive jaundice and in presence of increased intracranial pressure.
- Drugs-digitalis, beta blockers, morphine and diltiazem also bring the heart rate down.

Management
- Underlying cause is treated.
- Drugs-Atropine-0.02-0.04 mg/kg.
    - Epinephrine-0.1-0.5 mg/kg/IV.
    - Isoproterenol-0.01-0.2 µgm/kg/min I/V.
- Temporary pacing

Sinus Node Dysfunction (SND) (Fig. 3.18)

- Sinus pause-momentary cessation of activity-momentary absence of P wave and QRS complex.
- Causes
  - Increased vagal tone, CHD-ASD, AVSD.
  - Focal myocarditis, cardiomyopathy
  - Drugs-Digoxin, anti-arrythmics.
  - Hypoxia, hypothyroidism
  - Surgical-atrial operations-commonest in children.

Fig. 3.18: Sinus node dysfunction-ECG showing a sinus pause with a ventricular escape beat after 4s

- Diagnosis
  - Sinoatrial exit block
  - Sinus bradycardia, pause or arrest.
  - Tachycardia-due to atrial re-entry.
  - Bradycardia-hard to define-age specific.
- Presentation- asymptomatic or may present with fatigue, dizziness, syncope, exercise intolerance.

Management

- Severe bradycardia
  - I/V atropine-0.04 mg/kg.
  - I/V isoproterenol-0.05-0.5 µg/kg, but medical therapy not effective in chronic cases.
- Permanent pacemaker implantation-treatment of choice.
- Prevention-improved surgical technique to save guard anatomy, blood and nerve supply of SA node.

The decision to recommend treatment is straight forward when symptoms are documented during sinus node dysfunction (SND). The hemodynamic effect of a slow heart rate depends on how different it is from the patient's usual heart rate. Sudden decrease in rate may be poorly compensated by increases in stroke volume, particularly in those with poor cardiac function. All blocks, especially when symptoms are life threatening as with syncope or near-syncope, treatment decisions are complicated as also when symptoms either are absent or are difficult to document during SND.

1. Recommendations are somewhat controversial for asymptomatic patients.

    Moderate sinus bradycardia is normal in children and it rarely necessitates treatment. Underlying causes, such as hypothyroidism should be corrected.

    Acute medical treatment is indicated when severe sinus or functional bradycardia or frequent sinus arrest results in loss of consciousness. Regardless of cause, I/V atropine 0.04 mg/kg or Isoproterenol 0.05-0.5 µg/kg/min usually increases the heart rate.
2. When these drugs do not increase heart rate to a satisfactory level, a temporary transvenous or external pacemaker is indicated.[8]

    Chronic medical treatment has not been accepted as standard treatment for SND. Several pharmacologic agents are available, but success is variable and side effects prevalent.

    Patients with 3rd degree AV block (complete heart block) and those with severe sinus node dysfunction may require permanent cardiac pacing. In all cases, the occurrence of symptoms such as syncope, exercise intolerance, or dizziness prompts evaluation of pacing.

    Patients with persistent complete AV block as a result of cardiac surgery generally require pacing, even in the absence of symptoms.[11]

    Prophylactic cardiac pacing may be recommended in completely asymptomatic patients, with complete congenital atrioventricular block if daytime average heart rates fall below 50, and if at night rates are below 30, or if long pauses (>3 seconds) are recorded on Holter monitoring,[12] then these patients are at greater risk for progressing to syncope (Stokes-Adams attacks) or sudden cardiac death and therefore prophylactic cardiac pacing is indicated.

    When treatment is indicated, for infants, and children with SND, the accepted mode is permanent pacemaker implantation. The pace maker choices for SND include following types of multiprogrammable pacemakers: ventricular demand (VVI), atrial demand (AAI), universal (ODD, WIR and AAIR).

    Arrhythmias due to SND can be slow, fast or irregular. Sinus arrhythmias can be exaggerated in SND. Bradycardia is hallmark of SND. Bradycardia is hard to define, but on the basis of Holter monitoring studies suggest that heart rate below 40 in over 12 years is abnormal at anytime including sleep.

Atrioventricular Block (A-V conduction) Disturbance (Fig. 3.19)

AV block-disturbance in conduction between normal sinus impulse generation and ventricular response.

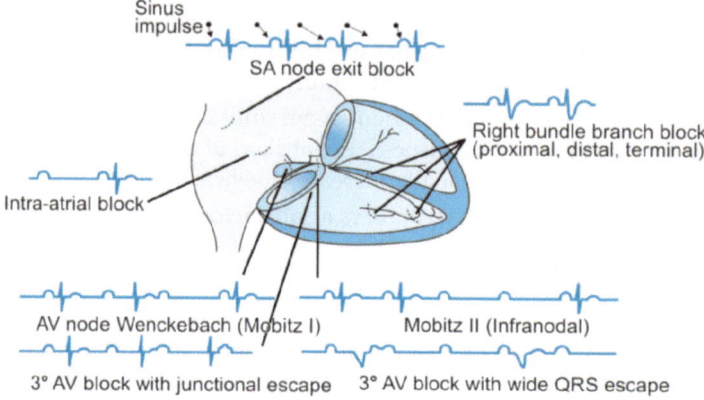

Fig. 3.19: Diagram of different levels of conduction block. Sinoatrial (SA) node exit block, intra-atrial block, Mobitz I and II atrioventricular block, and three levels of right-bundle-branch block are illustrated

First Degree Atrioventricular Blockm (Fig. 3.20)

First degree AV block is when PR interval is greater than established norms. This interval is more age dependent than rate dependent, so determination of normal intervals are based on the patients age. The PR interval is shorter than 160 ms in infancy rising to a maximum of 180 ms in adolescents. Generally structural heart lesions that produce first degree AV block are thought to do so by stretching the atria in the area of the AV node. First degree AV block has also been reported

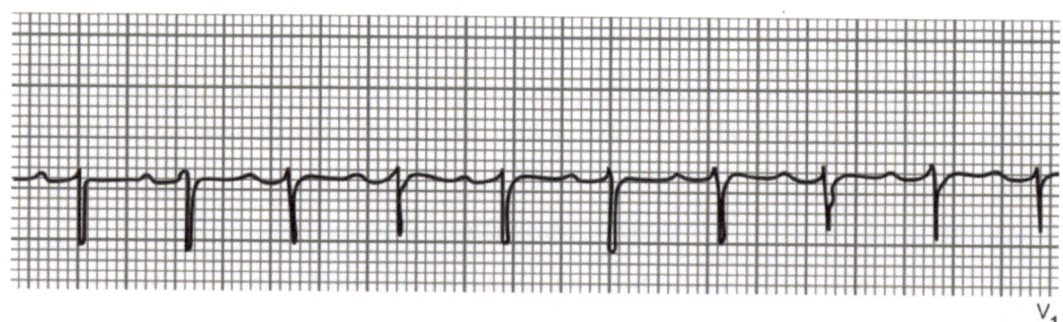

Fig. 3.20: Delay in conduction of impulse from SA to AV node

in up to 6% of neonates (Narula et al) when PR interval is >0.24 sec. There is no clinical significance of first degree AV block. It can be present in acute rheumatic fever, hypothermia digitalis effect, Ebstein's anomaly, etc.

Second Degree Atrioventricular Block

In 1907, Wenckebach described second degree AV block by timing jugular venous pulsations and associating atrial beats with blocked ventricular beats, Mobitz Type I (Wenckebach Block) block is at the level of AV-node where there is decrease in PP interval with increasing P-R interval and subsequent QRS complex being dropped (Fig. 3.21). Vagal dominance in normal children, myocarditis, cardiomyopathy, digitalis toxicity, endocardial cushion defects, Ebstein's anomaly etc may be the causes. The underlying cause should be treated. The block does not progress to complete heart block.

Mobitz Type II Atrioventricular Block (Fig. 3.22)

Second degree AV block is caused by intermittent loss of AV conduction without preceding lengthening of the PR interval. AV conduction is either normal or complete heart block. Block is at level of bundle of His-mostly progresses to complete heart block. The underlying cause has to be treated. Prophylactic pacemaker implantation may be indicated.

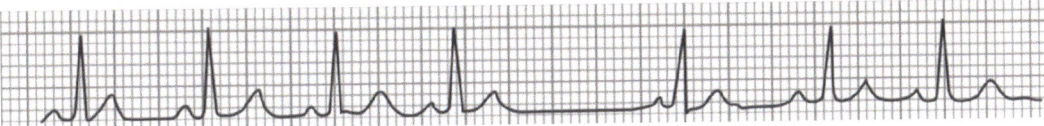

Fig. 3.21: Mobitz type I (Wenckebach phenomenon)

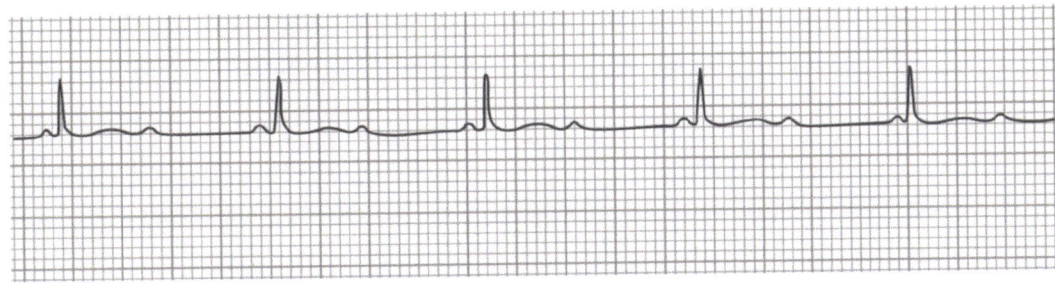

Fig. 3.22: Mobitz type II AV block

All types of heart blocks are worrisome from a clinical point of view because of its significance and the likelihood of sudden death. Clearly the first degree AV block does not carry this concern. Type I is mostly an incidental finding of little long term significance. The clinical significance of type I or II block also may depend on whether there is a wide QRS complex. Second degree AV block in the presence of intraventricular conduction delay usually is associated with Mobitz type II and may have an ominous prognosis. Therefore differentiating type I from type II is a useful clinical exercise.

Third Degree AV Block (Fig. 3.23)

Complete heart block occurs when the atrial impulse cannot propagate to the ventricles. It is usually congenital or occurs after surgery. The incidence is 1/22,000 live births. It is found in association with structural heart lesion especially congenitally corrected transposition. It may be associated with anti-RO antibodies in the mothers, but the exact mechanism by which these antibodies affect the His bundle is not known. There is a relationship of SLE in the pregnant mother with complete heart block in the fetus. There is great variation in symptoms in children with complete heart block from exercise-intolerance, syncopal attacks (Stokes-Adam's syndrome) when the heart rate is < 40 bpm congestive heart failure and even sudden cardiac death to a total lack of symptoms. An ECG is all that is required to make a diagnosis. P waves regular (regular PP interval), Q-R complexes regular (R-R interval regular) but P-R interval keeps varying. The diagnosis can be made antenatally with fetal echocardiography.

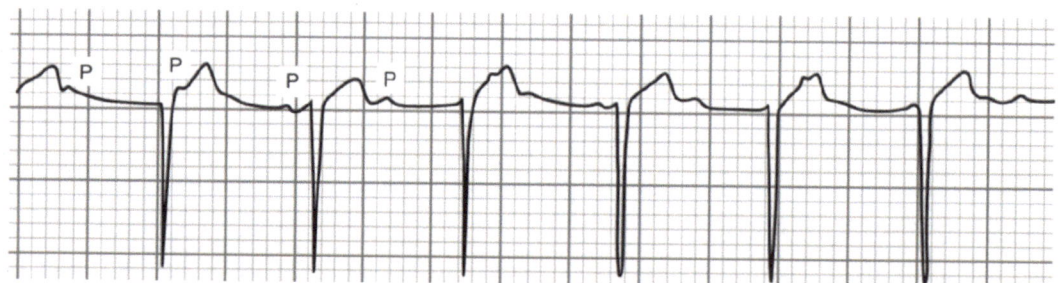

Fig. 3.23: Complete heart block, atrial rate of 80/min and ventricular rate of 39/min

Management

Medical

Acute medical treatment is indicated when severe sinus or functional bradycardia results in frequent sinus arrest which result in loss of consciousness. I/V atropine/0.04 mg/kg) or I/V isoproteronol (0.05-.5 mg/kg) usually increase heart rate. When these drugs fail, temporary transvenous ventricular pacemaker implantation in those awaiting permanent pacemaker which is the ultimate treatment.

Guidelines for Radiofrequency Energy Catheter Ablation of SVT

Abnormal Heart with SVT

Indications
1. Drug resistant arrhythmia (postoperative patients).
2. Long term treatment with antiarrhythmic agents with significant side effects.
3. Ventricular dysfunction because of prolonged drug therapy.

Normal Heart with SVT

Indications
1. Athlete with SVT.
2. Syncope due to SVT.
3. Tachyarrhythmia induced ventricular dysfunction.
4. Over 2 years with recurrent SVT on drug therapy.

Asymptomatic WPW

Indications: Athelete in whom an EP (electrophysiologic) study shows short antegrade effective refractory period of the accessory correction.

Bundle Branch Blocks

Bundle branch blocks-represent abnormal depolarization through Bundle of His and Purkinje System-abnormally wide QRS complexes due to delayed depolarization of intraventricular conduction tissues.

Right Bundle Branch Block (RBBB)

RBBB delays activation of right ventricle, commonly seen in Ebstein's anamoly or following Ventriculotomy.

Left Bundle Branch Block (LBBB)

- Much rarer condition.
- May be due to hypertrophic cardiomyopathy.

It may be seen in those children following TOF surgery-there may be co-existent left anterior hemiblock with RBBB.

Pacemaker Therapy[13]

A pacemaker is a device that delivers battery supplied electrical stimulus through electrodes-inserted into the heart, either directly over epicardium or transvenously.

Power Source-Lithium-iodine battery and an electronic circuit regulates the timing and characteristics of the stimuli.

In older children and adolescents, the pacemaker generator is implanted in the subpectoral region with leads attached to endocardium by transvenous route.

In infants and small children-pacemaker generators are implanted in the abdomen with leads attached to epicardial surface of heart. Here, pacemaker leads may be attached to a single chamber or to both atria and ventricles depending upon the rhythm of bradycardia. The generator is programmed to provide sufficient rate and rhythm support.

Table 3.3: Information on antiarrhythmic drugs mentioned in text (all drug doses are given as total daily dose unless otherwise stated)

Drug	Dose	Notes
Quinidine	IV quinidine gluconate is given 6-10 mg/kg kg at the rate of 0.3 to 0.5.mg/kg/min	Used to terminate SVT and VT atrial flutter and fibrillation, because of its side effects newer drugs have taken over.
Procainamide	Oral 30 to 60 mg/kg in 3, 4, 6 hr equally divided doses, IV infusion of up to 20 mg/kg loading dose at the rate of 50 mg/kg/min. A maintenance IV of of 30 to 60 mg/kg/min with normal renal function	Drug of choice in atrial fibrillation with WPW syndrome used in atrial, AV nodal and ventricular tachyarhythmia
Adenosine	Rapid IV bolus-initially 0.05 mg/kg increasing by 0.05 mg/kg to a maximum of 6.25 mg/kg	Used to terminate SVTs that involve the atrioventricular node as part of the re-entry circuit. Can also be used diagnostically to differentiate broad complex SVT from a ventricular

Contd...

Contd...

Amiodarone	Oral maintenance-150 mg/m IV infusion 5 mg/kg over 1 hr followed by 10 mg/kg/d	tachycardia. Can also reveal atrial flutter or primary atrial tachycardias by causing transient AV block. Has a broad antiarrhythmic spectrum. Rarely used as first line treatment. Useful in SVT, atrial and ventricular arrhythmias. Long term use is complicated by corneal micro-deposits, rashes, deranged thyroid function and other less common side-effects. Interacts with many drugs, but particular care should be taken if patients are already on digoxin.
Atropine	IV bolus 15-20 µg/kg	Used to increase heart rate in sinus node dysfunction or heart block.
Bretylium	IV 5 mg/kg over 3-5 min	Used for ventricular fibrillation or tachycardia resistant to lignocaine.
Digoxin	Maintenance 8-10 µg/kg (5-10 µg/kg in preterm) loading-IV or oral 25-35 µg/kg (20 µg/kg in preterm) give 1/2 dose followed by 1/4 dose 8h and 16 h later	Used to control paroxysmal SVT. Atrial flutter and fibrillation, avoid in atrial flutter or fibrillation with an accessory pathway as may predispose to ventricular tachycardia/fibrillation. For this reason not recommended in children over 1 year.
Mexiletine	50-l00 mg/kg 8 hrly. IV therapy is not available easily and is associated with high incidence of side effects	Ventricular arrhythmias.
Disopyramide	Oral 10-20 mg/kg in three divided doses (two divided doses in using slow release preparation)	Used principally to treat SVT but also effective in atrial flutter/fibrillation and ventricular arrhythmias.
Esmolol	IV-600 µg/kg over 1 min	Very short acting β-blocker useful in the emergency treatment of atrial tachyarrhythmias or ventricular tachycardia due to tricyclic poisoning.
Flecainide	Oral 3-6 mg/kg in two or three divided doses	Used to treat SVT and ventricular arrhythmias as second line treatment.
Isoprenaline	IV infusion 0.02-0.2 µg/kg/min	Used to increase heart rate in sinus node dysfunction or heart block.

Contd...

Contd...

Lignocaine	IV bolus 1 mg/kg IV maintenance 20-50 µg/kg/min	Used as emergency treatment of life threatening ventricular arrhythmias.
Phenytoin	IV loading 20 mg/kg over 30 min. Oral loading 15 mg/kg in four divided doses Day 1. 75 mg/kg in four divided doses Day 2. Oral maintenance approx. 5 mg/kg in two divided doses	Used to control ventricular arrhythmias in patients with structural heart disease or postoperatively. Plasma, drug levels should be 12-15 mg/L.

Table 3.3 gives the summary of all the antiarrhythmic drugs in the text.

REFERENCES

1. Prince J Kannankeril, Frank A. Fish-Disorders of cardiac rhythm and conduction in Hugh D Allen, DJ Driscoll, Robert E, Shaddy Timothy E, Feltes in Moss and Adams Heart Disease in Infants, Children and adolescents. 7th Ed., Lippincoll, Williams and Wilkins, 2008;293-343.
2. Ludomirsky, Garson A Jr. Supraventricular Tachycardia. In: Garison A Jr. Bricker JT, McNamara DG eds. The Science and Practice of Pediatric Cardiology, Philadelphia Lee and Febiger 1990;1809-49.
3. Michael J Silka. Bundle Branch Block. In: Garison A Jr, Bricker JT. McNarnara DG eds. The Science and Practice of Pediatric Cardiology, Philadelphia. Lee and Febiger 1990;2034-45.
4. Anita Khalil, Sandeep Kapoor. Cardiac Arrhythmias and Cyanotic spells. In: Sachdev HPS, Puri RK, Bagga A. Principles of Pediatric and Neonatal emergencies, Jaypee, 1994;92-103.
5. Ruaciman M, Arrhythmias in Archer N Burch M, Pediatric cardiology. An introduction Chapman and Hallmedical 1992;137-61.
6. Ko JK, Deal BJ, Strasburger JF, Benson DW Jr. Supraventricular tachycardia Mechanism and their age distribution in Pediatric Patients. Am J Cardiol 1992;69:1028-32.
7. Schwartz PI. Moss AJ. Vincent GM. Diagnostic Criteria for Long QT syndrome. Circulation 1993;88:782-4.
8. Benson DW Jr. Transoesophageal electrocardiography and cardiac pacing: State of the art. Circulation 1987;75:86-90.
9. Mehta A V, Sanchez GR, Riordan AC. Amiodarone therapy in children with refractory tachydysrrhythmia. In: Proceedings of the Second World Congress of Pediatric Cardiology. New York. Springer-Verlag. 1985.
10. Cast Investigators. Preliminary report: Effect of Encainide and Flecainide on mortality in a randomized trial of arrhythmia suppression after Myocardial infarction. N Engl J Med 1989;321,406-12.
11. B. Veltria Er. Mirowski M, Rad P. Clinical Efficacy of the Automatic Implantable defibrillator, 6 years clinical experience. Circulation 1986; 7: (Suppl 2) 109.
12. Nakamura F, Nadas A. Complete Heart Block in Infants and Children. N Enlg J Med 1964;270:1261-8.
13. Karpawich PP et al. Congenital Complete atrioventricular block: Clinical and electrophysiologic Predictors of need for pacemaker insertion. Am J Cardiol 1981;48:1098-1102.

CHAPTER 4

Pacemakers in Children

A pacemaker is a small battery powered medical device designed to electrically stimulate the heart muscle in an effort to restore the heart rhythm towards normal.[5]

A pacemaker system consists of two main parts:

The pulse generator and pacing leads. The pulse generator houses the lithium iodine battery and electronic circuits (like small computer). These circuits contain timers that regulate how often the pacemaker must send impulse to stimulate the heart.[2]

The pulse generator is small, measuring approximately 2" x 2" x 1/4" (45 mm x 45 mm x 6 mm) and weighing less than 2 ounces (20-30 gm). The pacing leads are flexible, insulated wires that connect to the pulse generator and carry the electronic impulse to the heart. In addition the leads also carry signals back from the heart to the pulse generator allowing the latter to sense the hearts natural electrical activity.[5]

By sensing the patient's natural rhythm, the pacemaker will only pace the heart whenever it is necessary.

The normal heartbeat originates in the heart's natural pacemaker called the 'sinus node'. The sinus node is usually located in right atrium, though this location can be different in the setting of some congenital heart defects. When the sinus node fires, a wave of electricity sweeps across the upper chambers of the heart (atria) causing the upper chambers to contract. The electrical impulse then travels from atria to lower chambers of the heart (ventricles) through "A-V node" located in center of heart resulting in ventricular contraction, which allows the blood to be pumped to the body (Figs 4.1A and B).

PACEMAKER THERAPY[3]

In general, the pediatric conditions that require pacemaker implantation are:
1. Symptomatic bradycardia → on medications
2. Recurrent bradycardia – tachycardia → sick sinus syndrome
3. Congenital A-V block → congenital complete heart block
4. Postoperative prolonged second on third degree A-V block or surgically acquired heart block which lasts for more than 7 days after surgery.
5. Others – Those with leaking valves, hypertrophic cardiomyopathy, dilated cardiomyopathy.

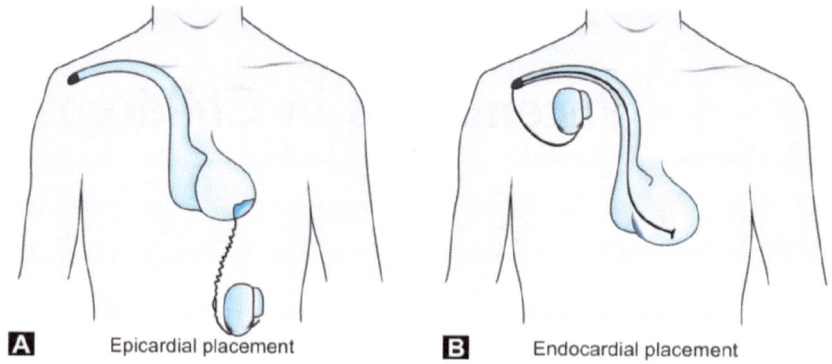

Figs 4.1A and B: Pacemaker attachment. (A) leads attached to the outer surface. (B) leads attached to the inner surface

Indications for Permanent Pacing in Children and Adolescents (American College of Cardiology/American Heart Association)

Guidelines for implantation of Cardiac Pacemakers and anti-arrhythmia devices.[3,4]

Class I Pacemaker Implantation – Necessary and Beneficial

1. Advanced second or third degree A-V block with symptomatic bradycardia, CCF or low cardiac output.
2. Sinus node dysfunction – Age appropriate bradycardia.
3. Postoperative advanced second or third degree A-V block that persists 7 days after cardiac surgery.[8]
4. Congenital third degree A-V block in an infant – ventricular rate < 50 beats/min or congenital heart disease < 70 beats/min.[1]
5. Sustained pause dependent ventricular tachycardia with/without prolonged QT.
6. Congenital third degree A-V block with a wide QRS escape rhythm or ventricular dysfunction.

Class II A Pacemaker Implantation–may be Beneficial

1. Bradycardia-Tachycardia syndrome with anti-arrhythmic treatment.[6]
2. Congenital third degree A-V block beyond 1st year – average heart rate of < 50 beats/minute.
3. Long QT syndrome with 2:1 AV block or third degree AV block.
4. Asymptomatic sinus bradycardia in a child with complex congenital heart disease with a resting heart rate of < 35 beats/minute.

Class II B Pacemaker Implantation–Usefulness Less Well Established

1. Transient postoperative third degree A-V block that reverts to sinus rhythm with residual bifascicular block.
2. Congenital third degree A-V block in an asymptomatic neonate, child or adolescent with an acceptable rate, narrow QRS complex and normal ventricular function.
3. Asymptomatic sinus bradycardia in an adolescent with congenital heart disease with heart rate < 35 beats/min.

Class III Pacemaker Implantation – not useful

1. Transient postoperative AV block with return of normal AV conduction within 7 days.
2. Asymptomatic postoperative bifascicular block with or without first degree A-V block.[9]
3. Asymptomatic type I second degree AV block.
4. Asymptomatic sinus bradycardia in an adolescent with the longest RR interval < 3 seconds and a minimum heart rate > 40 beats/minute.

Pacemaker - Types

1. Single chamber pacemakers use a single lead attached to either the atrium or to the ventricle.
2. Dual chamber pacemakers – use two leads, one attached to the atrium and other to the ventricle. Leads can be attached either to the inside surface (endocardium) or outside surface (epicardium) of the heart leads attached to the endocardium can be placed through a transvenous route that communicates with the heart. The leads are positioned within the heart with the help of fluoroscopy.[5]

Leads attached to the epicardium require surgical exposure of the heart by using an incision through the xiphoid process in a neonate or small infant. The pulse generator is positioned under the skin (sometimes under the muscle) in the upper chest near the collar bone or in the abdominal area depending upon age and size of the patient.

The cardiologist, cardiac surgeon and the nurse looking after the child can reprogramme the pulse generator with a special pacemaker programmer.

Lithium anode batteries of the iodide types are used exclusively. Battery longevity depends on battery size, stimulation frequency and output per stimulation. Battery life varies from 3 years (dual chamber) to 15 years (large single chamber device).

Postoperative Precautions

1. Following the procedure, certain activities will be restricted for days to a week.
   - Wound care – aseptic precaution of the incision – to be kept dry and clean.

- Pacemaker malfunction – The concerned doctor to be consulted for dizziness, excessive fatigue, fainting, difficulty in waking up breathless, palpitation and persistent hiccups. For infants – poor feeding and irritability should be a cause for concern.[7]
- Exercise–After the wound heals, the child should be active but should avoid contact sports, e.g. football, Karate, boxing, judo – where pacemaker may be damaged.

Precautions

1. Magnetic resonance imaging – is not allowed.
2. The pacemaker may set off some types of alarms at metal detectors at airports – the pacemaker identity card should be shown.
3. Mobile Phones should not be placed over pacemaker site.
4. Microwave ovens, most cordless and cellular phones and X-rays are safe.

CONCLUSIONS

Pacemaker installation should not greatly affect a child's school life, as long as instructions listed above are borne in mind and followed.

REFERENCES

1. Aellig NC, Balmer C, Dodge Khatami, Rahn M, et al. Long term follow up after pacemaker implantation in neonates and infants – Ann Thorac Surg 2007;83(4):1420-23.
2. Celikar A, Baspian O, Karagoz T. Transvenous cardiac pacing in children: Problems and complication during follow up – Anadolir Kardijoe Derg 2007;7(3):292-97.
3. Epstein AE, DiMarco JP, Freedman RA, Gettes LS, Gregorates G, et al. ACC/AHA/HRS 2008 guidelines for device based therapy of cardiac rhythm abnormalities: a report of the ACC/AHA Task force on practical guidelines – J Am Coll Cardiol 2008;52(21):1-62.
4. Gregorates G, Cheitlin MD, Conill A. ACC/AHA guidelines for implantation of cardiac pacemakers and anti-arrhythmic devices. J Am Coll Cardiol 1998;31:1175-1209.
5. Pacemakers in children in Pediatric Cardiology for Practitioners. Ed. Myung K Park (5th ed). Published by Mosby. Inc. 2008.
6. Silver ES, Pass RH, Hondof AJ, Liberman L. Paroxymal AV block in children with normal cardiac anatomy as a cause of syncope – Pacing clin Electrophysist 2008;31(3):322-26.
7. Silveth MS, Drago F, MArcora S, Rava L. Outcome of Single chamber ventricular pacemakers with transvenous leads implanted in children – Europace 2007;9(10):894-99.
8. Stephenson EA, Kaltman JR. Current state of Art for use of pacemakers and defibrillatiors in patients with congenital cardiac malfunctions.. Cardiac young 2006;16(3):151-56.
9. Thou T, Shen XQ, Zhow SH, Fang ZF, et al. Atrioventricular block: A serious complication in and after transcatheter closure of perimembranous ventricular septal detects. Clin Cardiol 2008;31(8):368-71.

CHAPTER 5

Cardiac Imaging

Imaging plays a critical role in the diagnosis and therapy of cardiovascular diseases in children. Its role has been strengthened even more by the development of percutaneous techniques for the treatment of both congenital and acquired abnormalities. The differential diagnosis of congenital heart disease was formerly made on the basis of plain films and esophagography. Cardiac catheterization and angiography were used for definitive diagnosis and precise depiction of cardiovascular anatomy. Development in cardiac imaging during 1980s and 1990s included the emergence of non-invasive and semi-invasive imaging techniques such as
- Echocardiography
- Color flow Doppler sonography
- Computed tomography (CT) and magnetic resonance imaging (MRI)

The purpose of this chapter is to give an indepth overview of principles and methodology of echocardiography, and magnetic resonance imaging.

ECHOCARDIOGRAPHY

Echocardiography is an extremely useful, safe and non-invasive method for diagnosis and management of heart diseases. Echo studies, which use sound waves, provide anatomic diagnosis and functional information. It includes M-mode (motion Mode), 2D (Two dimensional), Doppler studies and it also includes color flow studies. Before we go in to details of each one of them, little description about the various echocardiographic windows and the planes in which transducer is directed is mentioned below:

Echocardiographic Windows

These are the areas where transducer can be placed to get the ice pick view of the heart (Fig. 5.1).

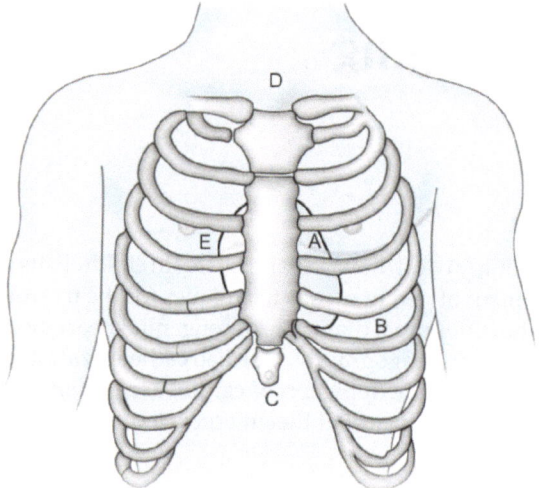

Fig. 5.1: Standard windows for echo examination.
A = parasternal window; B= apical window;
C = subcostal window; D = suprasternal window;
E = right parasternal window

Parasternal Windows

This is the area of the heart, which is not covered by the lungs. This is roughly a triangular area, which extends from the left second to fourth intercostal space in a normal individual. In patients with emphysema or obstructive airway disease the diaphragm is low and the window may extend lower down to fifth or even sixth space. Patients with enlarged hearts as in congestive cardiomyopathy are easy to examine as the dilated heart displaces the lungs laterally. The various planes in which the transducer is directed to get different views of the heart are:

1. *Parasternal sagittal plane or long axis view PLA (Fig. 5.2):* The patient lies on the left side in a semi-lateral position with their left hand placed behind their head. This view is obtained by placing the transducer on 3rd or 4th left intercostal space, just lateral to the sternum with marker pointing towards the right shoulder. This is the most basic view and shows the left ventricular in-flow and out-flow tracts, left atrium, aortic valve, aortic root, ascending aorta and ventricular septum. Pericardial effusion, VSD, TOF, persistent truncus arteriosus and overriding of aorta are best visualized in this view. Aorta is imaged to the right and left ventricular cavity with mitral valve to the left of the screen, and the left atrium is, posterior to the aorta. Above the septa, varying portion of right ventricle and RVOT are seen.

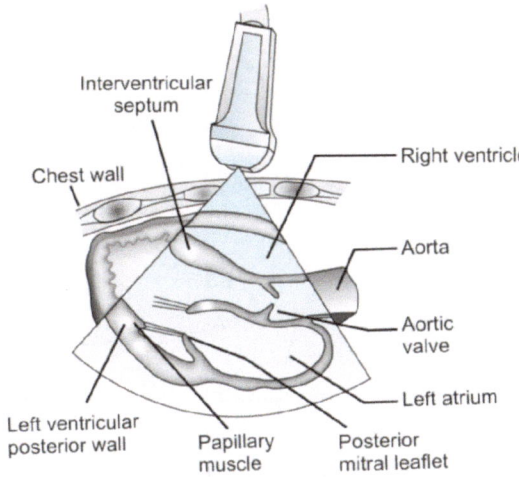

Fig. 5.2: Parasternal sagittal plane or long axis view

2. *Parasternal short axis view (Fig. 5.3):* This is the projection that provides cross sectional images of the heart and great arteries at different levels. Rotating the transducer from the long axis, clockwise at 90° from long axis of aorta, cross sectional images of the semi-lunar valves, mitral valve and papillary muscle can be examined.

   The circular aorta with its three cusps is displayed; in the mid portion of the screen with crescent-shaped RVOT above it. Angling the transducer superiorly, it demonstrates pulmonary valve just anterior and left of the aorta.

   These views are important in the evaluation of the aortic valve (bicuspid or tricuspid) pulmonary valve, pulmonary artery and its branches. RVOT, LVOT, PDA are visualized in a modified plane similar to Fig. 5.3B:

3. *Subxiphoid window and views:* The transducer is placed just right of the xiphoid process below the costal margin. In children excellent images of the heart and the great vessels can be obtained from the subxiphoid window. The subcostal four chamber view (Fig. 5.4) demonstrates atrial and ventricular septa and chambers, AV valves and drainage of systemic and pulmonary views. It is the best view for the evaluation of ASD. Also, with turning the transducer 90°, both the ventricular outflow tracts and the great arteries can be imaged.

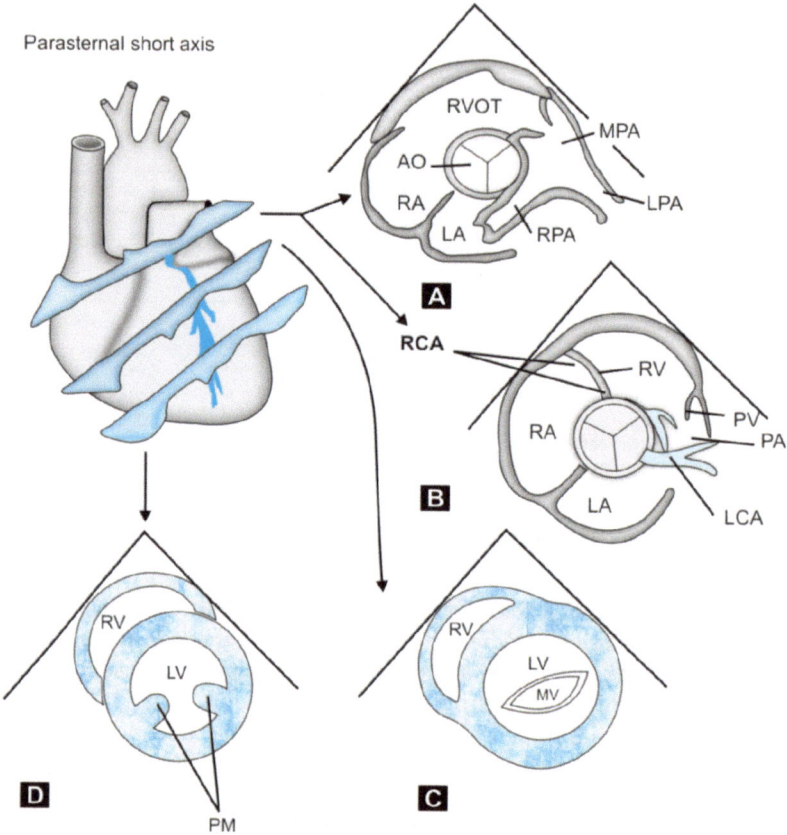

Fig. 5.3: Diagrammatic illustration of important two-dimensional echo view obtained from the parasternal transducer position. Parasternal short-axis views obtained at various levels: (A) and (B) the semilunar valve and great artery level (C), the mitral valve level (D), and the papillary muscle level. AO, Aorta; MV, mitral valve; LCA, left coronary artery; RPA, right pulmonary artery; PM, papillary muscle; RCA, right coronary artery

4. *Suprasternal window and views (Fig. 5.5):* This window is useful to obtain the superoinferior diameter of the left atrium. The suprasternal notch, when the neck is extended, accommodates the transducer, through which the cardiac structures can be imaged. Suprasternal, long axis (Fig. 5.4) and short axis help in the evaluation of anomalies in ascending and descending aorta aortic arch, size of the pulmonary arteries and anomalies of the systemic and pulmonary veins.

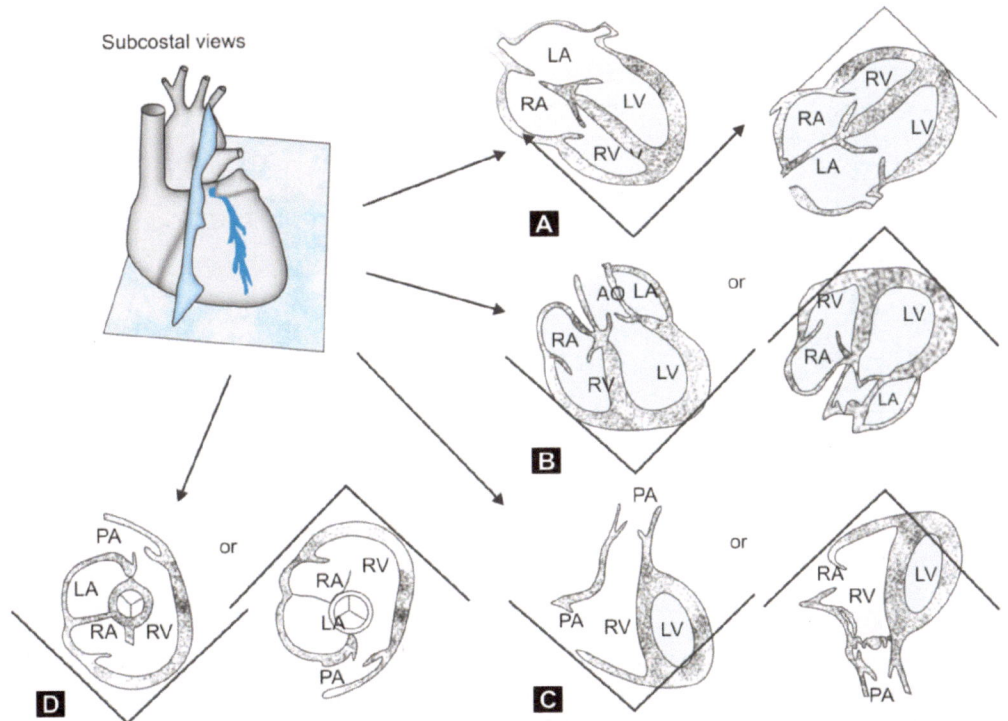

Fig. 5.4: Diagrammatic illustration of two-dimensional echo views obtained with the transducer at subcostal position. Both the apex-down and apex-up images are shown. (A) Subcostal four-chamber view. (B) Showing the LV outflow tract and the proximal aorta (Subcostal "five chamber" view). (C) View that shows the RV outflow tract and the proximal MPA. (D) Subcostal short-axis view

5. *Apical windows:* The transducer is kept over the apex and directed medially and superiorly, where lungs do not cover it. The apical four-chamber view (Fig. 5.6), evaluates the atrial and ventricular septa, AV valves, pulmonary veins, identification of anatomic RV and LV. Detection of pericardial effusion, endocardial cushion defect, is well imaged in this view.

Recommendations established by the American Society of Echo-cardiography-state that left sided structures of a patient's heart as we view the patient from the left hip should appear at the right of the television monitor, while the right sided structures should appear on the left.

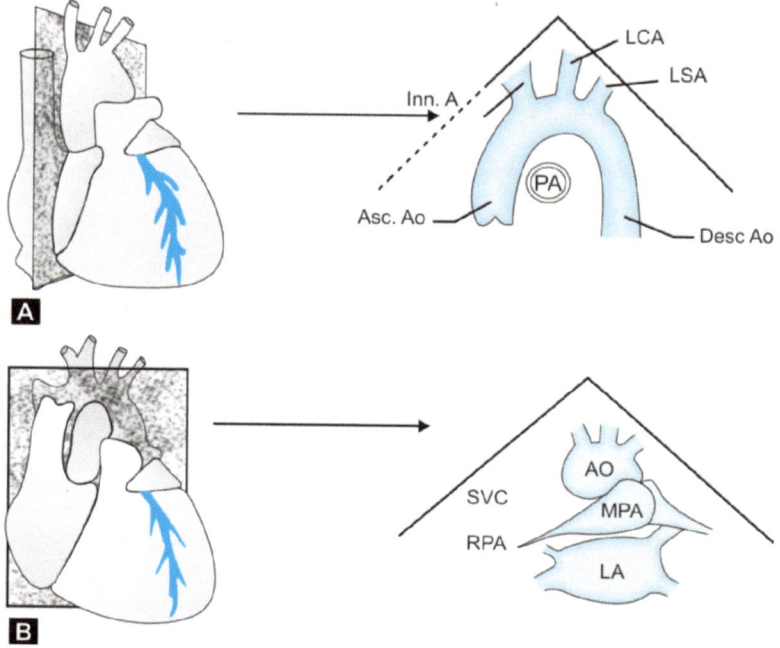

Fig. 5.5: Diagrammatic drawing of suprasternal notch two-dimensional echo views. (A) Long-axis view. (B) Short axis view, AO, Aorta; Asc Ao, ascending aorta; Desc Ao, Descending aorta; Inn A, innominate artery; LCA, Left carotid artery. LSA, left subclavian artery

All subsequent description of the 2-D echograms will be according to the patients anatomic relationship and not according to the image position on the screen. Also, the structures, which are closest to the transducer will appear at the top or apex of the image while those farthest away are at the bottom (Fig. 5.5).

Echocardiographic Studies

There are 4 basic modes:

B-mode, M-mode, Doppler and Color Flow imaging

B (brightness) mode is called as 2-D echo where the images are displayed real time in various shades of grey depending on their echo reflection. Doppler's mode helps to evaluate the velocity of blood

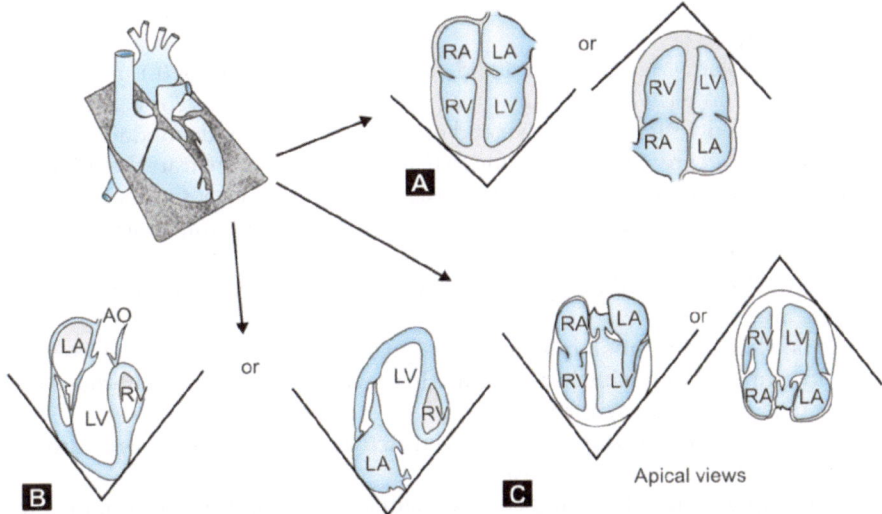

Fig. 5.6: Diagrammatic illustration of two-dimensional echo views obtained with the transducer at the apical position. Both the apex-down and apex-up images are shown. (A) apical four chamber view. (B) apical four-chamber view with LV outflow tract (apical "five-chamber" view). (C) apical long-axis view

across valves and in blood vessels. Color flow imaging uses the Doppler's principles where the direction of blood is easily identified by color coding. If the blood flows towards the transducer, it is coded red and if it moves away it is coded blue (Blue Away Red Towards-BART). Color flow imaging also demonstrates whether the flow is laminar or turbulent (disturbed). M mode refers to recording of movement of cardiac structures at a particular plane in single dimension. Each mode is not mutually exclusive but complementary to each other. Higher the frequency of ultrasound, higher the resolution power and lower is the tissue penetrating capacity. Most of the children with a thin chest wall have a good echo window and hence a transducer frequency of 8-12 MHz is ideal. For older or obese patients, transducer with a lower frequency is selected.

Sedation Protocol

A well-sedated or a quiet child is essential for complete echocardiographic assessment.

Neonate or young infants (< 6 months) – breastfeeding is good enough to keep the child sedated.

In children–(1) Oral chloral hydrate is an ideal non-toxic sedative given at 50-100 mg/kg, maximum being–1.5 gm. It takes 30-40 minutes for onset of action which remains till 90 minutes.

(2) Midazolam–most commonly used drug–Intranasal spray is given for rapid onset of action at a dose of 0.2-0.3 mg/kg.

Intravenous midazolam–May be needed and can be given in a dose of 0.1 mg/kg – but it is best avoided because its hypotensive effect may precipitate a cyanotic spell. The echocardial laboratory should be well equipped with investigative and emergency therapeutic modalities.

1. *Two dimensional echocardiography (B-mode):* It allows us to demonstrate the spatial relationship of structure for more accurate anatomic diagnosis of abnormalities of the heart and great vessels. It provides the tomographic images of the heart by directing the transducer along the various planes described earlier.

   Indications for 2-D Echocardiography are increasing with their increasing diagnostic accuracy. Some of these are:
   a. To screen newborns and small infants who appear to have cardiac defects.
   b. To rule out cyanotic congenital heart disease in newborns with clinical findings of PPHN and persistent fetal circulation syndrome.
   c. To diagnose PDA or other heart defects or ventricular dysfunction in a premature infant who is on a ventilator for pulmonary disease.
   d. To confirm diagnosis in infants and children with atypical findings of certain defects.
   e. To rule out important cardiac conditions that are indicated by other routine examination, chest X-ray or ECG.
   f. To follow up on any condition that may change with time and/or treatment (e.g., before and after indomethacin treatment for PDA in premature infants, evaluation of drug therapy for CHF or LV dysfunction, follow up of CHD).
   g. Before cardiac catheterization and angiocardiography.
   h. To replace cardiac catheterization and angiography in uncomplicated VSD, PDA, ASD.
   i. To evaluate cardiac function before any surgery.

2. *M-mode (motion mode echocardiography):* It has many important applications although 2-D echo has replaced many roles of the M-mode echo. They are:
   a. Measurement of the dimensions of cardiac chambers and vessels, thickness of the interventricular septum and free walls.
   b. Left ventricular systolic function.
   c. Study of the motion of cardiac valves, e.g. mitral valve prolapse (MVP), mitral stenosis, pulmonary hypertension and the interventricular septum.
   d. Detection of pericardial fluid.
   e. Dimension of the cardiac chambers and the aorta increase with increasing age.

   The mean values and ranges of common m-mode echo measurements according to the patients' weight are given in Table 5.1.

Table 5.1: Mean values and ranges of common m-mode echo measurements according to patients weight

	0 to 25 lb	26 to 50 lb	51 to 75 lb	76 to 100 lb	101 to 125 lb	126 to 200 lb
RV dimension	9 (3 to 15)	10 (4 to 15)	11 (7 to 18)	12 (7 to 16)	13 (8 to 17)	13 (12 to 17)
LV dimension	24 (13 to 32)	34 (24 to 38)	38 (33 to 45)	41 (35 to 47)	43 (37 to 49)	49 (44 to 52)
LV free wall (or septum)	5 (4 to 6)	6 (5 to 7)	7 (6 to 7)	7 (7 to 8)	7 (7 to 8)	8 (7 to 8)
LA dimension	17 (7 to 23)	22 (18 to 27)	23 (19 to 28)	24 (20 to 30)	27 (21 to 30)	28 (21 to 37)
Aortic root	13 (7 to 17)	17 (13 to 22)	20 (17 to 23)	22 (19 to 27)	23 (17 to 27)	24 (22 to 28)

Modified from Feigenbaum H: Echocardiography; ed 4. Philadelphia, 1986, Lea and Febiger.
It is obtained by following formula:

$$EF\% = \frac{(Dd)^3 - (Ds)^3}{(Dd)^3} \times 100$$

Normal mean ejection fraction is 74% with 95% prediction limits of 64-83% (Fig. 5.7).

3. *LV systolic function:* LV systolic function is evaluated by the fractional shortening, ejection fraction and systolic time intervals. Serial determination of these functions and measurements are important in conditions in which LV-function may change (e.g., in patients with acute or chronic myocardial disease or with chemotherapy induced LV-dysfunction where Dd is end diastolic dimension and Ds is end systolic dimension.

$$\text{Fractional shortening (FS)} = \frac{(Dd - Ds)}{Dd} \times 100$$

This is a reliable index of LV function. Mean normal value is 36% with 95% prediction limits of 28 to 44%. Fractional shortening is decreased in poorly compensated LV regardless of etiology (e.g. pressure overload, volume, overload, primary myocardial disorders, doxorubicin cardiotoxicity, etc.).

It is increased in compensated LV function such as volume over load lesions (e.g. VSD, PDA, AR, MR) and pressure overload lesions, e.g. moderately severe aortic stenosis, HOCM, coarctation of aorta, etc.

Ejection Fraction

It relates to the change in volume of the left ventricle with cardiac contraction.

4. *Systolic time intervals:* The systolic time interval of the ventricle includes the pre-ejection period and the ventricular ejection time (Fig. 5.7). The pre-ejection period (from onset of Q wave of ECG to the opening of semilunar valve) usually reflects the rate of pressure rise in the ventricle during isovolumic systole (i.e. dp/dt). The ventricular ejection time is measured from cusp opening of semilunar valve to the cusp closing. Although the pre-ejection period and ventricular ejection time are affected by the heart rate, the ratio of pre-ejection period (PET) to ventricular ejection time (VET) for both right and left sides is little affected by changes in heart rate. The method of measuring left pre-ejection period (LPEP) and left ventricular ejection time (LVET) is shown in Figure 5.6 in lower right panel.

5. *Doppler echocardiography:* The Doppler principle is applied to blood flow within the heart and the direction and velocity of blood flow can be determined by examining the movement of red blood cells by ultrasound beam. The Doppler effect is a change in the observed frequency of sound that results from motion of the source or target. When the moving object or column, of blood moves towards the ultrasonic transducer, the frequency of the reflected sound wave increases (i.e., a positive Doppler shift) and vice versa. Doppler ultrasound equipment detects a frequency shift and determines the velocity and direction of red blood cells flow with respect to the ultrasound beam.

Flow disturbances are seen with shunt lesions, stenosis or regurgitation of the cardiac valves or narrowing of the blood vessels. By convention the velocity of the red blood cells moving towards the transducer are displayed above the zero base line and those moving away from the transducer are displayed below the zero base line. Normal Doppler velocity is less than 1.0 m/sec., for the tricuspid and pulmonary valves and may be up to 1.6 m/sec for the ascending and descending aortas.

Modes of Doppler echocardiography: The way in which the Doppler ultrasound beam is emitted and detected has a significant bearing on the results obtained. The two different modes are:

a. Pulsed Doppler
b. Continuous Wave Doppler

Pulsed Doppler: Pulsed Doppler (PD) transducers have only one crystal, which acts as a transmitter and a receiver of ultrasound. This transducer emits a short burst of ultrasound first and then acts as a receiver for the returning signals. The advantage of pulsed technique is that a Doppler signal can be obtained from a specific area of cardiovascular system such as mitral valve level.

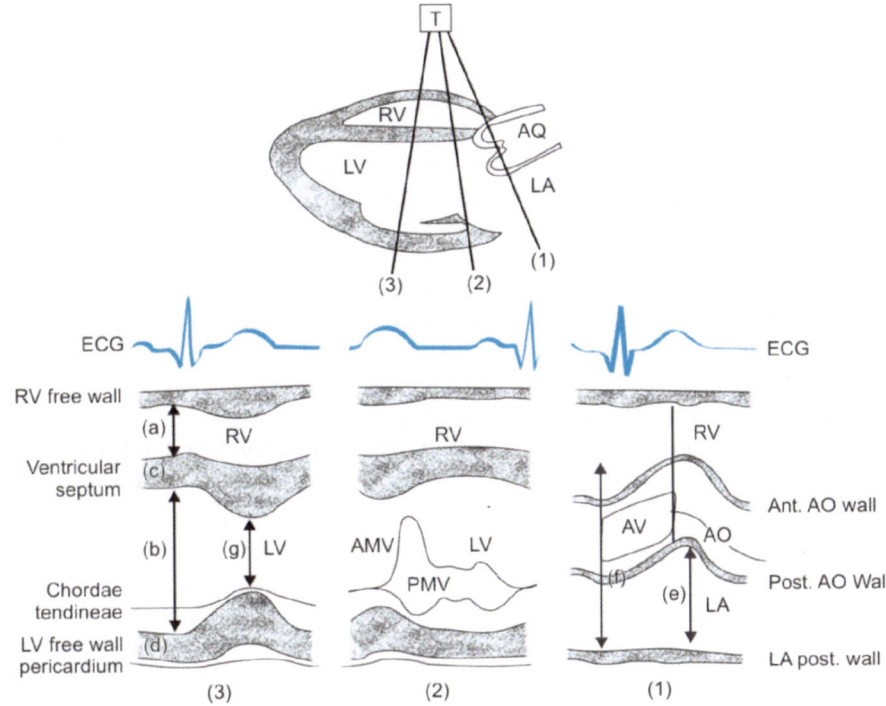

Fig. 5.7: A cross sectional view of the left side of the heart along the long axis (top) through which "ice-pick" views of the M-mode views are possible, but only three are shown in this figure. The dimension of the aorta (AO) and left atrium is measured along the line (1) Systolic time intervals for the left sides are also measured at the level of the aortic valve (AV). The line (2) passes through the mitral valve. Measurements made at this level are not useful in pediatric patients. Measurement of chamber dimensions and wall thickness of right and left ventricles is made along the line (3). Normal values of these measurements are shown in Table 5.1. (a) RV dimension; (b) LV diastolic dimension; (c) interventricular septal thickness; (d) LV posterior wall thickness; (e) LA dimension; (f) aortic dimension; (g) LV systolic dimension; AMV, anterior mitral valve; LVET, left ventricular ejection time; PEP, pre-ejection period PMV, posterior mitral valve

Continuous wave Doppler: To get information on blood velocity and direction, the ability to transmit and receive ultrasound is essential. For continuous wave (CW) ultrasound blood flow velocity and direction is achieved by two crystals in the head of a small transducer, one crystal to transmit and the other to receive (Figs 5.8A and B). A major limitation to CW technique is lack of discrimination of the many blood velocity components returning to the transducer e.g. when measuring blood velocity in the left ventricular outflow tract by CW technique, the returning signal cannot provide information about the location of peak velocity displayed. Using the duplex, Doppler and two-dimensional echo techniques, both imaging and blood velocity information can be obtained.

Information that can be obtained from Doppler spectrum includes:
  a. Velocity of blood through a sample volume (PW Doppler) or along entire beam path (CW Doppler).
  b. Direction of flow relative to transducer.
  c. Timing of flow events during cardiac cycle.
6. *Color flow mapping:* In pulsed and CW Doppler, ultrasound is emitted in a single direction. In color flow mapping, the ultrasound beam is rotated through an arc and recording of Doppler frequency shift are made throughout the arc.

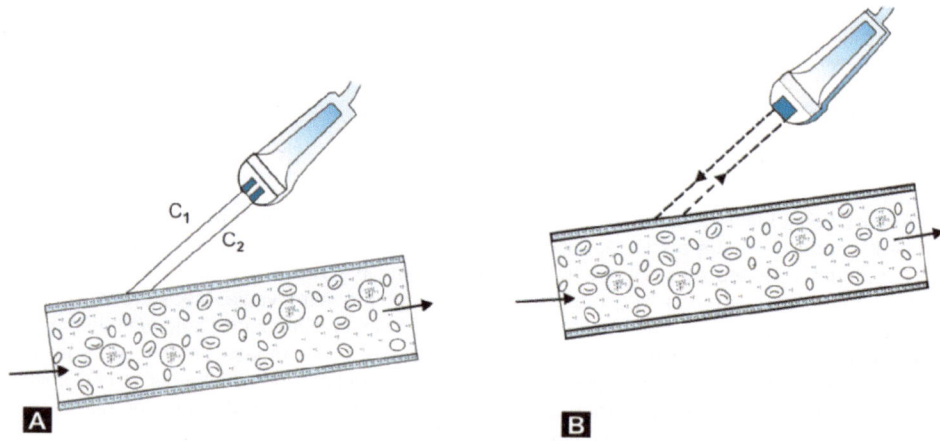

Figs 5.8A and B: Doppler transmission and reception. (A) Continuous wave Doppler signal. Note the two crystals, one for transmitting (C_1) and one for receiving (C_2); (B) Pulsed wave Doppler using a single crystal for transmitting and receiving

A color coded Doppler provides images of the direction and disturbance of blood flow super imposed on the echo-structural image. Red is used to indicate flow towards the transducer and blue is used to indicate flow away from the transducer (BART). Color may not appear when the direction of flow is perpendicular to the ultrasound beam. The turbulent beam is color coded as either green or yellow.

Contrast echocardiography: Injection of indocyanine green, dextrose in water, saline or the patients blood on to a peripheral vein or central vein produces microcavitations and creates a cloud of echoes on the echocardiogram. Structures of interest are visualized and recorded by M-mode or 2D echo at the time of injection. This technique has been replaced by color flow mapping and Doppler studies.

Other Echocardiographic Techniques

Fetal Echocardiography

Fetal echocardiographic structures can be visualized to help *in utero* diagnosis of cardiovascular anomalies. The transducer is placed in various positions on maternal abdominal wall. The effect of cardiovascular abnormalities and abnormal cardiac rhythms *in utero* are studied and the assessment for therapeutic interventions done.

Indications for fetal echo
a. A parent with congenital heart disease.
b. History of CHD in previous children.
c. Presence of fetal cardiac arrhythmias.
d. Presence of diabetes mellitus or collagen vascular disease in mother.
e. Presence of chromosomal anomalies.
f. Presence of extracardiac anomalies, e.g. diaphragmatic hernia, hydrops, polyhydramnios or oligohydramnios.
g. History of exposure of mother to certain drugs, e.g. progesterone, anti-convulsants, amphetamine and addictive drugs.

Transoesophageal Echocardiography (TEE)

If satisfactory images of the heart and blood vessels are not obtained from the usual transducer positions, e.g. due to obesity, chronic obstructive pulmonary disease then the physician may use TEE.

A two-dimensional transducer is placed at the end of flexible endoscope and high quality 2D images are obtained through esophagus. Pediatric use of this technique is limited to intraoperative use or in obese adolescents with complicated heart defects on whom risk of anesthesia or sedation is not worth taking for the expected benefits of this procedure.

Intravascular Echocardiography

The ultrasonic transducer can be placed in a small catheter so that vessels can be imaged. Useful in detecting atherosclerotic arteries in adults and coronary artery stenosis or aneurysms in children who had Kawasaki's disease.

Diagnostic steps of echocardiography-approach to a patient: It is essential to have accurate information on the clinical status, X-ray and ECG findings. It is possible to refer patients for treatment on the basis of echocardiographic/Doppler findings without doing the cardiac catheterization or angiograms. The key to accurate diagnosis in congenital heart disease is in following the rule of sequential chamber analysis starting from the atrial arrangement, followed by atrioventricular connection and finally ventriculoarterial connection. Then the associated malformations and their severity are described in detail. Some useful information before proceeding to perform echocardiography helps in diagnosing the heart disease.

1. Is the patient cyanosed?
   The presence of cyanosis makes the diagnosis of normal heart incompatible in the absence of lung disease.
2. Are the femorals palpable?
   Coarctation of aorta can be missed if one does not have prior information on this finding.
3. What is the situation of pulmonary blood flow?
   Normal, decreased or increased, this would be evident only with prior knowledge of clinical and X-ray findings.

Echocardiographic examination: The sequential chamber analysis should be adhered to even in the simplest form of CHD. The actual steps at echocardiographic examination start with identification of atrial arrangement. Trying to identify the morphological right atrium (RA) does this. The connection of pulmonary vein is variable and it cannot be assumed to be a marker for the left atrium (LA). The morphology of the atrial appendage, the site of the inferior vena-cava (IVC) and the coronary sinus connection are the main markers of the right atrium.

1. *Normal atrial arrangement or situs solitus:* The IVC and coronary sinus are connected to the right-sided right atrium and its appendage has all the features of a right atrial appendage.
2. *Mirror image atrial arrangement or situs inversus:* The IVC, coronary sinus are connected to the left-sided right atrium and its appendage resembles the morphological right atrium.

   2-D echo identifies the IVC/pulmonary veins. The atrial chamber that is connected to the IVC is the RA and the atrium that receives pulmonary veins is the LA.

3. *Localization of the ventricles:* By 2-D echocardiography the anatomic right ventricle (RV) and left ventricle (LV) are identified by the facts that the tricuspid valve leaflet usually inserts in the interventricular septum in a more apical position than the mitral septal leaflet and that the LV is invariably attached to the mitral valve and the RV to the tricuspid valve. A ventricular chamber that has two papillary muscles is the LV.
4. *Localization of the great arteries:* One can accurately determine the relationship between the two great arteries and also the relationship of the great arteries to the ventricles non-invasively through echo. There are four types of relationships between the two great arteries (Figs 5.9A to D).
   a. Solitus
   b. Inversus
   c. D-Transposition.
   d. L-Transposition
5. *Dextrocardia and mesocardia:* Dextrocardia is a condition in which heart is located on the right side of the chest. Mesocardia indicates that the heart is located in the midline of thorax approximately. These terms express the position of the heart but do not signify the segmental relationship of the heart.

    Normally formed heart that is displaced to the right side "of the chest secondary to hypoplasia of the right lung" is termed as dextroversion.

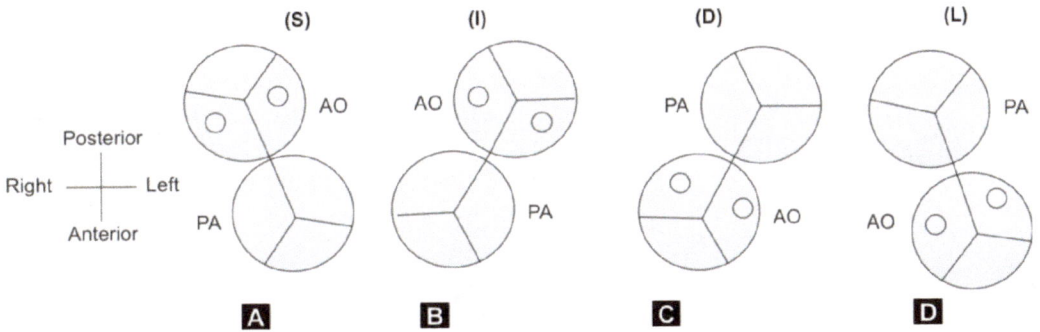

Figs 5.9A to D: Four types of relationships between the great arteries, viewed in the horizontal section. A, Solitus (S) relationship is present when the aortic valve is posterior and rightward to the pulmonary valve: B, In Inversus (I) relationship, the aortic valve is posterior to and left of pulmonary valve (mirror image). C, Complete transposition (D) is present when aortic valve is anterior and to right of pulmonary valve. D, congenially corrected transposition (L) is present when aortic valve is anterior and to left of the pulmonary valve

Four common types of heart in the right chest are
a. Classical mirror image dextrocardia (Fig. 5.10A).
b. Normal heart displaced to the right side of the chest (Fig. 5.10B).
c. Congenitally corrected TGA with situs solitus (Fig. 5.10C).
d. Single ventricle or differentiated cardiac chambers (situs-ambiguous with splenic syndromes) (Fig. 5.10D).

With chest X-ray and ECG, one can deduce the location of the atria and the ventricles in dextrocardia and mesocardia. More conclusive diagnosis of the segmental relationship can be made with the help of 2-D echo and angiocardiography.

MAGNETIC RESONANCE IMAGING

The ability of magnetic resonance imaging is to acquire anatomic and functional information about the cardiovascular system, is the central aspect of modern cardiology. Also, the knowledge regarding the metabolic characteristics and tissue composition of cardiovascular system will be taking an increasing importance. Magnetic resonance imaging (MRI), in cardiovascular system is used as an adjunct for the clinical assessment of the cardiovascular anatomy and function, metabolism and tissue composition.[1]

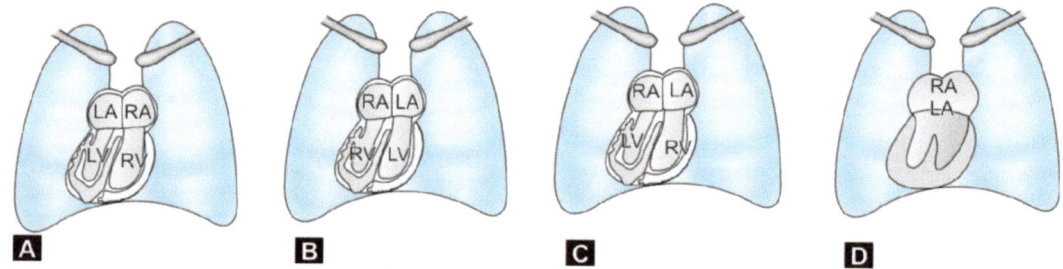

Figs 5.10A to D: Examples of common conditions when the apex of the heart is in the right chest. A, classic mirror-image dextrocardia. B, normally formed heart shifted toward the right side of the chest. C, L-TGA with sinus solitus. D, Situs ambiguous seen with splenic syndromes. (From Park MK, Guntheroth WG: How to read pediatric ECGs, ed 3, St Louis, 1992, Mosby)

Indication of Magnetic Resonance Imaging–Evaluation of Congenital Heart Disease

Cardiovascular magnetic resonance (CMR) is increasingly used in concert with other imaging modalities (echocardiography) for assessment of cardiac anatomy and functional measurements of blood flow, tissue characterization and for evaluation of myocardial perfusion and viability.
1. When transthoracic echocardiography cannot provide the required diagnostic information.
2. When clinical assessment and other diagnostic tests are inconsistent.
3. As an alternative to cardiac catheterization with its associated risks and higher costs.
4. To obtain diagnostic information for which CMR offers unique advantages.

Anatomical Evaluation

Contrast between flowing blood and the myocardial and blood vessel walls provide the basis for CMR in cardiovascular imaging.[2] In comparison to echocardiography, the contrast coloring is reversed i.e., in MRI the blood vessels and cardiac chambers have a high signal intensity and myocardium and blood vessel walls appear dark. Because of excellent spatial resolution, MRI facilitates measurement of chamber dimensions and wall thickness. The visceral and cardiac positions are readily apparent on MRI (Fig. 5.11).

The structures that are difficult to characterize by echocardiography are well defined by MRI, e.g delineation of great vessel anatomy, ascending and descending aorta, distal pulmonary arteries, systemic and pulmonary veins, right ventricular cavity and anterior wall of left ventricle. The gross structure of the cardiac valves can be ascertained by MRI, but because of their rapid motion and because they are normally very thin, the fine details of cardiac valve structures are not well defined. The presence of small defects in fossa ovalis and atrioventricular septum are difficult to ascertain because normal septal thickness in these areas approach the limits of resolution of MRI at present. Flow disturbances caused by small atrial and ventricular septal defects are apparent in flow sensitive MRI.

Evaluation in Specific Cardiovascular Disorders

Anomalies of the Aorta (Figs 5.12 and 5.13A and B)

MRI can depict the aorta and the aortic tree, when images are of good quality and common normal variant branching patterns of the aortic arch are also readily detected. Postoperative follow up in interrupted aortic arch anomalies can be very well seen. MRI also demonstrates malformation in which left pulmonary artery originates from the right pulmonary artery and courses posterior to the trachea and anterior to the esophagus.

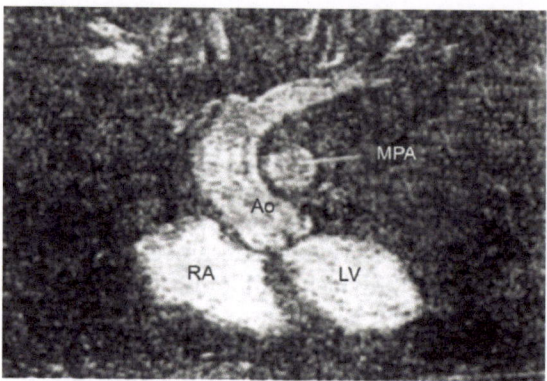

Fig. 5.11: MRI evaluation of normal cardiac chambers and blood vessels

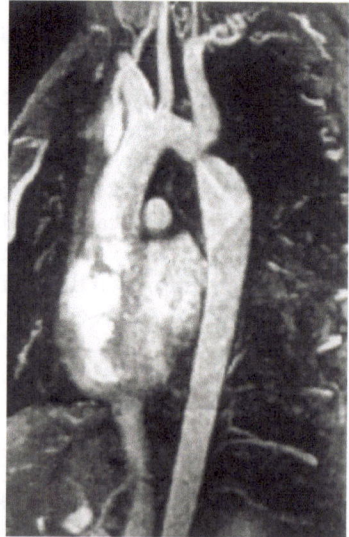

Fig. 5.12: Maximal intensity projection Gd enhanced 3-D MRA in a patient with severe aortic coarctation

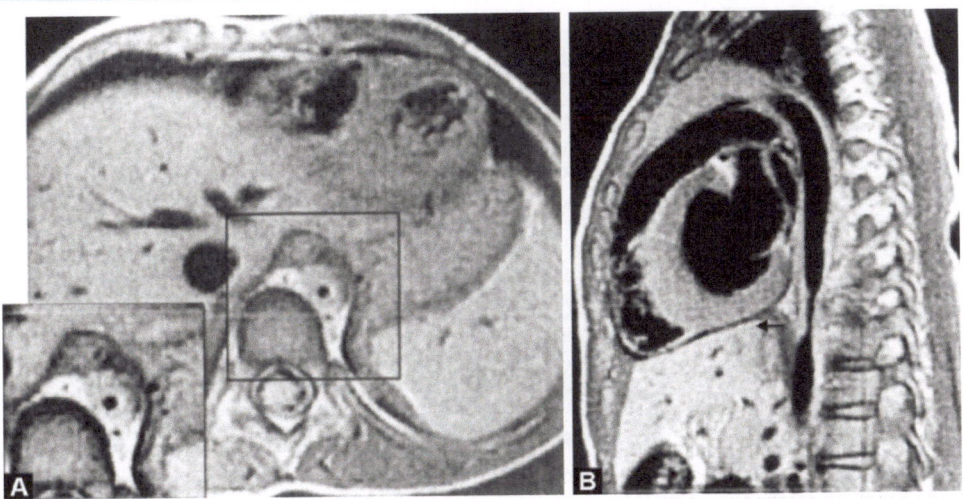

Figs 5.13A and B: Fast (turbo) spin echo imaging showing severe long segment abdominal coarctation in a patient with Takayasu: arteritis. (A) Sagittal view. (B) Axial (transverse) view showing marked thickening of aortic wall

Besides demonstrating coarctation of the aorta, before and after treatment,[3] MRI also assists in the evaluation of coarctation site and the degree of ventricular hypertrophy. For ventricular septal defects, though MRI is not particularly helpful for membranous defects, inlet, outlet though trabecular defects can be detected, and the velocity patterns of blood flow by MRI help to quantify the shunting in these patients (Figs 5.14A and B).

Detection of sinus venosus, fossa ovalis and ostium primum atrial septal defects by MRI have been described. It also rules out pulmonary venous anomalies associated with atrial septal defects (Fig. 5.15).

In Tetralogy of Fallot, high quality definition of distal pulmonary arteries are obtainable in MRI which helps in pre and postoperative assessment of patients. This is also useful in patients with pulmonary atresia and aorticopulmonary shunts.[4] It clearly demonstrates the origins of aorta and pulmonary artery and the relationship of these vessels to one another. It also helps to evaluate the associated anomalies, both pre and postoperatively in transposition of great arteries and tricuspid atresia.[5] MRI clearly shows systemic venous abnormalities, persistence of left superior vena cava and also abnormalities in pulmonary venous connections.[6] Partial anomalous pulmonary venous connections in childhood and adolescence are always associated with an atrial septal defect of the sinus venosus type and pulmonary veins and their connections are best depicted in transverse and

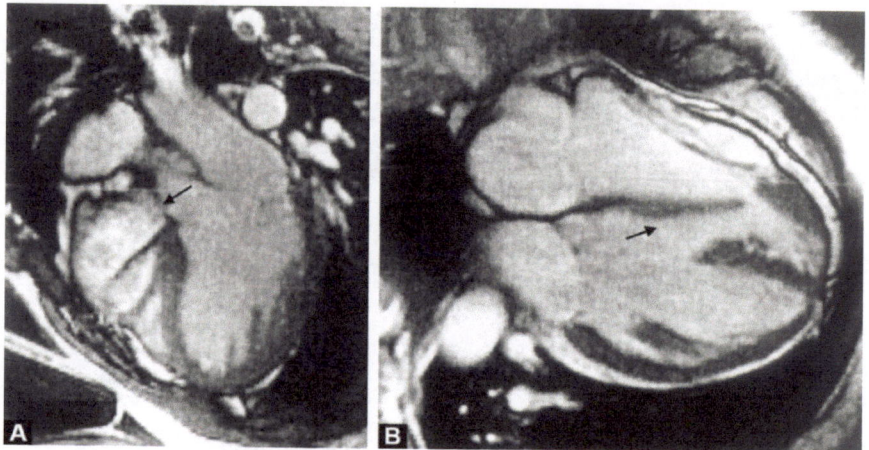

Figs 5.14A and B: ECG-triggered, breath-hold, cine steady-state free precession imaging of ventricular septal defect. (A) Small membranous ventricular septal defect (arrow). (B) Large muscular ventricular septal defect (arrow)

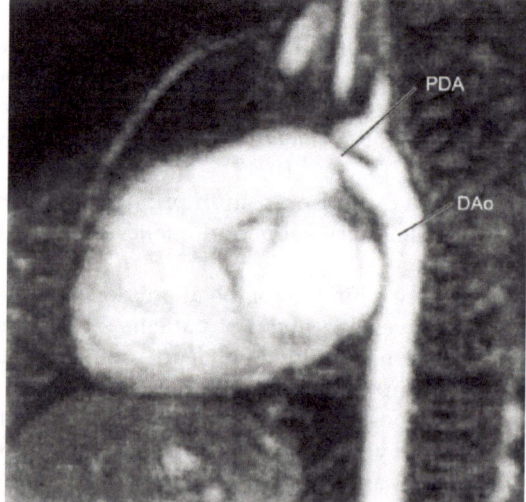

Fig. 5.15: Maximal intensity projection Gd-enhanced 3-D MRA in patient with patent ductus arteriosus

coronal planes. Quantitative gradient echo techniques help to quantify the velocity and flow in individual pulmonary veins. MRI helps to visualize atrioventricular septal defects and its associated anomalies such as coarctation of aorta, pulmonary artery stenosis, pulmonary and systemic venous anomalies and related ventricular hypoplasia.[7] It is also helpful in identifying complex congenital cardiovascular anomalies like heterotaxy syndrome which is difficult to delineate by echocardiography and angiography.[8]

Magnetic resonance imaging provides a better resolution of intracardiac and extracardiac mediastinal tumors. Enchancement with gadolinium and multiphasic cine MRI techniques help in evaluation of cardiac tumors.[9] Pericardium is normally visualized by standard echocardiography but when it is thickened in chronic constrictive pericarditis,[10] the vena cavae are dilated and the ventricles are small, pericardial effusion may also be demonstrated by MRI.[11] It is also possible to decide whether the pericardial fluid is transudate or exudate, chylous or hemorrhagic. MRI measurement of left ventricular hypertrophy correlates well with echocardiographic and angiographic determinations. It has a particular role in evaluating right ventricular hypertrophy because the right ventricle is well defined by MRI but is difficult to evaluate by echocardiography.

The presence of dilated cardiomyopathy is readily detected by MRI. Cardiac chamber sizes as well as volume determinations are well evaluated and correlated well with other methods but evaluation of segmental cardiac dysfunction and intracardiac thrombus is better evaluated by MRI as compared to echocardiography. In cardiac transplantation, MRI has a definitive role. Recent investigational studies in animals and humans suggest that in "MRI enhancement with gadolinium could facilitate detection of transplant rejection."[12] MRI could monitor the cardiac transplant patients for rejection and thus reduce the need for cardiac biopsies.

Cardiac Functional Assessment by MRI

Qualitative evaluation of overall ventricular function is made by systolic and diastolic short axis, long axis or four chamber images. Left and right ventricular ejection fractions can be calculated from sets of systolic and diastolic images. Many investigators believe that MRI is the clinical gold standard for ventricular volume, mass and ejection function. Regional cardiac wall motion abnormalities are evaluated with multiphasic MRI techniques. In a study by Young et al using myocardial tagging, the patients with hypertrophic cardiomyopathy had diminished regional three dimensional myocardial shortening in comparison to normal subjects.[13]

Factors Determining MRI Images

1. Infants and young children are given oral chloral hydrate for sedation for proper image which is less effective in children beyond 4 years of age.[14] Therefore intravenous sedation is required for uncooperative patients and sedation is rarely required for children beyond 8 years of age.

2. Synchronization of MRI signal acquisition with cardiac rhythm is essential. When this does not occur images are of poor quality.
3. Patients should be instructed to breathe as regularly as possible. Breath holding, may be effective in minimizing respiratory motion artefacts. Automatic respiratory synchronization techniques may be very valuable to improve cardiovascular images.
4. Major factor to determine the image quality is the signal to noise ratio.
5. Artefacts created by metals or other ferromagnetic images may degrade MRI images. Contrast may be maximized or minimized by appropriate manipulation of MRI parameter.

These parameters are effective on two commonly used imaging sequence-spin echo and fast imaging and steady precision (FISP).

MRI Angiography

Because flowing blood has different MRI characteristics than stationary tissues, it is possible to produce MR images that demonstrate regions containing flowing blood as areas of high signal intensity against a dark background in a projective format similar to angiography.

There are multiple techniques for producing MRI angiograms. However, these techniques fall in two major categories: time of flight (TOF) angiography and phase contrast angiography (PCA). TOF angiographic techniques are most widely used methods for obtaining magnetic resonance angiograms. The fundamental concepts of TOF magnetic resonance angiography is to increase the contrast between flowing blood and surrounding tissues by making magnetization of blood large and tissue magnetization small. TOF MR angiography is widely used in the study of the carotid arteries and intracranial vessels. It is also used for evaluation of the femoral and popliteal arteries.

The second category of techniques for performing MR angiography are phase contrast methods.[15] These techniques are based on principles that flowing spins moving through a magnetic field gradient change their phases in proportion to their velocity and to the time that the gradient is applied. Phase contrast MR is just beginning to be applied in clinical studies. The venous system is particularly well demonstrated by phase contrast MR angiography.[16]

Clinical Cardiac MR Spectroscope

Investigational studies of the human myocardium with MRI spectroscope are just beginning. A great deal of technical development will be necessary before MRI spectroscope can be routinely applied in a clinical setting. Conway et al studied patients with aortic valve disease with cardiac magnetic resonance spectroscope. They found that the myocardial PCr/ATP ratio was substantially lower in patients who were being treated for heart failure than in other patients or in controls. They suggested that measurement of the myocardial PCr/ATO ratio could be useful in determining optimal time for aortic valve replacement in these patients.

Multiple investigations with 31 PNMR spectroscopes have noted abnormalities in skeletal muscle metabolism in experimental animals and in patients with congestive cardiac failure.

Pediatric Cardiac MRI Spectroscopy

The above studies are encouraging in that they demonstrate the feasibility of human cardiac MRI spectroscope. At present, however, localized human, cardiac spectroscopic studies are restricted to the anterior ventricular walls and cardiac apex because of limitations in the localization techniques used. Furthermore, current cardiac spectroscopic studies are lengthy and cannot feasibly be combined with comprehensive imaging and flow studies in standard clinical settings.

The third problem is that the static magnetic field of the scanner may activate the pacemaker resulting in a synchronous pacing. There is also a possibility that MRI might damage the pacemaker requiring its replacement.

Pregnancy is a relative contraindication to MRI studies, although the magnetic fields used in clinical images have no effects on the embryo and patients have undergone MRI during all trimesters of pregnancy without ill effects on mother, fetus or resultant infant. However when maternal and fetal health considerations require diagnostic studies, MRI is preferable to other methods, such as computed X-ray, tomography or angiography.

Hazards and Contraindications of MRI

Millions of patients have undergone MRI studies without any noticeable immediate or long term sequelae. The standard clinical imaging magnet attract ferromagnetic objects, extreme caution should be used in approaching magnets with objects containing iron or other ferromagnetic materials. The non electronic intravascular devices are compatible with MRI images. Prosthetic cardiac valves manufactured after 1964, contain little ferromagnetic material. Patients having these valves can be routinely studied. Heart valves manufactured before 1964 have substantial ferromagnetic material. The presence of cardiac pacemaker is an absolute contraindication to MRI studies.

Another problem that can arise when pacemaker is subjected to MRI scanning is interference with sensing function of the pacemaker.

CONCLUSIONS

MRI facilitates the diagnostic evaluation of congenital and acquired cardiovascular disease in many ways. Present MRI techniques provide excellent anatomical and functional definition of many aspects of cardiovascular disease and may greatly increase the clinician's ability to evaluate the cardiovascular system.

REFERENCES

1. Jonston DL, Rockey R, Okada RD. Principles of cardiovascular nuclear magnetic imaging. In: Clinical Cardiac Imaging, Miller DD, Bums RJ, Gill JB, Ruddy TD, eds. New York, McGraw Hill, 1998;103-125.
2. Naazarian GK, Julsrud PR, Ehrman Rl et al. Correlation between magnetic resonance imaging of the heart and cardiac anatomy. Mayo Clin Proc 1987;62:573-83.
3. Mohiaddin RM, Kilner JP, Rees et al. Magnetic resonance volume flow and jet velocity mapping in aortic coarctation. J Am Col Cardiol 1993;22:1515-21.
4. Vick GW III, Rockey R, Huhta JC et al. Nuclear magnetic resonance imaging of the pulmonary arteries, subpulmonary region and aortopulmonary shunts: A comparative study with two-dimensional echocardiography and angiography. Am Heart J 1990;119:1103-10.
5. Fletcher BD, Jacobstein MD, Abraniowsky CR et al. Right atrioventricular valve atresia: anatomic evaluation with MR imaging. AIR 1987;148:671-4.
6. Oxer RA, Singh S, LaCorte MA et al. Cardiac magnetic resonance imaging in children with congenital heart disease. J Pediatr 1986;109:460-4.
7. Persons JM, Baker EJ, Anderson RH et al. Morphological evaluation of atrioventricular septal defects by magnetic resonance imaging. Br Heart J 1990;74:701-4.
8. Geva T, Vick GW III, Wendt RE et al. Role of spin echo and cine magnetic imagine in pre-surgical planning of heterotoaxy syndrome. Comparison with echocardiography and catheterization. Circulation 1994;74:701-4.
9. Fukuzama S, Yamomoto T, Shimade K et al. Hemangioma of the left ventricular cavity: Presumptive diagnosis by magnetic resonance imaging. Heart vessels 1993:8:211-4.
10. Masui T, Finck S, Higgins CB. Constrictive pericarditis and restrictive cardiomyopathy: Evaluation with MR imaging. Radiology 1992;182:369-73.
11. Rockey R, Vick GW III R et al. Assessment of experimental pericardial effusion using nuclear magnetic resonance imaging techniques. Am Heart J 1991;121:1161-9.
12. Mousseaux E, Farge D, Guillemain R et al. Assessing human cardiac allograft rejection using NMR with Gd-D OTA. J Comput Assist Tomogr 1993;17:237-44.
13. Yound AA, Kramer CM, Ferrari VA et al. Three-dimensional left ventricular deformations in hypertrophic cardiomypathy. Circulation 994;90:854-67.
14. Greenberg SB, Faerber Em, Aspinall CL. High dose choloral hydrate sedation for children undergoing MR imaging: Safety and efficacy in relation to age. AJR 1993;11:939-41.
15. Sheppard S. Basic concepts in magnetic resonance angiography. Radiol Clin North Am 1995;33:911-3.
16. Nghiem HV, Winter IC Ill, Mouintford MC et al. Evaluation of the portal venous system before liver transplantation: Value of phase contrast MR angiography. AIR 1995;164:871-8.

CHAPTER 6

Congenital Heart Disease: General Aspects

Congenital heart disease (CHD) is defined as the structural, functional or positional abnormality of the heart, in isolation or in combination, present from birth, but may manifest any time after birth or may not manifest at all.

Congenital heart disease may be encountered by many types of physicians who help a patient over a lifetime, but the specialty of medicine which the physician practices greatly influences the type of cardiac problems seen. The neonatologist and the pediatric cardiologist see acutely ill newborns with a large proportion of cyanotic congenital heart disease who present with heart failure, hypoxemia, acidosis and variety of other acute problems. The general pediatrician sees a population of less acutely ill patients in whom most of the life threatening cardiac problems have either been effectively treated or the more devastating lesions have already succumbed.

By the time, the adult cardiologist sees the patient with congenital heart disease, the population has changed even more because most of the patients with cyanotic heart disease have either died or have had surgical correction of the underlying lesion done. Whereas, ventricular septal defect which is the most common congenital cardiac defect seen in infancy and childhood, has in all possibility spontaneously closed by this time. On the other hand, atrial septal defect and bicuspid aortic valve which were not picked up in infancy may be detected in adulthood when they start manifesting clinically.

Congenital heart diseases are not fixed anatomic defects that appear at birth but instead a dynamic group of anomalies that originate in fetal life and changed considerably during postnatal development. The majority of congenital anomalies of the heart are present six weeks after conception and most anomalies compatible with six months of intrauterine life permit live offsprings at birth.

INCIDENCE

The importance of congenital heart disease can scarcely be over-emphasized. Until the last two decades, it was believed that rheumatic heart disease was the commoner form of heart disease in children, but now-a-days with the decline of rheumatic fever more in the developed countries and even in the developing ones, congenital heart disease are diagnosed more because of presence of more and more advanced diagnostic modalities. No accurate figures are available but the incidence of CHD varies worldwide between 4-8/1000 live births and are much higher in still births and abortuses which are independent of geographical distribution. The eight most common cardiac anomalies account for 80% of all lesions (Table 6.1) and the rest 18-20% have complex anomalies. A study on 11,000 consecutive live births in a tertiary care hospital in Delhi gave an incidence of CHD as 3.9/1000 live births[1] whereas in another study on autopsies from Chandigarh, the incidence was as high as 7.5/1000 births, alive or dead (Table 6.1).

On summarizing the global figures, an average prevalence of CHD is 9/1000 in aggregate, and 3/1000 for serious heart defects. It can be estimated that 1.2 million affected babies are born worldwide every year with congenital heart anomalies, of whom 400,000 babies are severely affected.[2-4]

Table 6.1: Common congenital anomalies[2]

Acyanotic	- VSD (32%)	Cyanotic	- Tetralogy of Fallot	-6%
	- PDA (12%)			
	- Pulmonic stenosis–8%		- Transposition of great arteries	-5%
	- ASD–6%			
	- Coarctation of aorta–6%			
	- Aortic stenosis–5%			

ETIOLOGY

The etiology of congenital heart disease is largely unknown and so prevention is almost impossible (Table 6.2). A multi-factorial inheritance is gaining ground which includes genetic and environmental interaction in 90% and solely of genetic origin in 8%, (chromosomal in 5% and single mutant gene 3%). There are certain environmental factors (2%) which include intrauterine infections, e.g. Rubella, drugs, alcohol intake, narcotic drugs and irradiation which are potentially teratogenic in nature in producing congenital cardiac defects especially when they act between 5th-8th weeks of gestation. There are certain defects, e.g. aortic stenosis, coarctation of aorta, TGA, TOF, etc which are more commonly seen in males whereas atrial septal defect (ASD) and PDA are more commonly seen in females. Those patients living at high altitude and hilly areas also manifest more with heart defects common ones being ASDs and PDAs. Maternal obesity reports an increased risk for conotruncal abnormalities in the offspring.[6] Heart defects consistently associated with maternal diabetes include situs inversus, heterotaxy, conotruncal defects like complex-transposition of great arteries and obstructive hypertrophic cardiomyopathy which ultimately resolve. The rising rate of diabetes underscores the need for action to help prevent diabetes related heart defects.[5]

Table 6.2: Congenital heart disease-etiology

- Largely unknown
- Maternal
  - Age and parity
  - Systemic illnesses
    - Diabetes mellitus — TGA, VSD, HOCM
    - Systemic lupus erythematosus (SLE) — Complete heart block (CHB)
    - Pre-eclampsia — Intrauterine growth retardation (IUGR)
    - Phenyl Ketonuria — VSD, ASD, PDA.
- Intrauterine infections — 5-8th week of gestation.
  - Rubella — PDA, peripheral pulm. art. stenosis.
  - Mumps, varicella — Endocardial fibroelastosis.
  - Coxsackie B — myocarditis (late pregnancy)
  - Cytomegalovirus — myocarditis
- Drug intake/Addictions
  - Alcohol–fetal alcohol syndrome — VSD, PGA, TGA
  - Cigarette smoking, nicotine — IUGR
  - Amphetamine — VSD
  - Hormones
  - Insulin, thyroid, oral Contraceptives- — TGA, TOF, VSD.
  - Lithium — Ebstein's anomaly
  - Anticonvulsants
  - Phenytoin — PS, AS, COA
  - Antimetabolites
  - Steroids
  - Barbiturates, salicylates
  - Vitamins
    - Vitamin D — Supravalvular aortic stenosis
    - Vitamin A (Retinol) — TGA
- High altitude — Increased incidence of ASD and PDA
- Sex
  - Males — Bicuspid aortic valve, AS, COA, TGA, TOF.
  - Females — ASD, PDA.

Maternal pregestational diabetes is an established teratogen, which affects not only developing heart but also numerous extra cardiac organs.[7] Heart defects consistently associated with maternal diabetes include situs inversus and several conotruncal defects (transposition of great arteries) and some left ventricular outflow obstructive defects (obstructive hypertrophic cardiomyopathy). Risk for diabetic embryopathy can be considerably reduced by strict glycemic control before conception, thus providing an important opportunity for primary prevention.[8]

The findings relating maternal obesity with heart defects in the offsprings is inconsistent, but some studies report conotruncal anomalies[9] with risks typically associated with BMI > 29, with unrecognized diabetes. Heart defects in congenital rubella syndrome include most commonly peripheral pulmonic artery stenosis, patent ductus arteriosus and rarely tetralogy of Fallot.[10]

If febrile illnesses in the first trimester cause an increased risk for heart defects, avoidance of all contacts and pre-conceptional immunization before flu season may be effective. Periconceptional use of multivitamin supplements may be associated with a reduced risk of congenital heart defects associated with febrile illnesses.[11]

Maternal phenyl ketonuria (PRU) patients have high levels of phenyl–alanine during pregnancy, and have a high likelihood of having children with microcephaly, mental retardation and high incidence of left sided cardiac defects (e.g. coarctation of aorta, hypoplastic left heart syndrome, and patent ductus arteriosus).[12] Thalidomide is a major teratogen and may be responsible for pulmonary stenosis.

Vitamin A occurs in two forms, β carotene and retinol. β Carotene is safe and does not give rise to heart defects but retinol in high doses (>10000 IU) is associated with increased risk for heart defects, especially α-transposition of great arteries.[13]

Alcohol is an established human teratogen and causes a wide range of structural malformations which include ventricular and atrial septal defects.[14]

Lack of intake of vitamins during pregnancy, e.g. folic acid, multivitamin, vitamin C etc, increases the risk for low birth weight and preterm birth. One study reports an increased risk for conotruncal anomalies and e.g. transposition of great vessels, especially in those women who did not use vitamin supplements especially in the periconceptional period.[15]

Chromosomal abnormalities e.g. Down's syndrome in which almost 40-50% manifest with congenital-heart disease. These include endocardial cushion defect followed by ASD secundum and VSD. Turner's syndrome is almost always associated with coarctation of aorta and trisomy[13-15] with VSD and PDA. There are a number of extracardiac anomalies associated with selected CHDs which are listed in Table 6.3.

Table 6.3: Extracardiac anomalies as pointers towards specific CHDs

Extra-cardiac anomaly	Most likely CHD
Polydactyly with syndactyly	VSD
Arachnodactyly	ASD
Moon facies and hypertelorism	PS
Down's syndrome (Trisomy 21)	Endocardial cushion defect, VSD, ASD secundum
Turner's syndrome	Coarctation of aorta, AS
Noonan's syndrome	PS, dysplastic PV, Peripheral PS
Rubella syndrome	PDA, branch pulmonary artery stenosis
Ellis-Van-Creveld syndrome	ASD, Single atrium
Holt Oram syndrome	ASD 2°
Marfan's syndrome	Aortic aneurysm, AR, MVP.
Hurler's syndrome	AR, MVP
Trisomy 13	VSD
Trisomy 18	VSD, PDA

DIAGNOSTIC EVALUATION OF A CHILD WITH CONGENITAL HEART DISEASE

Does the Child have Heart Disease? (Flow chart 6.1)

Assessment of a child for the presence of heart disease is facilitated by Nadas's criteria (Table 6.4) which are divided into major and minor criteria.

I. *Major criteria*
   a. *Systolic murmur grade III or more in intensity:* A systolic murmur of grade III or more in intensity and if associated with a thrill, always indicates the presence of underlying heart disease. Systolic murmurs may be pansystolic or ejection systolic in character.
   A pansystolic murmur is always abnormal and indicates the presence of:
      i. Ventricular septal defect
      ii. Mitral regurgitation
      iii. Tricuspid regurgitation.
   An ejection systolic murmur if associated with a thrill, is suggestive of organic heart disease. Almost 50% of children below the age of 5 years have a soft ejection systolic murmur which may be because of anemia or other hyperkinetic circulatory states. These murmurs usually disappear as the child grows older.
   b. *Diastolic murmurs:* Presence of diastolic murmurs are always indicative of the presence of heart disease, if severe systemic hypertension and hyperkinetic circulatory states have to be excluded.

Flow chart 6.1: Clinical approach to diagnosis of CHD in a newborn[2]

- **Cyanosis**
  - 1. TGA
  - 2. Rt. sided obstruction
  - Severe PS
  - Pulmonary atresia, Tricuspid atresia
  - → Duct dependent heart disease

- **CVS collapse (shock like state)**
  - 1. Hypoplastic left heart syndrome (HLHS)
  - 2. Critical aortic stenosis
  - Coarctation of aorta
  - → Duct dependent heart disease

- **Mild cyanosis + CCF**
  - 1. TAPVC
  - 2. Truncus arteriosus
  - → Critical heart disease
  - → Refer to pediatric center for management

- **Arrhythmia**
  - Heart rate >200 Tachy-arrhythmia
  - Heart rate >60 complete heart block
  - → Refer to pediatric cardiac center for evaluation and management

- **Late onset CCF (>2 weeks of age)**
  - -VSD
  - -AVSD
  - -PDA
  - -Cardiomyopathy
  - -ASD+PAPVC
  - → Refer to pediatric cardiac center for evaluation and management

- **Asymptomatic**
  - Peripheral pulmonary artery stenosis (innocent)
  - Small VSD, Mild PS
  - → Non-urgent heart disease
  - → For diagnostic evaluation

Table 6.4: Nadas's criteria

Major	Minor
Systolic murmur > grade III	Systolic murmur < grade III
	Abnormal S_2
Diastolic murmur	Abnormal ECG
Cyanosis	Abnormal X-ray chest
Congestive heart failure	Abnormal BP

Presence of one major or two minor criteria suggest the presence of heart disease.

c. *Cyanosis:* Cyanosis may occur due to:
   i. Right to left shunt (R-L shunt).
   ii. Pulmonary parenchymal disease.
   iii. Low cardiac output.
   iv. Methemoglobinemia.

   Cyanosis due to R-L shunt is called "central cyanosis" which can also result from pulmonary venous desaturation due to lung disease. Central cyanosis is characterized by arterial oxygen desaturation, normal saturation being 98% and also the presence of carboxyhemoglobin being more than 5 g%. Cyanosis due to pulmonary venous desaturation tends to disappear on giving oxygen whereas cyanosis due to R-L shunt is unaffected (Hyperoxia test).

   Cyanosis resulting from low cardiac output is due to increased extraction of oxygen by the tissues which are inadequately perfused due to low cardiac output, and the resulting cyanosis is referred to as peripheral cyanosis.

   Methemoglobinemia is a systemic disorder, where the hemoglobin gets reduced to methemoglobin by certain chemicals, e.g. nitrate. It can be clinically separated from true cyanosis since it is not associated with clubbing. In addition, all the other additional features e.g. physical examination, chest roentgenogram and electrocardiogram are normal.

d. *Congestive cardiac failure (CCF):* Presence of congestive cardiac failure is indicative of underlying cardiac disease at any age. Anemia may precipitate CCF in a child with underlying heart disease, which on it's own to produce CCF has to be very severe.

II. *Minor criteria:* Presence of two minor criteria is necessary to indicate presence of heart disease. The significance of murmurs has been dealt with in the "major criteria" above. Though pansystolic murmur always indicates presence of underlying heart disease, it is however possible to have a pansystolic murmur of mitral or tricuspid regurgitation if the left or right ventricles are dilated due to myocardial disease.

a. *Systolic murmur < grade III*

b. *Abnormal second heart sound:* Presence of abnormal second sound almost always indicates presence of heart disease. Correct interpretation of second sound abnormalities helps in identifying the presence of heart disease and also coming to a precise diagnosis.

c. *Abnormal electrocardiogram:* In CHD evaluation, the maximum use of the electrocardiogram is for the purpose of determining the electrical axis, identifying the presence or absence of right/left ventricular hypertrophy. If the clinical assessment of child is normal, with a normal chest skiagram, then an abnormal electrocardiogram is not enough to give the clinical diagnosis of the CHD (Figs 6.1A and B).

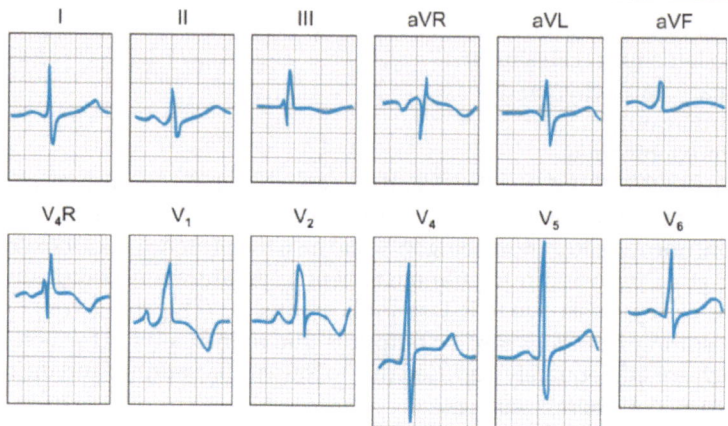

Fig. 6.1A: ECG of patient with right ventricular hypertrophy. RVH in the QRS complex

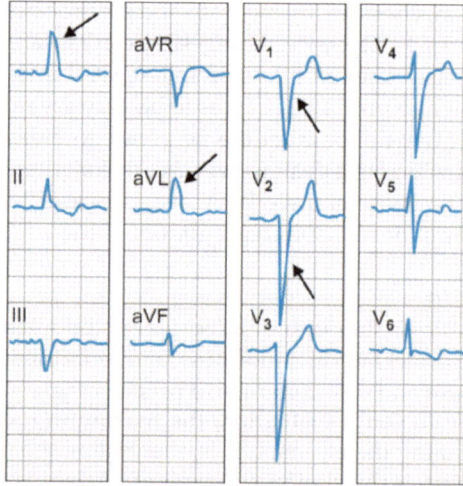

Fig. 6.1B: ECG of patient with left ventricular hypertrophy. A - Arrow showing interventricular conduction delay, Arrow - ST segment depression and T wave inversion

Abnormal Chest Roentgenogram

Presence of cardiomegaly only in a good inspiratory film is suggestive of heart disease. Secondly, below the age of 2 years, presence of a normal thymic gland shadow in continuation with the cardiac border may give a false impression of cardiomegaly. A lateral chest skiagram or a fluoroscopy can help in separating the thymic shadow from the cardiac silhouette. The chest skiagram helps in diagnosing certain congenital cardiac defects, e.g. TOF, TGA and TAPVR (Figs 6.2A and B).

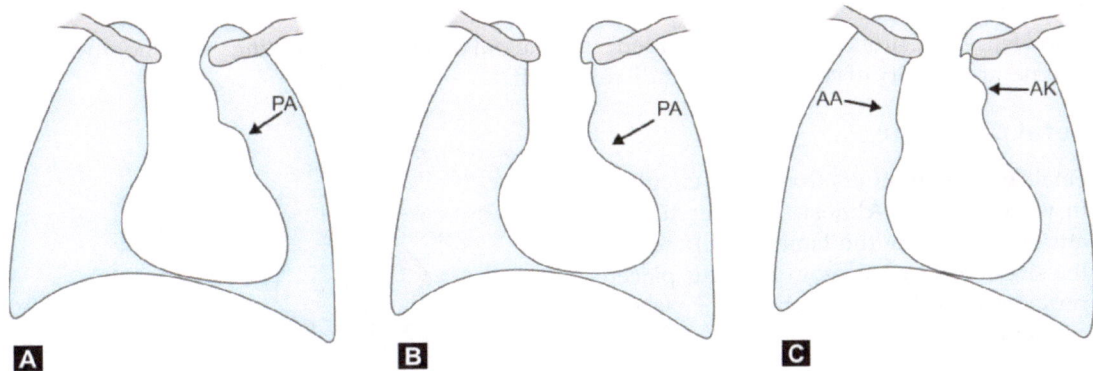

Fig. 6.2A: Abnormalities of great arteries. (A) Prominent MPA (PA) segment as seen in PAH; (B) Concave PA segment as seen in PS; (C) Dilatation of aorta–as dilated ascending aorta (AA) or prominence of aortic knob (AK)

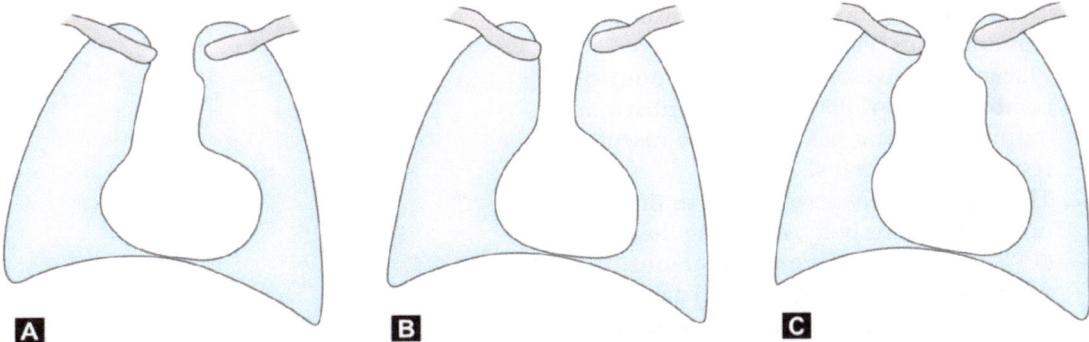

Fig. 6.2B: Abnormalities of cardiac silhouette. (A) "Abnormal boot shaped heart" seen in TOF; (B) "Abnormal egg shaped heart" seen in TGA; (C) "Snowman" sign seen in TAPVR

Abnormal Blood Pressure

Correctly recorded high blood pressure indicates systemic hypertension and the cause may be coarctation of aorta, aorto-arteritis or other renal causes. In infants the measurement of blood pressure is difficult because the right sized blood pressure cuff may not be available. The cuff should cover at least two thirds of the circumference as well as the length of the arm and pressure should be recorded using a mercury sphygmomanometer.

Fetal and Perinatal Circulation

Knowledge of fetal and perinatal circulation is an integral part of understanding the pathophysiology and natural history of congenital heart disease (CHD).

Fetal Circulation

Fetal circulation differs from adult circulation in various ways. Almost all differences are attributable to the fundamental difference in the site of gas exchange. In the fetus placenta provides the site where exchange of gases and nutrients take place.

Course

There are four shunts in fetal circulation- placenta, ductus venosus, foramen ovale and ductus arteriosus (Fig. 6.3).
1. Placenta receives the largest amount of combined (i.e. right and left) ventricular output (55%) and has the lowest vascular resistance in the fetus.
2. The superior vena cava (SVC) drains the upper part of the body, including the brain (15% of combined ventricular output) whereas inferior vena cava (IVC) drains the lower part of the body and placenta (70% of combined ventricular output). Since the blood is oxygenated in the placenta, the O_2

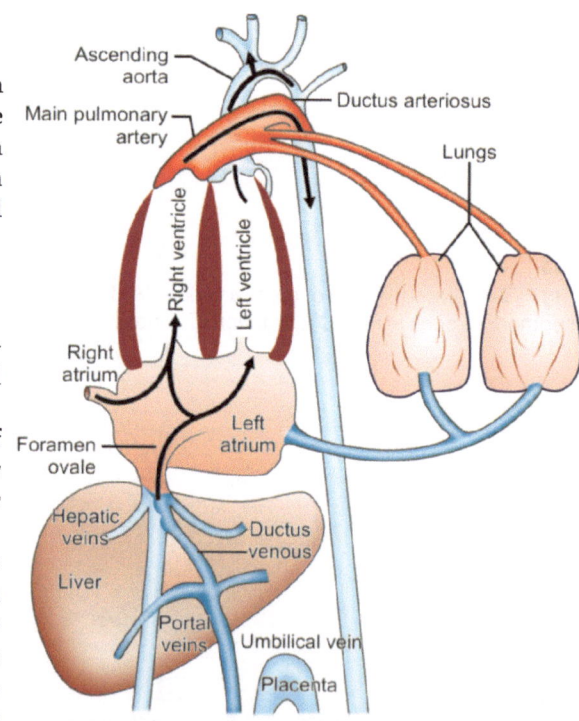

Fig. 6.3: Fetal circulation showing 4 sites of shunt

saturation in IVC (70%) is higher than that in SVC (40%). The highest PO_2 is found in the umbilical vein (32 mm Hg).
3. Most of the SVC blood goes to the right ventricle (RV). About one third of the IVC blood with higher oxygen saturation is directed by the crista dividens to the left atrium (LA) through the foramen ovale, whereas the remaining two thirds enters the RV and main pulmonary artery (MPA). The result is that the brain and coronary circulation receive blood with higher oxygen saturation (PO_2 of 28 mm) than the lower half of body (PO_2 of 24 mm Hg).
4. Less oxygenated blood in the pulmonary artery flows through the widely open ductus arteriosus to the descending aorta and then finally to the placenta for oxygenation.

Dimensions of Cardiac Chambers

Since the lungs receive only 15% of combined ventricular output, the branches of the PA are small. This is important in the genesis of the pulmonary flow murmur of the newborn.

Also, the RV is larger and more dominant than the left ventricle (LV). The RV handles 55% of the combined ventricular output whereas LV handles only 45%. In addition the pressure in RV is identical to that in LV (unlike in the adult). This fact is reflected in the electrocardiogram of the newborn, which shows more RV force than that of the adult (Fig. 6.4).

Fetal Cardiac Output

Unlike the adult heart, where the stroke volume is increased when the heart rate goes down, the fetal heart is unable to increase stroke volume when the heart rate falls. Therefore the fetal cardiac

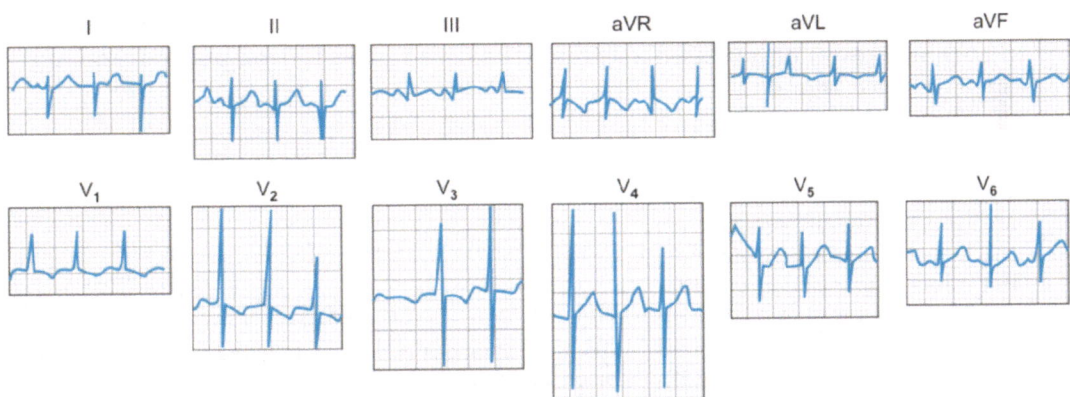

Fig. 6.4: Normal ECG of newborn-RV predominance

output depends on the heart rate. In fetal distress when the heart rate drops, a serious fall in cardiac output results.

Changes in Circulation After Birth

The primary change in circulation after birth is a shift of blood flow for gas exchange from the placenta to the lungs. The placental circulation disappears and the pulmonary circulation is established.

1. *Clamping of the umbilical cord results in*
   a. An increase in systemic vascular resistance (SVR) as a result of the removal of the very-low-resistance placenta.
   b. Closure of the ductus venous as a result of lack of return of blood from the placenta.
2. *Lung expansion results in the following:*
   a. A reduction in the pulmonary vascular resistance (PVR), an increase in pulmonary blood flow (PBF) and a fall in PA pressure (Fig. 6.5).
   b. Functional closure of the foramen ovale occurs as a result of increased pressure in the LA in excess of right atrial (RA) pressure. The LA pressure increases as a result of the increased pulmonary venous return to the LA and the RA pressure falls as a result of closure of ductus venosus.
   c. Closure of patent ductus arteriosus (PDA) as a result of increased arterial oxygen saturation.

Clinical Features

1. *Cyanosis:* Presence of cyanosis is an important manifestation when the lips and nails become blue, but it has to be decided whether the cyanosis appeared at birth or later. Transposition of great arteries (TGA) manifests with cyanosis at birth whereas in TOF,

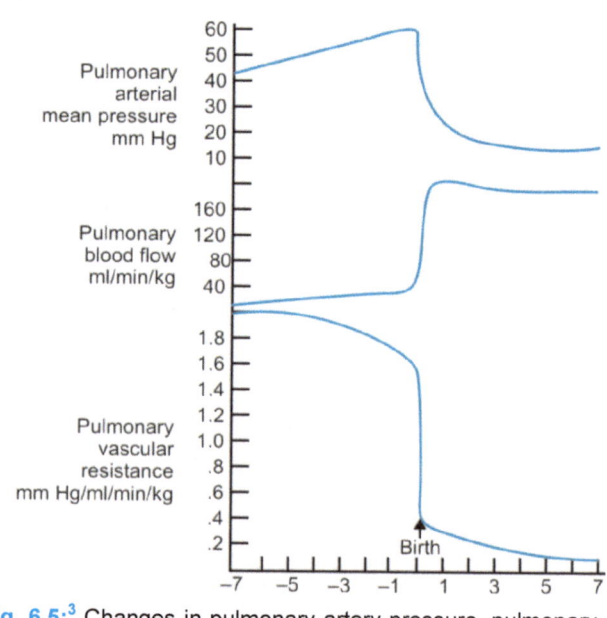

Fig. 6.5:[3] Changes in pulmonary artery pressure, pulmonary blood flow and pulmonary vascular resistance preceding birth, at birth and after birth

it appears after 6-8 weeks. If the cyanosis appears in an infant after a feed or while crying, then it suggests that the shunt temporarily reverses, which can happen in a large VSD.

Even when the cyanosis is severe, clubbing does not appear before about 3 months of age and is first visible as a fullness at the base of the thumb nail.

Differential diagnosis of cyanosis due to right to left shunt:

2 As - Aortic atresia, pulmonary atresia with normal aortic root.
5 Ts - Transposition of great arteries (TGA)
Tetralogy of Fallot (TOF)
Tricuspid atresia (TA)
Total anomalous pulmonary venous return (TAPVR)
Truncus arteriosus

2. *Tachypnea:* When the resting respiratory rate is > 50/minute with associated feeding difficulty and early fatiguability-these signify an underlying large L-R shunt, which ultimately leads on to a state of "failure to thrive".
3. *Frequency of respiratory infections:* Large shunts are associated with increased pulmonary blood flow (PBF) and are more predisposed to repeated chest infections.
4. Persistent sweating indicates an underlying large L-R shunt.
5. *Murmurs:* A heart murmur heard within a few hours of birth indicates a stenotic lesion (PS, AS) or a small L-R shunt (VSD, PDA). A soft systolic murmur with no radiation is usually innocent in nature.
6. *Chest pain:* Chest pain of cardiac origin is not sharp but rather a deep heavy pressure or a feeling of choking or a squeezing sensation and it is usually triggered by exercise. It is not associated with breathing except that of pericarditis. Cardiac conditions that may cause chest pain include:
   - Severe aortic stenosis (AS).
   - Pulmonary vascular obstructive disease.
   - Mitral valve prolapse (MVP).
   - Pericarditis.
   - Kawasaki's disease.
7. *Palpitation:* Palpitation is a subjective feeling of rapid heart beats which may suggest supraventricular tachycardia or premature ventricular beats.
8. *Respiration:* Respiration may be loud which masks the heart sounds. Rapid shallow respiration indicates metabolic acidosis, commonly seen in TOF following an episode of a cyanotic spell.
9. *Neurologic symptoms:* A history of stroke suggests embolization or thrombosis secondary to cyanotic CHD with polycythemia or infective endocarditis.

10. *CCF associated with respiratory infections:* More so in infants when the chest infection is fulminating. The CCF may be difficult to distinguish from pneumonia and chest infection usually precipitates CCF.
11. *Edema:* It is usually in the periorbital area or on the dorsum of feet.
12. *Congestive cardiac failure (CCF)*
    Classified in order of age:
    - During first week
        - Aortic atresia
    - One week to one month
        - Coarctation of aorta, transposition of great vessels
    - One month to 3 months
        - Transposition of great vessels, endomyocardial disease, coarctation of aorta, ventricular septal defect.
    - 3 months to 6 months
        - Endomyocardial disease, transposition of great vessels, ventricular septal defect, total anomalous pulmonary venous return, coarctation of aorta.
    - If the child survives infancy-6 common lesions are
        - Atrial septal defect, patent ductus arteriosus, ventricular septal defect, tetralogy of fallot, pulmonary stenosis, coarctation of aorta.

Management

Congenital heart disease may be broadly classified into 2 main groups, cyanotic and acyanotic. Once a diagnosis of congenital heart disease has been made in any age group, then the strategies for immediate and long term management of the patients have to be planned out. The medical management of any congenital cardiac disorder[16] whether cyanosed or otherwise would be on following lines:
1. Congestive cardiac failure
2. Cyanosis
3. Treatment of infective endocarditis.
4. Catheter intervention procedure.

Medical Management

I. *Congestive heart failure:* Care of infants with heart failure must include careful consideration because the underlying structured, functional, biochemical or physiological properties of young heart differ considerably from those of its older counterparts. The young heart contains fewer myofilaments to generate force with and to shorten during contraction. In addition, the chamber stiffness of the young heart is greater than that in later life.

The general aims of treatment are to achieve an increase in cardiac performance, augment peripheral perfusion and decrease pulmonary and systemic venous congestion. The initial therapy is aimed at stabilizing an infant's condition for diagnostic ultrasonography or angiographic study as soon as possible. In almost all situation, the decision to intervene surgically or to routine medical management requires a definitive anatomical diagnosis.

Treatment
a. *General interventions*
- Rest–occasional sedation
- Temperature and humidity control
- Oxygen inhalations
- Diet–high protein, low sodium load, calorie dense formula (0.8 Kcal/ml)–by nasogastric route.
- Treatment of infection, if present.

b. *Specific interventions*

A. Preload manipulation
- Volume infusion to increase venous return.
- Diuretics
  - Loop diuretics — Furosemide, torsemide
  - Thiazides — hydrochlorothiazide, metolazone
  - Aldosterone Antagonists — spironolactone, eplerenone.
  - Vasodilators — Angiotensin converting enzyme inhibitors – ACE - Inhibitors
    - Captopril, enalapril
  - Angiotension receptor blockers (ARB) – Losartan

B. Afterload reduction
- Facilitate ventricular emptying by reducing wall tension.
- Drugs–Arteriolar dilators–Hydralazine.

c. *Inotropic stimulation*
- Improve physical and metabolic milieu
  - pH, PaO_2, glucose, calcium, hemoglobin
- Control rhythm disturbances–Beta blockers–Metoprolol, carvedilol
- Inotropic drugs–digitalis
  - Dopamine, dobutamine
  - Amrinone, milrinone.

d. *Others*
   - Mechanical ventilation
   - Prostaglandin manipulation
   - Peritoneal dialysis.
e. Interventions (Catheter directed manipulations)

II. *Cyanosis:* Cyanosis in infants often presents as a diagnostic emergency necessitating prompt detection of the underlying cause. Cyanosis may occur due to:

a. Right to left shunt–Central cyanosis.
b. Low cardiac output–Peripheral cyanosis.
c. Pulmonary disease–Leading to defective oxygenation.
d. CNS disease–Meningitis/Encephalitis.
   - Decreased respiratory effort
e. Systemic–Methemoglobinemia.

Cyanosis due to R-L shunt (Central cyanosis) is characterized by arterial oxygen desaturation in presence of carboxyhemoglobin being more than 5 gm%. Cyanosis due to pulmonary venous desaturation tends to disappear on giving oxygen whereas cyanosis due to R-L shunt is unaffected (Hyperoxia test).

Failure of hyperoxia test makes cyanotic congenital heart disease a possible diagnosis although infants with severe respiratory disease and those with persistent pulmonary hypertension will also fail. Failure of hyperoxia test using a pulse oximeter (failure to increase oxygen saturation to 90% or more) is significant and may be of value in confirming the clinical diagnosis of cyanotic congenital heart disease in the absence of echocardiographic examination.

Cyanosis resulting from low cardiac output is due to increased extraction of oxygen by the tissues which are inadequately perfused due to low cardiac output–and the resulting cyanosis is referred to as peripheral cyanosis.

Methemoglobinemia is a systemic disorder, where the hemoglobin gets reduced to methemoglobulin by certain chemical, e.g. nitrates. This does not give rise to arterial oxygen desaturation and also it does not manifest with clinical features of cyanosis, e.g. clubbing, etc.

Cyanotic Congenital Heart Disease

Most cases of cyanotic congenital heart disease that require early intervention for cyanosis have a resting saturation of less than 80% and do not increase saturation to above 90% by 100% oxygen administration. Some cases of common mixing, e.g. TAPVC and double inlet ventricle have higher saturations.

Treatment

Following parameters have to be clarified to plan the treatment.
1. Assess if the cyanosed infant has any other congenital anomaly.
2. Antibiotics have to be started–if infection is suspected.
3. Consent for early surgery to be obtained.
4. Prostaglandins–use to be evaluated.

Prostaglandin E Series

These groups of drugs are indicated in those cyanosed infants where ductus arteriosus has to be kept patent, which will increase the pulmonary blood flow. Today, the obstructed form of total anomalous pulmonary venous drainage is the only truly cardiac surgical emergency.

In all, the other duct dependant circulation in cyanotic congenital heart disease and left sided obstructive lesions, the ductal patency can usually be maintained with prostaglandin infusion to stabilize the patient so as to permit surgery on a semi-urgent basis. Some indications of prostaglandin infusion include duct dependant pulmonary circulation as in case of pulmonary atresia with intact ventricular septum, transposition of great arteries with intact ventricular and atrial septum and also neonates with hypoplastic left heart syndrome.

Prostaglandins will improve oxygenation and prevent deterioration in those with obstructed pulmonary blood flow. Prostaglandin E1 is available as intravenous infusion whereas prostaglandin E2 can be given orally as well as parenterally. Side effects include apnea and hypotension.

Use of Indomethacin or Ibuprofen

Oral or intravenous indomethacin has been used successfully for nonsurgical closure of patent ductus arteriosus (PDA). Results are gratifying when used in first 10 days after birth and also in premature infants. Second course may be indicated if the clinical signs of ductus reappear after the initial closure. Indomethacin should not be administered in infants with renal dysfunction, overt bleeding, shock, necrotizing enterocolitis or electrocardiographic evidence of myocardial ischemia. Ibuprofen is also being used with similar results.

Eisenmenger Syndrome–Management

Eisenmenger syndrome refers to patients with congenital heart defects who have a systemic level of pulmonary artery pressure and high pulmonary vascular resistance with right to left as bidirectional shunting. Congestive heart failure may occur which responds to digitalis and diuretics. Anticoagulants have been recommended to prevent *in situ* thrombosis in lungs. Hemoglobin concentration at 20 gm/dl gives a situation of polycythemia where repeated phlebotomies or erythropoiesis may be required. Oral iron therapy is required for hypochromia and microcytosis. Pregnancy is contraindicated because of high maternal and fetal morbidity and mortality.

Treatment of Intercurrent Infection

Intercurrent infections in children with congenital heart disease (lower respiratory tract infections in large L-R shunts, cerebral abscess in cyanotic congenital heart disease, infective endocarditis) have to be looked for and treated with specific antimicrobial therapy. Delay in accurate diagnosis could lead to fulminant progression of infection or worsening of hemodynamics. Prophylaxis for infective endocarditis should be given within 60 minutes prior to start of an invasive procedure and should be directed towards the common organisms involved.

III. Treatment of Infective Endocarditis

It is imperative that the selection of antibiotics regimen be guided by blood cultures to demonstrate persistent bacteremia as well as antibiotic sensitivity testing. Treatment should begin on clinical suspicion while awaiting results to treatment. The duration of therapy varies from 4-6 weeks depending on the organism isolated and on the underlying premorbid condition. Surgical intervention is necessary if there is progressive worsening of congestive heart failure, embolic episode, non-response to treatment of prosthetic valve dysfunction.

IV. Catheteric Intervention Procedure

Recent advance have allowed a variety of therapeutic procedure using specially modified catheters, to be used in a cardiac catheterization laboratory. These procedures may save the lives of critically ill infants who are awaiting surgery.

The following interventional procedures will be discussed:
1. Atrial septostomy (Balloon/blade)
2. Balloon valvuloplasty.
3. Balloon angioplasty.
4. Device closure techniques.

Atrial Septostomy (Balloon/Blade)

Balloon atrial septostomy remains the standard initial palliation before corrective surgery for TGA, TAPVC and in selected cases of tricuspid atresia and pulmonary atresia, where a large communication is required.

A special balloon tipped catheter is placed in left atrium (LA) from RA through PFO. The balloon is inflated with a contrast material and rapidly pulled back into RA, thereby creating a large opening in the atrial septum. This procedure is carried out in infants less than 6 weeks of age, but in those who are older than 6-8 weeks–the septum becomes too thick which has to be cut with a catheter tipped blade.

Balloon Valvuloplasty

This procedure is carried out with the help of balloons made of plastic polymers which are placed over catheters with guide wires which go beyond the valves which have to be dilated. The balloons (elongated sausage shaped) are positioned over the valves and inflated with a contrast material to relieve the obstruction at stenosed valve. This can also be used in neonates with critical PS. The procedure is more difficult and a little dangerous in aortic stenosis and is indicated only when peak systolic gradient is more than 50-60 mm Hg without significant AR. This procedure is associated with a number of life threatening complications. Balloon valvuloplasty has been very successful in rheumatic mitral stenosis but not in congenital mitral stenosis.

Balloon Angioplasty

Balloon catheters similar to those used in balloon valvuloplasties are used for the relief of stenosis of blood vessels. This is an extremely useful tool in the management of postoperative residual obstruction of coarctation of aorta–where the success rate is close to 80%. This procedure is less effective in native coarctation of aorta where 17% of them have been documented to develop aortic aneurysm. Surgery is a better choice than balloon dilatation for native coarctation. Hypoplastic or stenosed branches of pulmonary arteries can be dilated with balloons and immediate success rate is about 60%, but restenosis occurs in a significant number of patients. Modification of balloon technique using an intravascular stent may improve the long term success rate.

Device Closure Techniques

1. Patent ductus arteriosus–A double umbrella plug (RashKind device) is used to close PDA and closure is achieved in 95%.
2. ASD secundum–A double umbrella device (Lock Clamshell occluder) has been used successfully in closing ASD secundum.
3. VSD–Successful closure of muscular VSD has been achieved in selected patients by using double umbrella clamshell device.

Surgery

Indications for surgery are varied for different defects. They are indicated only in presence of growth failure, chronic hypoxemia or CCF. Details of each will be dealt in specific CHD defects.

Primary Prevention (Table 6.5)

Since the cause is not known, primary prevention is almost impossible.

Pre-conception care–Care should be taken for a period of 12 months which includes 3 months before conception-known as pre-conceptual period. This period together with at least first 2 months

Table 6.5: Prevention of congenital heart disease-guidelines

1. Multivitamin containing folic acid to be used daily before conception. Daily dose of folic acid—0.4 mg. The dose to be increased in those with previously affected pregnancy.
2. Preconceptional assessment of risk factors and maternal conditions—diabetes, maternal phenyl-ketonuria, smoking, alcohol, rubella immunization, chronic illnesses and medication.
3. Common exposures to be stopped—especially smoking and alcohol use before conception–avoid passive smoking. Family members to be made to understand the dangers of smoking.
4. Reassess medication use—target medications with teratogenic effect—e.g. epileptic medications—Valproic acid.
5. Avoid contact with individuals with febrile illnesses—associated with viral illnesses, e.g. Rubella.

of pregnancy, provides a crucial opportunity for promoting healthy cardiac structures which develop in the first 7 weeks post-conception (9 weeks following last menstrual period) during which time many women may be unaware of the pregnancy, potentially exposed to teratogens and with limited or no prenatal care.[17]

1. For the individual, pre-conceptional health includes:[18]
    a. Identifying and managing chronic illnesses or exposures to infection.
    b. Avoiding exposures to acute illnesses, alcohol and smoking.
    c. Taking a multivitamin daily containing folic acid.
2. Population based interventions include:
    a. Increasing health care access, improving health behavior.
    b. Refocussing health professionals on common preventable risk factors for heart defects, e.g. systemic maternal illnesses–diabetes, drug intake, smoking, X-ray exposure etc.
3. Specific to population based intervention
    - Monitoring and intervention to reduce health disparities.

REFERENCES

1. A Khalil, R Aggarwal, S Thirupuram, R Arora. Incidence of congenital heart disease among hospital live birth in India. Indian Pediatric 1994;31(5):519-27.
2. Hoffman JI, Kaplan S. The incidence of congenital heart disease. J Am Coll Cardiol 2002;39;1890-1900.
3. Jegnander E, Williams W, Johansen OT, et al. Prenatal detection of heart defects in a non-selected population of 30, 149 fetuses–detection rates and outcome. Ultrasound Obstet Gynecol 2006;27:252-65.
4. Hiraishi S, Agata Y, Nowatari M, et al. Incidence and Natural course of trabecular ventricular septal defect: Two-dimensional echocardiography and color Doppler flow imaging study. J Pediatr 1992;120:409-15.
5. Mokdad AH, Ford ES, Bowman BA, et al. Prevalence of obesity, diabetes and obesity related health risk factors. JAMA 2003;289:76-79.

6. Waller DK, Mills JL, Simpson JL, et al. Are obese women at higher risk for producing malformed offsprings? Am J Obst Gynecol 1994;170:541-48.
7. Berrera JE, Khonry MJ, Cordero JF, et al. Diabetes mellitus during pregnancy and the risks for specific birth defects: A population based case-control study. Pediatrics 1990;85:1-9.
8. Harris MI, Hagel KM, Cowie CC, et al. Prevalence of diabetes, impaired fasting glucose and impaired glucose tolerance in US adults. The Third National Health and Nutrition Examination survey. 1988–1994. Diabetes Care 1998;21:518-24.
9. Mikhail LN, Walker CK, Mittendorf R. Association between maternal obesity and fetal cardiac malformations in African Americans. JAMA 2002;94:695-700.
10. Reef SE, Redd SB, Abernathy E, et al. The epidemiological profile of rubella and congenital rubella syndrome in United States, 1998-2004: The evidence for absence of endemic transmission. Clin Infect Dis 2006;43(Supl 3):S126-32.
11. Botto LD, Mulinare J, Erickson JD. Do multivitamin or folic acid supplements reduce the risk for congenital heart defects? Evidence and gaps. Am J Med Genet A 2003;121:95-101.
12. Levy HL, Guldberg P, Guttler F, et al. Congenital heart disease in maternal phenyl Ketonuria: Report from maternal PKV collaborative study. Pediatric Res 2001;49:636-42.
13. Rothman KJ, More LL, Singer MR, et al. Teratogenicity of high vitamin A intake. N Engl J Med 1995;333:1369-73.
14. Institute of Medicine Ed. Committee to study Fetal Alcohol Syndrome, Diagnosis, Epidemiology, Prevention and treatment, Washington DC: National Academy Press 1996.
15. Shaw GM, Nelson V, Carmichael SL, et al. Maternal Periconceptional Vitamins: Interactions with selected factors and congenital anomalies? Epidemiology 2002;13:625-30.
16. Anita Khalil. Medical management of congenital heart disease–Ped. Today 2005;VIII (3):154-59.
17. Jenkins KJ, Correa A, Feinstein JA, et al. Non-inherited risk factors and congenital cardiovascular defects: Current Knowledge Circulation 2006;1.
18. Johnson K, Posner SF, Biermann J, et al. Recommendation to improve preconception health and health care–United States–MMWR Recomm Rep 2006:1-23.

CHAPTER 7

Congenital Heart Disease: Specific Lesions
Diagnostic Approach to Congenital Heart Disease

PART I

When evaluating a patient with congenital heart disease there is a tendency to think that task of identifying the specific congenital abnormality may be overwhelming because there are so many different types of congenital heart diseases. However it is reassuring to recognise that only twelve congenital cardiac lesions account for more than 90% of all congenital heart diseases. Furthermore these 12 lesions can be further divided into four categories with 3 lesions each which can be recognized from the clinical examination. It is true that the expertise of pediatric cardiologists and sophisticated technology will be needed to arrive at the correct diagnosis in some individuals, but in most cases a careful clinical evaluation can establish the diagnosis. Table 7.1 gives a detailed classification of all congenital cardiac lesions.

The clinical approach is based on whether the patient is cyanotic or acyanotic and whether there is shunt vascularity on chest X-ray or not. Once these determinations have been made the patient can be considered in one of four categories (Flow chart 7.1).

Table 7.1: Classification based on clinicopathological presentation

1. Acyanotic	-	(a) Volume overload – Shunt vascularity-(L-R shunt) Atrial septal defect Ventricular septal defect Patent ductus arteriosus
		(b) Pressure overload – Normal vascularity-Obstructive lesions Pulmonic stenosis Aortic stenosis Coarctation of aorta
2. Cyanotic	-	(a) Volume overload Shunt vascularity-(R-L shunt) Transposition of great arteries (TGA) Total anomalous pulmonary venous connection (TAPVC) Persistent truncus arteriosus
		(b) Pressure overload Decreased vascularity-(R-L shunt) Tetralogy of Fallot (TOF). Tricuspid atresia (TA) Ebstein's anomaly

Congenital Heart Disease: Specific Lesions

Flow chart 7.1: Congenital heart disease–clinical classification[14]

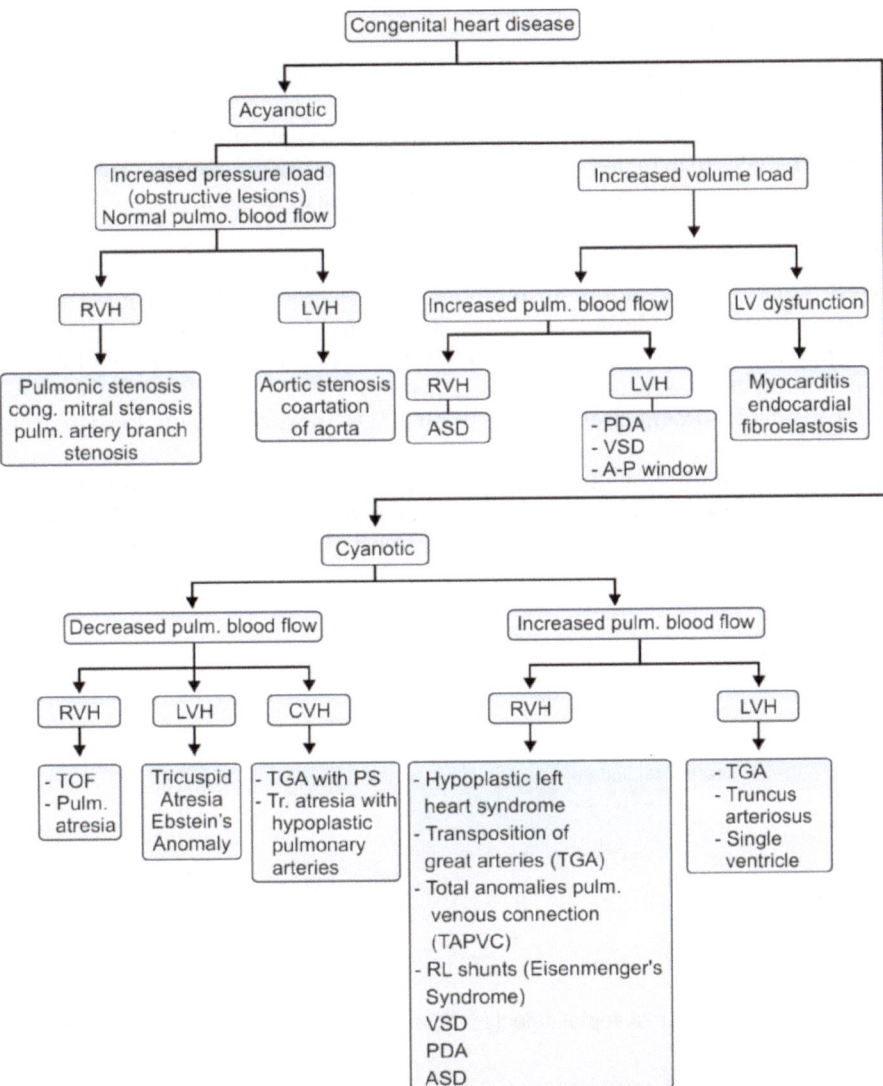

ACYANOTIC-VOLUME OVERLOAD L-R SHUNT

Atrial Septal Defect (ASD)

Any opening in the atrial septum, other than a competent foramen ovale is an atrial septal defect (ASD).

Ostium secundum defect (ASD) occurs as an isolated defect in 5-10% of all CHDs. It occurs twice as commonly in females than males[1]). ASD occurs in 1 child/1500 live births.[2] Holt and Oram noted the association between ASDs and anomalies of the upper extremities.[3]

Pathology

Three types of ASDs exist-secundum, primum and sinus venosus defects (Fig. 7.1).
1. Ostium secundum defect-commonest defect, accounting for 50-70% of all ASDs. This defect is present at the site of fossa ovalis-allowing left to right shunting of blood from LA to RA.
2. Ostium primum defects-30% of all ASDs.
3. Sinus venosus defect-occurs in about 10% of all ASDs, most commonly located at the entry of SVC into RA.

Defects at the level of fossa ovalis presumably result from deficiency, perforation or absence of septum primum. Because ostium secundum appears enlarged they are labeled as secundum type. In the setting of a large interatrial communication a chronic left to right shunt imposes a volume

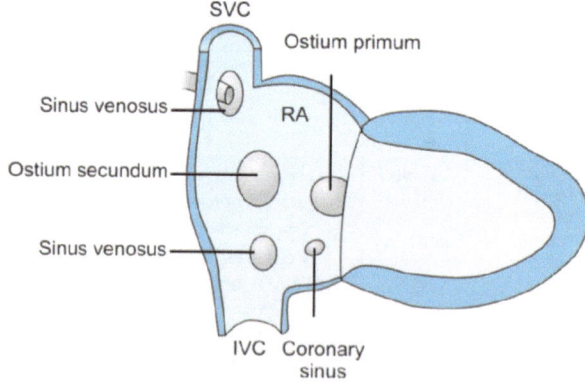

Fig. 7.1: Anatomy of atrial septal defects (ASDs) viewed with the right atrial wall removed

overload on the right sided cardiac structures and results in dilation of the right atrium and ventricle, where mural thrombus formation is distinctly uncommon. The chronic volume overload causes dilatation of the entire pulmonary vascular bed. Microscopically, the arteries, capillaries and veins are engorged. Medial hypertrophy is evident in the muscular pulmonary arteries and veins, although its extent is usually masked by vascular dilation. Muscularization of arterioles may also occur.[4] The direction in which the blood flows through the defect primarily is related to the relative compliances of the ventricle, resulting in less resistance to filling from the right atrium and in most situations, shunting in left to right. In infancy, the right ventricle is thick, stiff and not very compliant. Therefore, there is a minimal amount of left to right shunting. In the first few weeks of life, the pulmonary vascular resistance decreases, the right ventricle becomes more compliant and amount of left to right shunting increases.

Clinical Manifestations (Fig. 7.2)

1. Most infants with ASDs are symptomatic and the condition goes undetected. They may present at 6-8 weeks of life with a soft ejection systolic murmur and possibly a widely split and fixed S_2.
2. Older children with moderate left to right shunt are often asymptomatic and those with large shunts are likely to complain of fatigue and exertional dyspnea. Growth failure is uncommon.
3. Physical examination—Large L-R shunt—(older child)
   - Precordial bulge with a hyperdynamic cardiac impulse
   - Auscultation
     a. Wide and fixed splitting of second sound due to constant time interval between A_2 and P_2 throughout respiratory cycle.

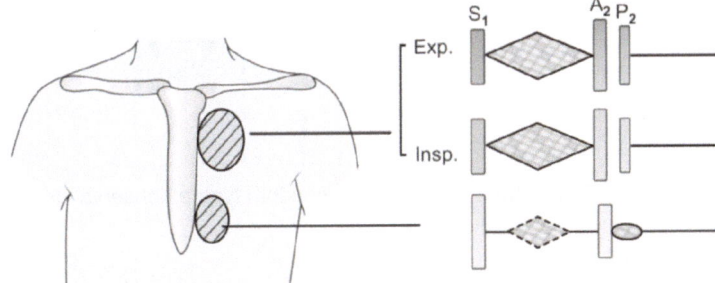

Fig. 7.2: Cardiac findings of atrial septal defects. Heart murmurs with solid borders are primary murmurs and those without solid borders are transmitted murmurs

b. Soft ejection systolic murmur at 2nd left intercostal space, due to increased blood flow across pulmonary valve.
c. Early to mid diastolic murmur at lower left sternal border due to increased blood flow across tricuspid valve producing a functional TS.
4. When significant PAH develops–the above mentioned characteristic findings disappear because of L-R shunt shrinks:
- Widely split P_2 can disappear and P_2 becomes louder
- Systolic murmur at upper left sternal border becomes shorter.
- Diastolic border disappears.

Electrocardiography (Fig. 7.3)

1. RAD + 90 to + 180 degrees
2. RVH and RBBB with VSR[1] are typical, consistent with right ventricular volume overload pattern in V_1.
3. P-R interval may be prolonged especially in older patients because of intra-atrial and sometimes H-V conduction delay resulting in first degree A-V block[5]
4. In about 50% of cases, tall P waves reflect right atrial enlargement.

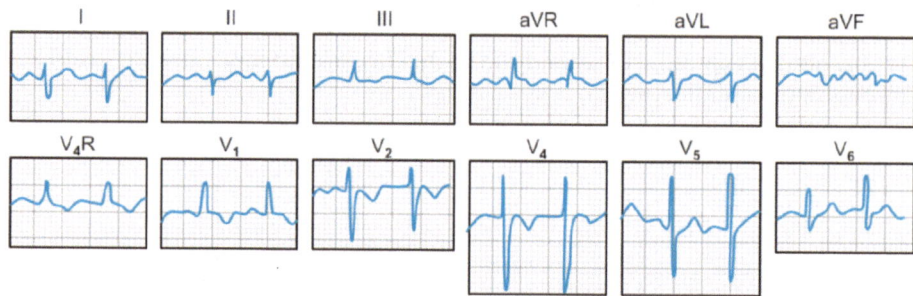

Fig. 7.3: Tracing from a child with secundum type atrial septal defect

X-ray Studies (Fig. 7.4)

1. Cardiomegaly with right atrial and right ventricular enlargement (cardiothoracic ratio > 0.5).
2. Prominent pulmonary artery seen in large shunts.
3. Prominent pulmonary vascular markings.

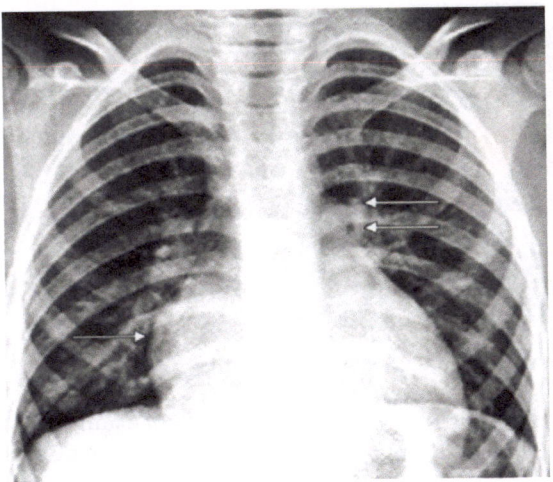

Fig. 7.4: Posteroanterior view of chest roentgenogram from a child with atrial septal defect. The heart is mildly enlarged with involvement of the right atrium and the right ventricle. Pulmonary vascularity is increased and the main pulmonary artery segment is likely prominent

Echocardiography (Figs 7.5A and 7.5B)

1. Echocardiography shows increased right atrial and right ventricular dimensions and defect in atrial septum which can be best seen in the subcostal four chamber view.
2. ASD secundum–dropout in mid atrial septum.
    - ASD primum–defect in lower atrial septum.
    - Sinus venosus ASD–deficiency in posterosuperior atrial septum.
    - Coronary sinus ASD–communication at the level of orifice of coronary sinus.

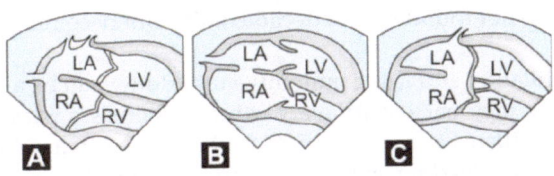

Fig. 7.5A: Diagram of 2-D echo of three types of ASD. (A) Sinous venosus defect, the defect is located at posterior superior atrial septum, usually just beneath the orifice of the SVC. (B) Secundum ASD defect is located in the middle portion of the atrial septum. (C) Primum ASD defect is located in the anterointerior atrial septum

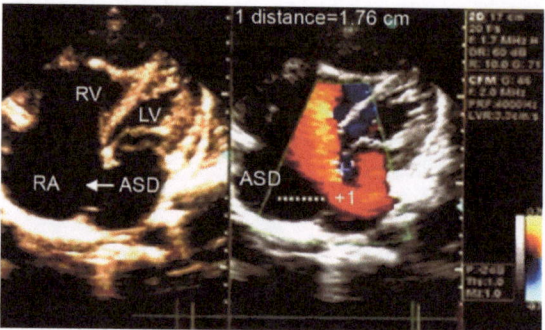

Fig. 7.5B: Echocardiogram showing large ASD secundum

3. Transoesophageal echocardiography (TEE) has become the most accepted mode of examination in older patients where associated partial anomalous pulmonary venous connection can also be diagnosed.
4. Pulsed Doppler examination–characteristic flow pattern with maximum left to right shunt occurring in diastole.
    - Color flow mapping–evaluates the hemodynamic status of ASD.
    - Doppler examination–estimates the systolic pressures in right ventricle and pulmonary artery from tricuspid and pulmonary valve regurgitation Doppler velocity waveforms.

Natural History

1. If ASD is less than 3 mm-spontaneous closure occurs in 100% before 18 months of age 87% of 3-5 mm (small) ASDs, 80% of 5-8 mm (medium) ASDs–also close spontaneously. But if the defect is >8 mm (large)-it rarely closes spontaneously.
2. Congestive heart failure not found in first decade of life, but becomes common beyond 40 years of age.[6]
3. The onset of atrial fibrillation and less commonly atrial flutter can be a hallmark in the course of patients with ASDs. The incidence of atrial arrhythmias increases with advancing age to as high as 13% in patients older than 40 years[7] and 52% in those older than 60 years of age.[8]
4. Pulmonary vascular disease leading on to pulmonary hypertension can occur in 5-10% of patients with untreated ASDs, predominant in females.[9] It usually occurs after 20 years of age.
5. Infective endocarditis does not occur in isolated ASDs, therefore prophylaxis against subacute bacterial endocarditis is unnecessary.

Management

Medical

1. No exercise restriction is indicated.
2. In infants-CHF should be treated urgently because it facilitates spontaneous closure.

Catheter Device Closure

Transcatheter techniques for closure of ASDs have been available for a number of years. In 1976, King et al[10] reported the first transcatheter closure of ASD secundum in humans with a double umbrella device. Since then there have been a number of devices, but problems were encountered which included residual shunts, embolization of device, hardware fracture, etc.

In December 2001, Amplatzer septal occluder (ASO) device became the only FDA approved device for transcatheter closure of ASDs. Reports of long term transcatheter closure with ASO–has been successful without any deaths or any other complications for an average of 6 years.

Erosion and thrombus formation have occurred with use of septal occluder devices. In a single center with a report of 40% patients where 9 different atrial septal occluder devices were used thrombus formation in right or left atrium was found in 1-2 % of patients, but ASD device had not brought about any thrombus formation.[11] Temporary AV blocks have been reported after the procedure, all resolving by 6 months.

Surgical

Prior to advent of interventional catheter procedure for major ASDs (left to right shunt with a QP/QS of > 1.5:1) in children and young adults, surgical repair was the treatment of choice.

Some consider a smaller shunt to be an indication because of danger of paradoxical embolization and cerebrovascular accident. High pulmonary vascular resistance (PVR) (i.e., > 10 units/m^2) is a contraindication to surgery.

Surgery is usually delayed till 3-4 years of age because of the possibility of spontaneous closure. In some patients with larger ASDs, closure is done at younger ages. There is no advantage in delaying repair much beyond this age and definite harm in delaying to teenage years, and because longstanding volume overload of the right atrium causes some irreversible changes that possibly contribute to atrial arrhythmias and premature death. But if CCF in infancy does not respond to medical management, then surgery is indicated and the defect is repaired under cardiopulmonary bypass with either a simple suture or a pericardial teflon patch.

Postoperative Follow Up

Atrial or nodal arrhythmias occur in 7 to 20% of the postoperative patients. Occasionally sick sinus syndrome may supervene especially when a sinus venosus defect is repaired. This eventuality may require anti-arrhythmic medication or pacemaker implantation.

Ventricular Septal Defect (VSD)

Ventricular septal defect is the most common form of congenital heart diseases if bicuspid aortic valve is excluded. Approximately 20% of patients with congenital heart disease have VSD as a solitary lesion.[12] Recent echocardiographic studies demonstrated an incidence of VSD in newborns to the 5-50/1000 live births.[13] VSDs are slightly more common in females.[14] In most patients (>95%) VSDs are not associated with a chromosomal abnormality. A multifactorial cause has been proposed in which interaction between hereditary predisposition and environment results in the defect.

Pathology (Figs 7.6A and B)

The ventricular septum may be divided into a small membranous portion and a large muscular portion. The muscular septum has 3 components–the inlet, the trabecular and the outlet (infundibular). Trabecular septum may be-central, marginal or apical.

VSD Classification

1. Perimembranous: most common 80% of surgical or autopsy series.[15]
2. Outlet–5.7% of surgical/autopsy series. Situated first beneath the pulmonary valve (Supracristal, infundibular, etc.)

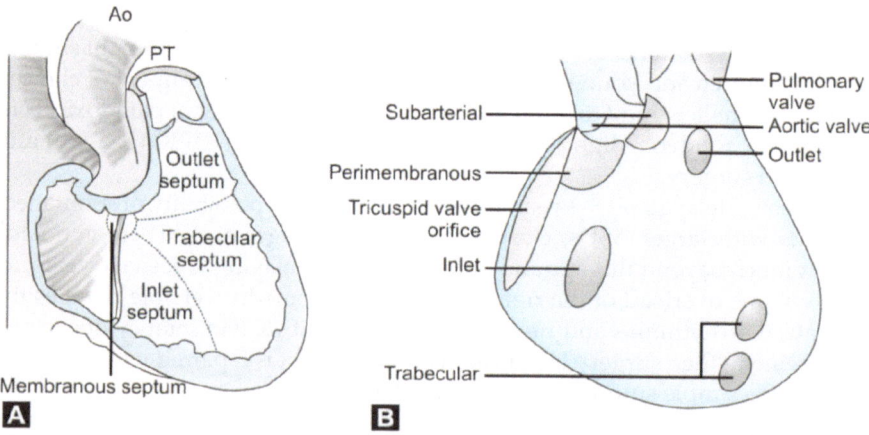

Figs 7.6A and B: The four major components of ventricular septum seen from the right ventricular aspect. The membranous septum is continuous with portion of the outlet septum, the trabecular septum and the inlet septum. (B) Possible sites of ventricular septal defects

3. Inlet–5.8%. Posterior and inferior to perimembranous defect etc.
4. Muscular–5–20%
   a. Central–mid muscular–may have multiple apparent channels on RV side and coalesce to single defect on LV side.
   b. Apical–multiple channels on RV side which coalesce to a single defect on LV side.
   c. Marginal–along RV septal formation
   d. "Swiss Cheese" Septum–large number of small muscular defects.

Clinical Manifestations (Figs 7.7 and 7.8)

History

1. Small VSD-patient is asymptomatic and growth is normal.
2. Moderate to large VSD
   - Repeated pulmonary infections
   - Easy fatigability
   - Decreased exercise tolerance, CCF
   - Failure to thrive
   - Pulmonary hypertension.
3. In unoperated VSD
   - Pulmonary hypertension
   - Reversal of shunt (Eisenmenger's syndrome)
   - Central cyanosis
   - Level of activity decreased.

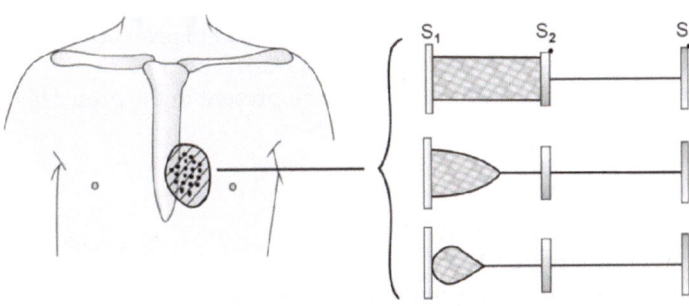

Fig. 7.7: Cardiac findings of a small ventricular septal defect. A regurgitant systolic murmur is best audible at the lower left sternal border. It may be holosystolic or less than holosystolic. Occasionally, the heart murmur is in early systole. A systolic thrill (dots) may be palpable at the lower left sternal border. The S_2 splits normally and the P_2 is of normal intensity

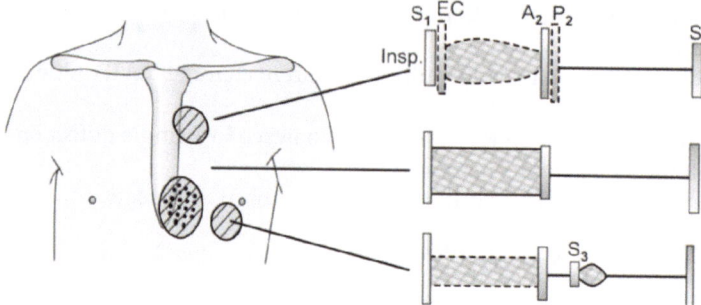

Fig. 7.8: Cardiac findings of a large ventricular septal defect. A classic holosystolic regurgitant murmur is audible at the lower left sternal border. A systolic thrill is also palpable at the same area (dots). There is usually a mid-diastolic rumble, resulting from relative mitral stenosis. Ejection click (EC) may be audible in the upper left sternal border when associated with pulmonary hypertension. The heart murmurs shown without solid borders are transmitted from other areas are not characteristic of the defect. Abnormal sounds are shown in black

Physical Examination

1. Small VSD — Child is well developed and acyanotic
   Moderate to Large VSD
   - Holosystolic murmur with thrill
   - Tachypnea, tachycardia
   - Repeated chest infection leading on to failure to thrive
   - CCF-enlarged liver
   - Reversal of shunt-cyanosis, respiratory distress (Eisenmenger's syndrome)
   - Hyperdynamic precordium
   - S_1 and S_2-well heard. P_2 may be single and loud in presence of PAH
   - Pansystolic murmur 3-5/6 heard at left sternal border.
   - An apical diastolic murmur may also be present in the presence of moderate to large shunt.

Electrocardiography (Fig. 7.9)

1. Moderate sized VSD-LVH with LAH–volume overload
2. Large VSD-combined ventricular hypertrophy (CVH)[16]
3. Eisenmenger's Complex–RVH–rSR′ pattern in v′ with slurring of upstroke of R wave.

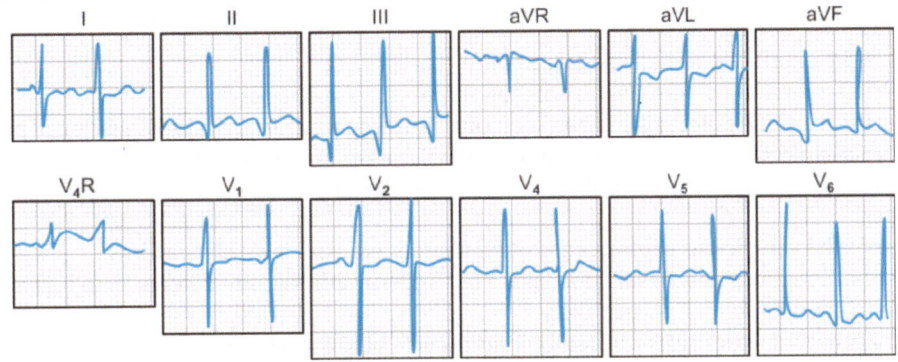

Fig. 7.9: ECG tracing from a child with ventricular septal defect

X-ray Studies (Fig. 7.10)

1. Cardiomegaly depending on the size of VSD and magnitude of L-R shunt.
2. When reversal of shunt takes place-hilar PA enlarges and peripheral lung fields become oligemic.

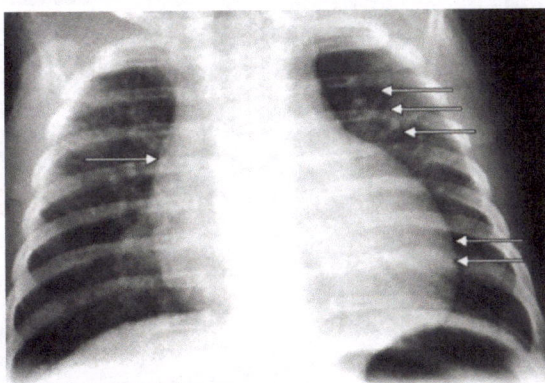

Fig. 7.10: X-ray chest of a patient with ventricular septal defect. There is a prominent thymic shadow (arrow). The heart is enlarged and the left contour is rounded suggesting a dilated left ventricle (double arrows). The pulmonary vascular markings are prominent indicating a left to right shunt (triple arrows)

Echocardiography (Figs 7.11A and B)

The echocardiographic criteria to determine the size of VSD[17]
1. Large VSD–when the defect size equals the diameter of aortic root.
2. Moderate size VSD–defect size is between one third to two thirds of the diameter of aortic root.
3. Small VSD–defect size is less than one third of diameter of aortic root.
4. Very small VSD–diagnosed usually by color Doppler and the defect size is less than 5 mm in diameter.

Whole of interventricular septum cannot be visualized from a single window.
1. Parasternal long axis and basal short axis views–perimembranous defects (Fig. 7.6) adjacent to aortic and tricuspid valve respectively.
2. Four chamber view (apical/subcostal)–inlet defects below both AV valves.
3. Basal short axis view–outlet defects adjacent to aortic and pulmonary valves.
4. Muscular (trabecular) VSDs can be seen in any of the long axis, short axis or four chamber views (Figs 7.11A and B).

Estimation of pulmonary and systemic flows can be derived from the product of time velocity interval obtained by pulse wave Doppler and cross sectional areas at the site of flow (aorta or pulmonary artery) (Fig. 7.12).

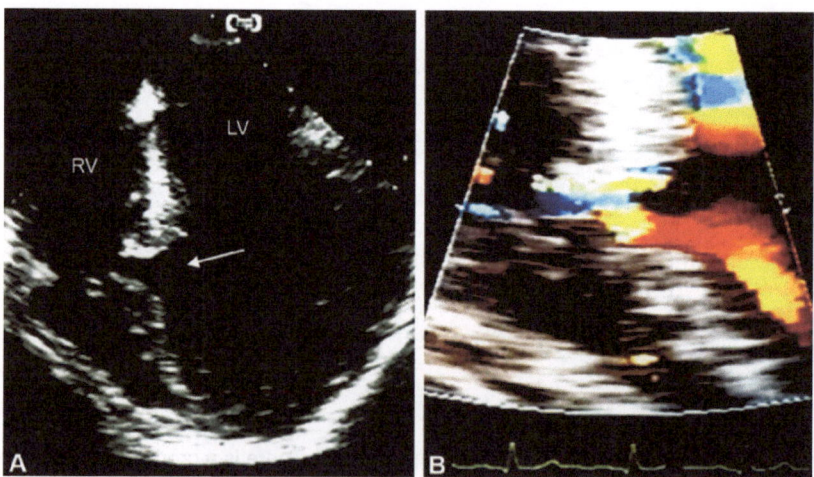

Figs 7.11A and B: (A) Muscular ventricular septal defect (arrow), (B) color flow mapping shows flow from left to right ventricle

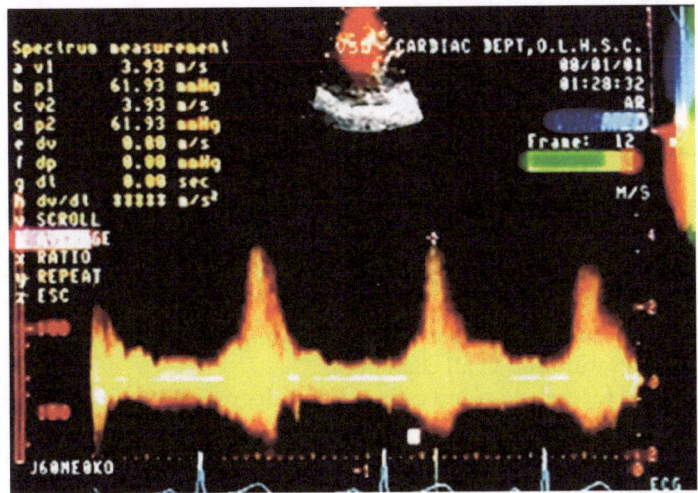

Fig. 7.12: Doppler profile of flow across VSD. It shows maximum velocity if flow across the VSD is about 4 m/s (which indicates a small VSD)

Interventricular pressure gradient is measured by modified Bernoulli equation from velocity of flow across the VSD[18]. The interventricular gradient is inversely proportional to the size of VSD and pulmonary arterial pressure. Echocardiography particularly 2-D echocardiography with color Doppler mapping has almost replaced cardiac catheterization and angiocardiography for routine diagnosis of VSD.

Main aim is to detect:
1. Size and location of VSD
2. Estimation of shunt flow (relative flow to systemic and pulmonary circulation)
3. Pressure gradient across VSD to know interventricular pressure difference.
4. Estimation of RV and PA pressure.
5. LA and LV diameter.
6. To determine ventricular systolic function.
7. To ascertain other associated defects.

Magnetic Resonance Imaging (MRI)

Gated MRI provides excellent anatomical diagnosis of VSD as well as other associated cardiac malformation. Cine MRI gives functional assessment of wall motion and shunt flow.

Radionuclide studies help in detecting left to right shunt and magnitude of pulmonary to systemic flow.

Cardiac Catheterization and Angiocardiography

Cardiac catheterization is not advised routinely and small VSDs do not require catheterization. The main indication for cardiac catheterization are:
1. To delineate the number and locations of VSDs.
2. Estimation of magnitude of shunt.
3. Estimation of pulmonary vascular resistance (PVR) for surgical risk assessment.
4. Estimate ventricular systolic function.
5. Document presence or absence of associated defects (e.g. left SVC).
6. Estimation of oxygen saturation in all chambers.
7. Aortogram is required for detection and estimation of degree of aortic regurgitation when present.

Differential Diagnosis in Infants

Presence of acyanotic shunt manifestations of CCF and a systolic murmur–the possibilities are:
1. Complete AV canal defect
2. AP window without PS
3. Single ventricle without PS (if acyanotic)
4. DORV without PS.
5. Large PDA

In Older Children

1. Pulmonary stenosis (mild to moderate).
2. Aortic stenosis (mild to moderate).
3. Innocent systolic murmurs.

Complications

Large VSD
1. Congestive heart failure
2. Arrhythmias
3. Infective endocarditis.
4. Eisenmenger's complex–reversal of shunt.

Natural History

1. Spontaneous closure in 30-40% of cases with small (5 mm) membranous and muscular VSDs.
2. CCF develops in large VSDs, after 8 weeks of age.
3. In a large VSD, pulmonary vascular obstructive disease may begin to develop as early as 6-12 months of age but the resulting reversal of shunt does not get established till the teenage years.
4. In large VSDs-infundibular stenosis may develop, which decreases the magnitude of L-R shunt (acyanotic TOF).
5. Pulmonary hypertension may develop by 10 years leading to Eisenmenger's complex.
6. Aortic regurgitation may set in between 2-10 years of age in about 5% of cases of high VSD (outlet type) due to improper support by one of the aortic cusps.
7. Arrhythmias in large VSDs.
8. Infective endocarditis is one of the principal hazards and life threatening complications of all types of VSDs.

MANAGEMENT

Medical

1. No exercise restriction in the absence of pulmonary hypertension.
2. Maintenance of good dental hygiene, antibiotic prophylaxis against infective endocarditis.
3. Treatment of CCF-decongestive therapy (digoxin and diuretics) and ACE-inhibitors if the shunt is large.
4. Frequent feeding of high calorie formula. Anemia-to be corrected by iron therapy or blood transfusion.
5. "Amplatzer" device for closure of selected muscular defects-is possible and is being done in some centers. There is a growing trend for catheter device closure of all types of VSDs with collaboration of both cardiologist and cardiac surgeon.

SURGICAL

Indications

1. Small defects–where QP/QS < 1.5:1, no need to operate because they close on their own.
2. Large VSDs-if CCF responds to decongestive therapy, then surgery is delayed. If CCF does not respond-then the VSD should be closed within the first 6 months of life.
3. After 1 year of age-significant L-R shunt with QP/QS of at least 2: 1 indicates surgical closure.
4. Older infants with large VSDs and increased pulmonary resistance should be operated immediately.
5. Surgery is contraindicated in presence of predominant R-L shunt or PVR/SVR >0.5.

Complications

1. Incomplete closure.
2. Different degrees of heart blocks-RBBB, left anterior hemiblock or even complete heart block.
3. Aortic regurgitation.

Patent Ductus Arteriosus

Patent ductus arteriosus (PDA) is the most common type of extracardiac shunt seen in clinical practice. It presents persistent patency of the vessel that normally connects the pulmonary artery and the aorta in fetus (Fig. 7.13). When the ductus remains patent even after birth in a term infant, it is called as persistent ductus arteriosus.

Patent ductus arteriosus occurs in 5-10% of all CHDs, excluding premature infants where it is a common problem. It is more common in females than males (M: F = 1:2). PDA is commonly seen in low birth weight infants (< 1.5 Kg), those born at high altitude and also in rubella syndrome.

Pathology

1. The ductus arteriosus is derived from 6th aortic arch. The ductus is interposed between the proximal portion of the left pulmonary artery and beginning of descending aorta, just distal to left subclavian artery.

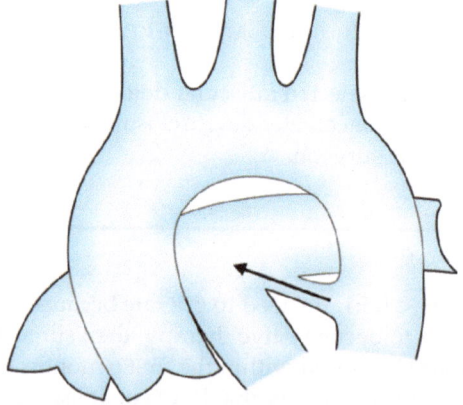

Fig. 7.13: Patent ductus arteriosus

2. There is persistence of patency of the ductus which is a communication between the left pulmonary artery and the descending aorta, 5-10 mm distal to the origin of the left subclavian artery.
3. The ductus is usually cone-shaped with a small orifice towards the P A, which is restrictive to blood flow. The ductus may be short or long, straight or tortuous ranging between 0.2–2 cm. The closure starts from pulmonary end, and aortic end is dilated–ductus ampulla. In fetal life, the diameter of ductus is equal to diameter of descending aorta and in neonatal period, it is half of it.

Mechanisms of Postnatal Closure

Postnatal closure of ductus arteriosus is effected in two phases:
1. At birth–Contraction and cellular migration of the medial smooth muscle in the wall of ductus arteriosus–produces shortening, increased wall thickness and protrusion into the lumen of the thickened intima resulting in functional closure.[19] This commonly occurs within 12 hours after birth in a full term infant.[20]
2. Second stage–completed by 2-3 weeks–produced by infolding of endothelium, disruption and fragmentation of the internal elastic lamina, proliferation of subintimal layers and hemorrhage and necrosis of subintimal region. Connective tissue formation replaces muscle fibers with fibrosis and permanent sealing of lumen to produce ligamentum arteriosum.
3. During fetal life, the partial pressure of oxygen (PO_2) to which the ductus arteriosus is normally exposed is 18 to 28 mm Hg.[21] An increase in PO_2, as occurs with ventilation after birth, constricts the ductus arteriosus in mature foetal animal.[22] Though in early pregnancy the ductus arteriosus does not respond to oxygen at high concentration but as gestation advances, the amount of constriction in response to increasing PO_2 is greater and the level of PO_2 required to initiate a response decreases.[23] Release of other vasoactive substances, e.g acetylcholine, bradykinine, other calecholamines may contribute to post-natal closure of ductus arteriosus.[24]
4. Prostaglandins, the cyclooxygenase mediated product of arachidonic acid metabolism, is involved in the overall physiology of the ductus arteriosus. Prostaglandins play an active role in maintaining the ductus arteriosus in a dilated state during fetal life.[25] PGE_2 and PGI_2 are formed intramurally in the ductus arteriosus and may extend their action locally on muscle cells. Endogenous PGI_2, production is almost tenfold than that of PGE_2 but the latter is more potent in keeping the ductus arteriosus open. The fetus has a high circulating concentration of prostaglandins, because they are produced in the placenta and decreased by being catabolized in the lungs.
5. At birth, the placental source is removed and a marked increase in pulmonary blood flow allows effective removal of PGE_2. Thus patency or closure of ductus arteriosus represents a balance between the constricting effects of oxygen and other vasoconstrictive substances and relaxing effects of several prostaglandins.

Clinical Manifestations (Fig. 7.14)

Patients are usually asymptomatic when the ductus is small. A large shunt PDA-is accompanied by tachypnea, hyperdynamic circulation and poor weight gain. It might be associated with repeated chest infections, and congestive cardiac failure.

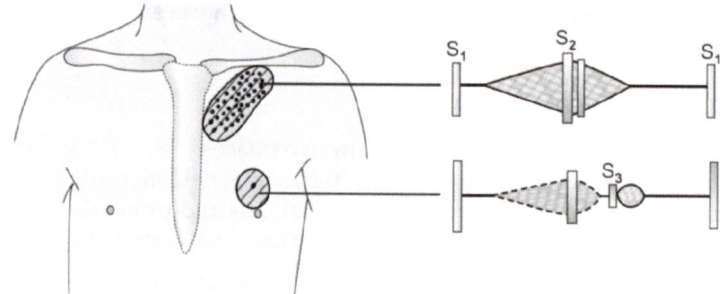

Fig. 7.14: Cardiac findings of patent ductus arteriosus. A systolic thrill may be present in the area shown by dots

Physical Examination

1. In presence of a large shunt-tachycardia and exertional dyspnea may be present.
2. Hyperactive pre-cordium with a systolic thrill at the upper left sternal border along with bounding peripheral pulses with wide pulse pressure.
3. On auscultation, P_2 may be loud in presence of pulmonary artery hypertension. S_3 is audible and loud and harsh 4/6 continuous machinery murmur is best heard at the left infraclavicular area with multiple sounds (eddies) heard during the continuous murmur–typical finding of PDA.

Electrocardiography (Fig. 7.15)

1. In small to moderate sized PDA-Normal or LVH.
2. Large PDA-combined ventricular hypertrophy.
3. In reversal of shunt-RVH develops.

X-ray Studies (Fig. 7.16)

The chest X-ray is normal when the shunt is small. Cardiomegaly with LV contour, LA enlargement and increased pulmonary vascularity (plethora) are usual features of PDA. The dilatation of main pulmonary artery (MPA) is the earliest radiological sign of PDA. Aortic knuckle is prominent.

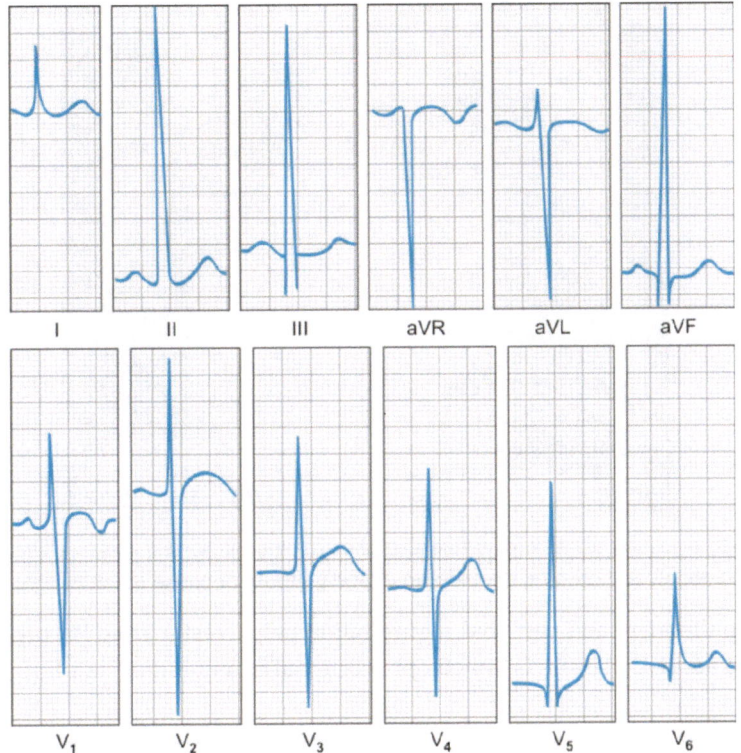

Fig. 7.15: Tracing from a patient of PDA showing left ventricular volume overload (deep S wave in V_1 with tall R in V_5) and q waves in $V_5 - V_6$

Echocardiography (Fig. 7.17)

1. PDA can be imaged in most of the patients by 2 D echo in a high parasternal or a suprasternal notch view.
2. The dimensions of LA and LV provide an indirect assessment of the magnitude of the left to right shunt.
3. Doppler-ductal shunt patterns-A continuous positive flow indicates a pure left to right shunt with the PA pressure lower than aortic pressure (Fig. 7.17).

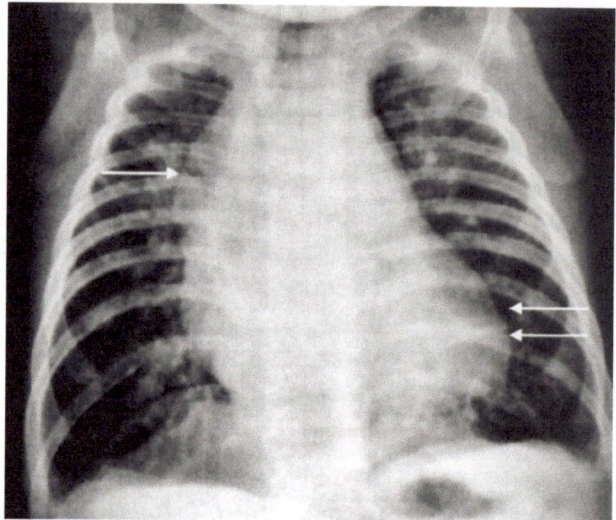

Fig. 7.16: X-ray chest of a large patent ductus arteriosus. The thymus is prominent (arrow). There is cardiomegaly (LV contour, double arrow) and plethora because of left to right shunt

4. Presences of pulmonary and tricuspid regurgitation help in estimating PA pressure.
5. Ratio of LA to aorta dimension is directly proportional to amount of shunt.

DIAGNOSIS

Small PDA

Patients are asymptomatic. The hallmark of diagnosis is a continuous murmur with longer diastolic component audible over upper left sternal border and infraclavicular area.

Large PDA

1. Possible history of heart failure in infancy and repeated chest infections since infancy.
2. Physical findings include manifestation of hyperdynamic circulation–high volume pulse with pulsatile precordium, cardiomegaly with continuous thrill over left infraclavicular area. There

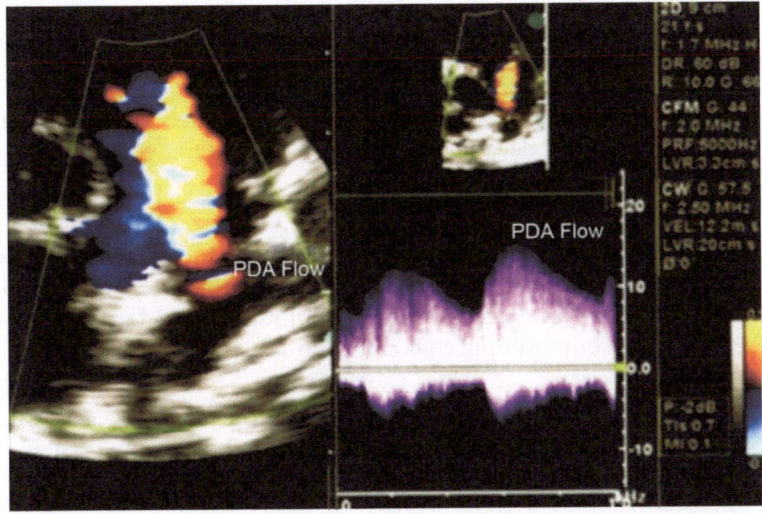

Fig. 7.17: Echocardiography of PDA, left panel showing color flow from descending aorta to pulmonary artery along its left margin and right panel showing continuous turbulence obtained from the same site

is a loud continuous murmur, rough in character, a crescendo-decreascendo murmur best heard in the infraclavicular area.
3. A prominent S_3 and also a mid diastolic flow murmur over the apex are often present in large shunts (Fig. 7.14).

Complications

1. Repeated chest infection
   - Severe form (bronchopneumonia)
2. Congestive cardiac failure
   - In premature infants with large PDA, CCF develops in first week of life.
3. Infective endocarditis–more common in adolescents.
4. Pulmonary hypertension and pulmonary vascular disease–due to large shunt through PDA.

Natural History

1. Unlike PDAs in preterms, spontaneous closure of the PDA does not occur in term infants because of structural abnormality of the ductal smooth muscle.
2. Reversal of shunt takes place if a large PDA remains untreated and pulmonary hypertension develops by the end of second decade.

Management

1. Indomethacin is ineffective in term infants, but helps in closing PDAs in preterms.
2. Non-surgical closure-Catheter closure of ductus with different devices. Stainless steel coils (Gianturco coils) are in an experimental stage. An optimum candidate for the device-the ductus should be 2.5 mm in size but multiple coils can close a ductus up to 5 mm.

TREATMENT

Premature Infant

1. Maintenance of adequate hematocrit (> 45%) and hemoglobin. A reduction in hemoglobin requires an increased cardiac output to maintain peripheral oxygenation and with a left to right shunt and an already compromised myocardium, anemia may further impair cardiac function.
2. For peripheral tissue oxygen delivery, fetal hemoglobin has to be replaced by adult hemoglobin by exchange transfusion.
3. Nutritional–glucose and electrolyte requirements have to be carefully maintained. For high caloric intake, intravenous alimentation may be required and Na^+ administration commonly restricted to low maintenance amounts.
4. In premature infants–digitalis is ineffective and is not used now. Supportive treatment for L-R shunt should be used and the shunt should be closed at the earliest.
   Non-surgical Closure
   Indomethacin therapy
   a. Oral or (lyophilized) intravenous indomethacin to constrict the ductus arteriosus has led to successful non-surgical closure in a large proportion of treated infants[26]–results are best when used before 10 days of age and in less mature infants.
   Dosage schedule varies
   1st dose–0.2 mg/Kg by nasogastric tube or intravenously
   Indomethacin–doses depend on age
   - If < 48 hours–the subsequent 2 doses are 0.1 mg/Kg
   - If 2-7 days–0.20 mg/Kg
   - If > 7 days–0.25 mg/Kg

A total of 2 doses are given 12-24 hours apart depending on urinary output.

If clinical signs reappear then a second course may be considered.

Administration of indomethacin to infants (birth weight < 1000 gm).[27] In these infants, treatment should be started immediately when the diagnosis is made, usually before 72 hours of age. Prophylaxis on the first day has no advantage because not all infants develop PDA.

b. *Ibuprofen*–evaluated as a possible alternative to indomethacin.[28]

Meta-analysis of some studies have shown a comparable rate of ductal closure after ibuprofen therapy.[29] Ibuprofen has shown less toxicity on kidneys, less effect on cerebral vasculature, but has not shown a decreased risk for intra-ventricular hemorrhage.[30] But when used for prophylaxis, there has been an increased risk of pulmonary hypertension.[31]

Contraindication for Indomethacin Therapy

a. Renal dysfunction–serum creatinine–> 1.6 mg/dl

   Blood urea nitrogen > 20 mg/dl

b. Overt bleeding

c. Shock

d. Necrotizing enterocolitis.

e. Electrocardiographic evidence of myocardial ischemia.

5. Early surgical ligation (< 10 days of age) reduces duration of stay, ventilator support and overall morbidity. Improved lung mechanisms have been confirmed in premature infants 26-29 weeks gestation after ligation showing an increase in dynamic compliance, tidal volume and minute ventilation. The benefit of surgical treatment in premature infants has been estimated to be fourfold as compared to medical treatment.[32]

6. If after 48-72 hours of adequate medical management–left ventricular failure is still uncontrolled, surgical closure is performed. Ligation or clip ligation are done instead of division of ductus arteriosus.

7. Regardless of size, PDA should be ligated if no reversal of shunt has taken place.

ACYANOTIC-PRESSURE OVERLOAD

Obstructive Variety Pulmonic Stenosis (PS)

Congenital heart disease with obstruction to right ventricular outflow tract is most commonly due to pulmonary valve stenosis.

Pulmonic stenosis occurs in 8-12% of all CHDs. About 1.1-2.1% of siblings also have been found to have pulmonary stenosis.[33]

Pathology

1. PS may be valvular, subvalvular (infundibular) or supravalvular.
2. In valvular PS, the pulmonary valve is thickened with fused or absent commissures and a small orifice (Figs 7.18A to C).
3. Isolated infundibular PS is rare; it is usually associated with perimembranous VSD with overriding of aorta.
4. Supravalvular PS-also called stenosis of the main pulmonary artery. It is seen in association with rubella syndrome.
5. Pulmonary valve dysplasia–seen in 10% cases. The valves have thickened cusps composed of myxomations tissue with no fusion. The valve annulus is hypoplastic. This is most commonly seen in Noonan's syndrome.
6. Secondary changes occur in right ventricle and pulmonary artery. The infundibular region of right ventricle, becomes diffusely hypertrophied producing subvalvular obstruction. At autopsy small areas of myocardial infarctions have been seen in the subendocardial area due to severe pulmonary stenosis.
7. Most patients develop post-stenotic dilatation of the pulmonary artery trunk, except in patients with dysplastic pulmonary valves.

Clinical Manifestations (Fig. 7.19)

1. In mild cases, the patient is asymptomatic. Easy fatigability and exertional dyspnea may be present in moderately severe cases and congestive heart failure and chest pain on exertion may develop in severe cases.

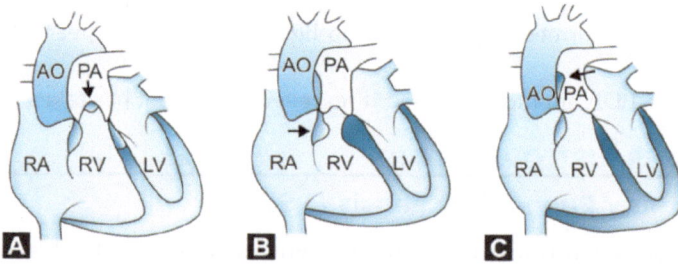

Figs 7.18A to C: Anatomic types of PS. (A) Valvular stenosis, (B) Infundibular stenosis, (C) Supraventricular PS (or stenosis of the MPA). Abnormalities are indicated by arrows

2. Most patients are acyanotic and well developed. Newborns with critical PS-are cyanotic and tachypnoic.
3. On examination-a parasternal heave may be present with a right ventricular tap at the apex, and also a systolic thrill may be present in the upper left sternal border (ULSB).
4. On auscultation-a systolic ejection click with a widely split S_2 and also with a soft P_2, depending on the severity of PS. An ejection systolic murmur (grade 2-5/6) is heard at the ULSB, again the loudness depends on the severity.

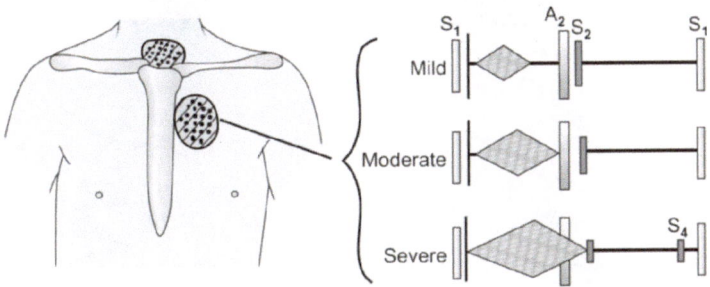

Fig. 7.19: Cardiac findings of pulmonary valve stenosis. Abnormal sounds are shown in black dots, represent areas with systolic thrill. EC, ejection click

X-ray Study (Fig. 7.20)

Heart size is usually normal but MPA segment is prominent (post-stenotic dilatation). In severe PS-pulmonary venous markings are decreased.

Electrocardiography (Fig. 7.21)

In moderately severe PS-RAD with RVH.
R wave in V_1 is >20 mm when there is systemic pressure in RV.

Echocardiography

1. Two-dimensional echo in parasternal short axis view-shows thick pulmonary valve cusps with restricted systolic motion (doming), MPA is often dilated (post-stenotic dilatation) (Fig. 7.22).
2. The Doppler study can estimate the pressure gradient and severity of pulmonary stenosis (Figs 7.23 and 7.24).

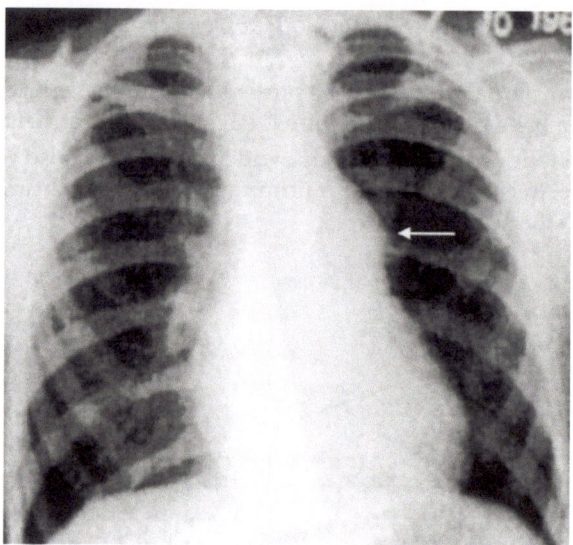

Fig. 7.20: Chest X-ray of PS showing RV contour, RA enlargement, arrow showing post-stenotic dilatation of pulmonary artery and decreased vascularity

3. The diagnosis of dysplastic pulmonary valve usually can be ascertained by echocardiography. Leaflets appear thickened and immobile, and pulmonary valve annulus is hypoplastic and supra annular narrowing of the proximal main pulmonary artery is often present.

MANAGEMENT

Medical

1. Restriction of activity is not necessary, except in severe cases of PS.
2. Antibiotic prophylaxis against SBE-is always indicated when dental or lower GIT or genitourinary interventions are done.
3. Balloon valvuloplasty is preferred to surgery for moderate PS (RV systolic pressure >50 mm Hg). It has been successful in severe PS in newborns also.
4. Critical PS in newborns-Prostaglandin E infusion helps in opening up of PDA-thereby decreasing hypoxia.
   Later on balloon valvotomy may be performed-if unsuccessful, surgery is indicated.

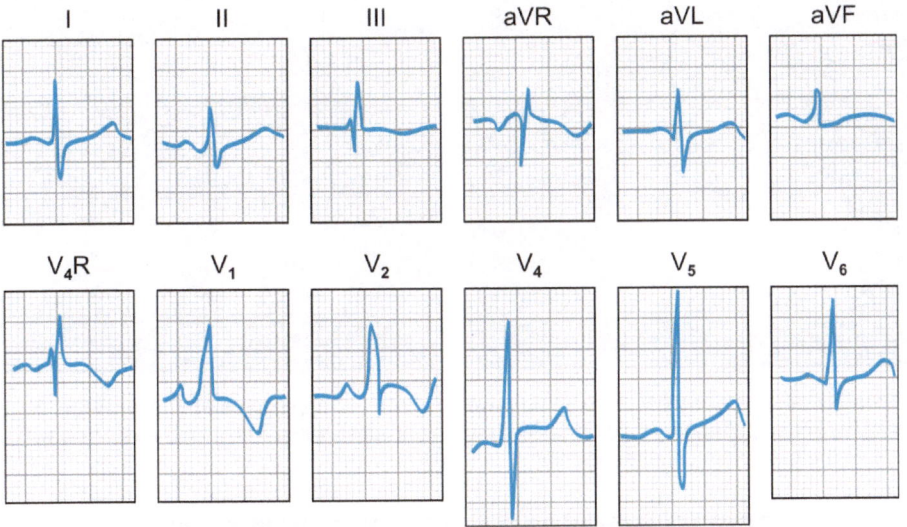

Fig. 7.21: ECG of patient with pulmonary valve stenosis with right ventricular hypertrophy. Arrows, RVH in the QRS complex and ST-and T wave in right ventricular strain in V_4R and V_1

Surgical

1. Valvular PS-when RV systolic pressure is >80 mm Hg and those in whom balloon valvuloplasty is unsuccessful (dysplastic valve)-surgery is indicated on an elective basis.
2. Infants with critical PS-require surgery on an urgent basis.

Aortic Stenosis (AS)

Congenital bicuspid aortic valve occurs in 1.3 % of the population.[34] Given that overall prevalence of congenital heart disease in infants is approximately 0.8% with aortic stenosis accounting for 3-8% of these lesions, it is clear that minor malfunctions of the aortic valve are frequently undetected early

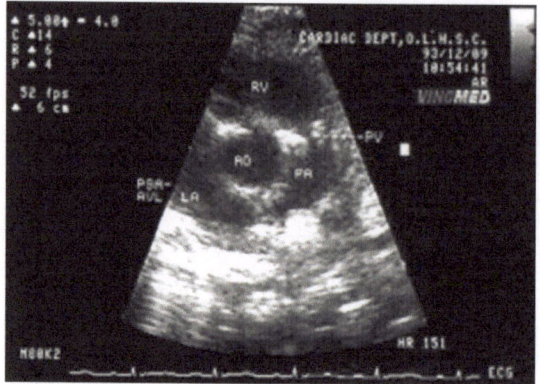

Fig. 7.22: Parasternal short axis view at the aortic valve level showing thickened pulmonary valve (PV) leaflets in systole. Note the restricted leaflet separation

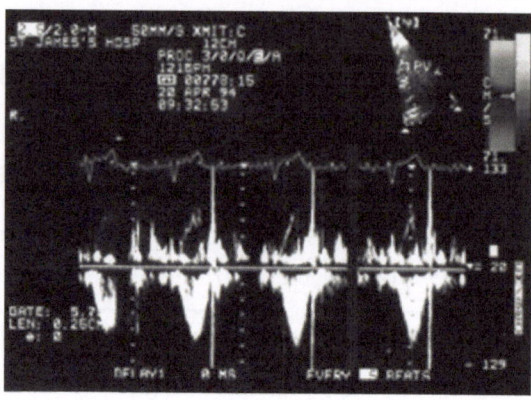

Fig. 7.23: Doppler profile of patient with mild pulmonary stenosis showing a slight increase in peak flow velocity

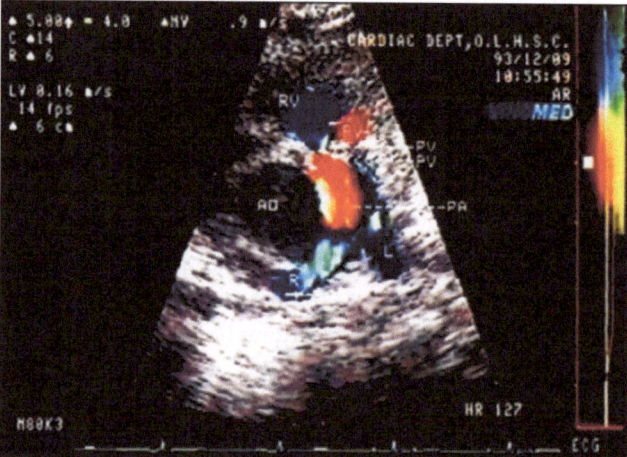

Fig. 7.24: Color flow mapping of pulmonary flow in a patient with pulmonary stenosis. Note the change in color code (Red/Mosaic) at the valve level

in life. Only 2% of the patients with congenitally abnormal aortic valve will experience significant stenosis or regurgitation by adolescence.[35] Males are affected more frequently than females, ratio reported to be in the range of 3:1 to 5:1.[36] Associated congenital heart defects occur in approximately 20% of patients with congenital aortic stenosis and most common associations are ventricular septal defect, coarctation of aorta and patent ductus arteriosus.[37] There is compelling evidence for a genetic link to aortic stenosis. Valvular aortic stenosis is associated with Turner syndrome and supravalvular aortic stenosis is associated with Edward's syndrome. In summary, it appears that congenital aortic stenosis arises from a complex interaction of environmental and genetic factors, which are not fully understood.

Pathology

Stenosis may be valvular, supravalvular and subvalvular (Figs 7.25 A to E).
1. Valvular AS may be of 3 types: (Figs 7.26A to C).
    - Unicuspid valve with one lateral attachment.
    - Bicuspid aortic valve-fused commissure and an eccentric orifice-commonest form of AS:
    - Tricuspid aortic valve-very uncommon-three unseparated cusps with a stenotic central orifice.
    - In some, congenitally abnormal aortic valve, medial necrosis leads to a weakened ascending aorta leading on to annular dilation or aneurysm of ascending aorta with risk of dissection or rupture and annular dilation is more commonly associated with aortic regurgitation.
2. Supravalvular AS-annular constriction above aortic valve at the upper margin of sinus of valsalva. Occasionally ascending aorta is diffusely hypoplastic.

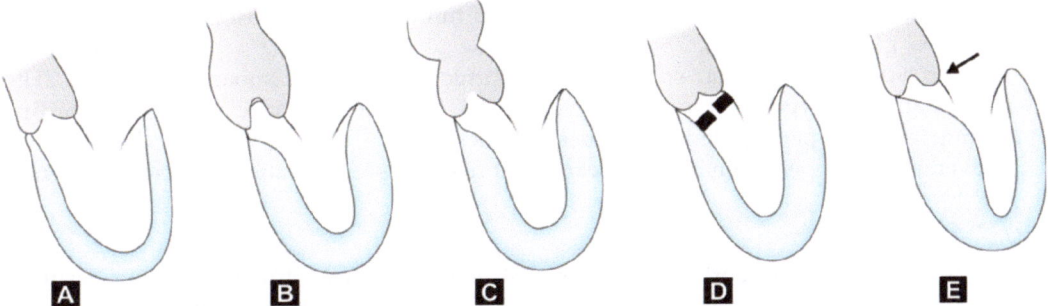

Figs 7.25A to E: Anatomic types of aortic stenosis. (A) Normal (B) Valvular stenosis (C) Supravalvular stenosis (D) Discrete subaortic stenosis (E) Idiopathic hypertrophic subaortic stenosis

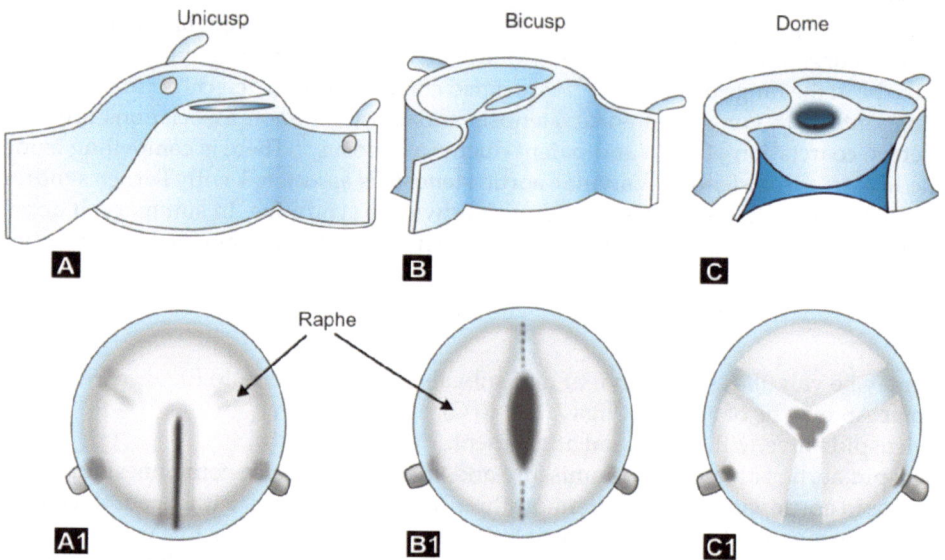

Figs 7.26A to C: Anatomic types of aortic valve stenosis. Top row is side view and bottom row is the view as seen in surgery during aortomy. (A) Unicuspid aortic valve. (B) Bicuspid aortic valve. (C) Stenosis of a tricuspid aortic valve. (From Goor DA. Lillehel CW: Congenital malformations of the heart. New York. 1975. Grune and Stratton)

3. Subvalvular AS (subaortic)-may be because of pressure of a membrane or diaphragm (discrete) which accounts for 10% of all AS cases or form a tunnel like fibromuscular narrowing (tunnel stenosis of LV out flow tract).

   Another type of subvalvular stenosis is idiopathic hypertrophic subaortic stenosis (IHSS)-a manifestation of hypertrophic cardiomyopathy, where the subaortic area of myocardium is asymmetrically hypertrophied to produce obstruction.
4. Left ventricular hypertrophy and myocardial fibrosis are seen in patients with aortic stenosis.

Physiology

The physiologic impact of aortic stenosis is obstruction of left ventricular outflow, resulting in increased left ventricular afterload. If stroke volume is normal, the magnitude of the pressure gradient reflects severity of the stenosis. Stroke volume, cardiac output, baseline heart rate and ejection fraction generally remain normal, although contractility is decreased and end diastolic volume and pressure are increased in those with severe symptomatic aortic stenosis. Left ventricular subendocardial ischemia and infarction may occur in patients with valvular aortic stenosis and unobstructed coronary arteries.[38]

Clinical Manifestations (Fig. 7.27)

1. Children with mild to moderate AS are usually asymptomatic. In severe cases-chest pain or dyspnea, easy fatigability and syncope may occur in infants with critical stenosis of aortic valve. They may also develop CCF in the first few months of life.
2. On examination-acyanotic with normal growth and development. In severe aortic stenosis-'anacrotic' pulse with narrow pulse pressure, systolic thrill over the upper right sternal border radiating to the carotid arteries. Pre-systolic tap indicates forceful atrial contraction over precordium.

On auscultation-in severe AS-an ejection click with paradoxical splitting of S_2. A harsh ejection systolic murmur heard over 2-3rd left intercostal space radiating to the neck.

In presence of aortic regurgitation, a decrescendo diastolic murmur may be present.

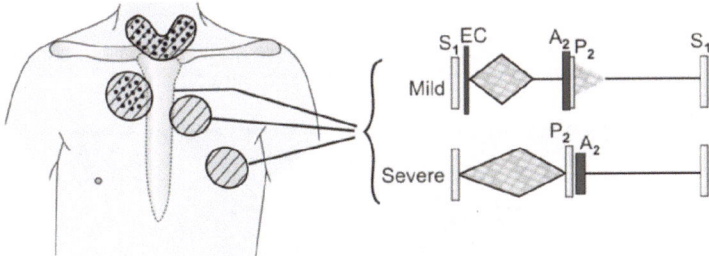

Fig. 7.27: Cardiac findings of aortic valve stenosis

Electrocardiography

1. Left ventricular hypertrophy (LVH) with strain in severe aortic stenosis (Fig. 7.28).
2. Exercise induced ischemic ST changes likely to reflect subendocardial ischemia owing to an imbalance in oxygen balance.

X-ray Studies (Fig. 7.29)

1. Cardiac size is usually normal.
2. If AR is also associated then cardiomegaly may develop.

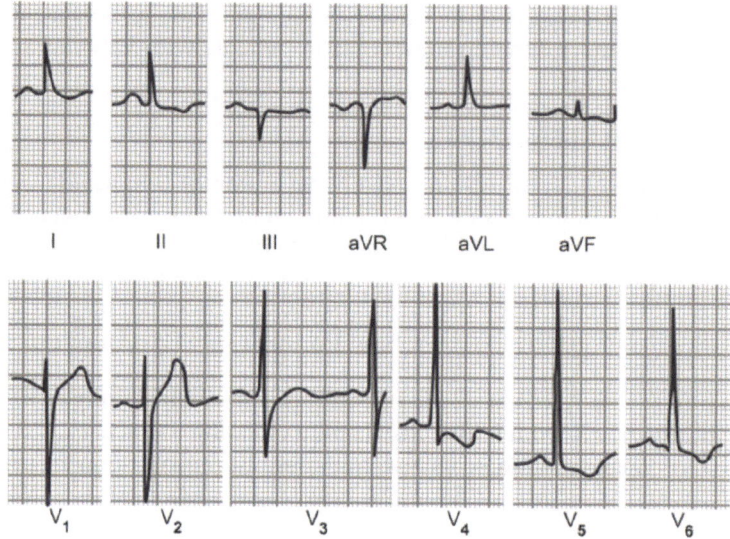

Fig. 7.28: Tracing from a child with severe aortic stenosis. It shows left ventricular hypertrophy with "strain pattern"

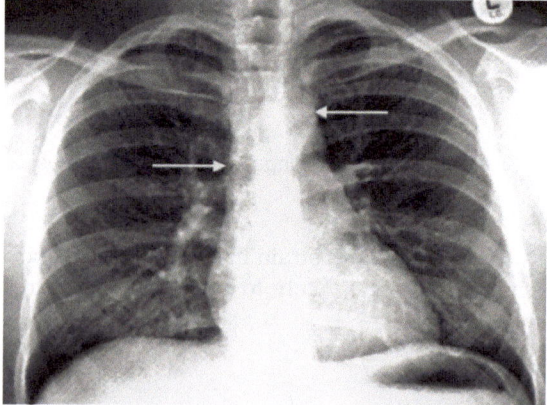

Fig. 7.29: Aortic stenosis. Note the prominent aortic shadows (arrows) indicating dilated ascending aorta, common in this condition

3. Left atrial enlargement suggests severe aortic stenosis.
4. Critical AS in newborns-generalized cardiomegaly with pulmonary venous congestion.
5. Ascending aortic enlargement common finding in older children.

ECHOCARDIOGRAPHY

Valvular AS

1. In parasternal short axis view (Fig. 7.30).
   In bicuspid aortic valve-the orifice appears as a non-circular (football shaped) opening in systole. In tricuspid aortic valve-centrally located small orifice with thickened commissures in systole and a heavy Y pattern in diastole.
2. In the parasternal long axis view-"doming" of the thick aortic valve with restriction to the opening is seen in systole.
3. Supravalvular AS-narrowing results from a discrete membrane in parasternal long axis view and apical long axis view. The diffuse hypoplasia of the ascending aorta is best seen in the suprasternal view.
4. Doppler studies-estimate the severity of stenosis (Fig. 7.31).[37]

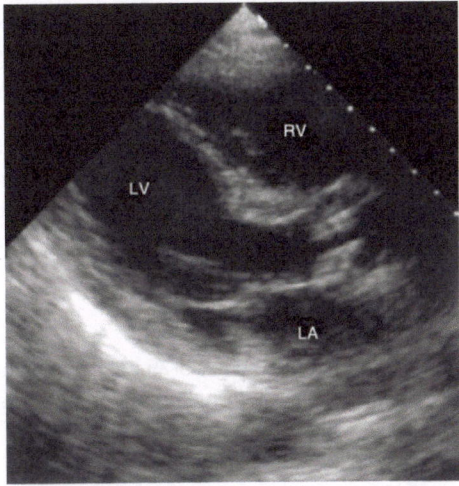

Fig. 7.30: Parasternal long axis view showing a heavily calcified aortic valve with doming of the leaflets

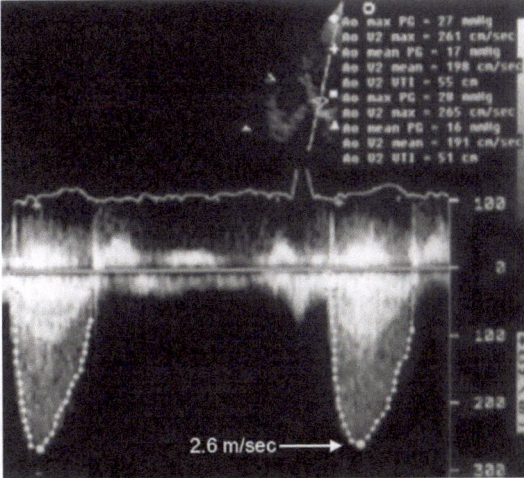

Fig. 7.31: CW Doppler profile of aortic flow in a patient with aortic stenosis ($V_{max} > 5$ m/s)

5. According to American Heart Association guidelines, in full grown adolescents, the normal aortic valve area is 3-4 cm^2, but in children it is 2 cm^2. In children, the aortic valve area should be normalized to body surface area. If aortic valve area in a child is > 0.5 cm^2–mild stenosis. For the aortic stenosis to be severe, the valve area has to be < 0.5 cm^2.[39]

MANAGEMENT

Medical

1. Management of good oral and dental hygiene and antibiotic prophylaxis against bacterial endocarditis is mandatory.
2. Children with moderate to severe AS should not perform sustained strenuous activities.
3. Percutaneous balloon valvuloplasty may be tried to relieve the stenosis, though the results are not good as those for PS and subsequent progression of stenosis or regurgitation is expected.

Surgical

1. Closed aortic valvotomy-using calibrated dilators or balloon catheters without cardiopulmonary bypass-may be performed in sick children-low mortality.
2. Other surgical procedures are performed under cardiopulmonary bypass-which include: Aortic valve replacement-required for unicuspid or severely dysplastic bicuspid aortic valve-by a porcine valve allograft or a pulmonary valve autograft. The prosthetic valve needs prolonged anticoagulation. Replacement with a prosthetic valve provides the most durable result though the prosthetic valve needs lifelong anti-coagulation which is a problem for small children.
3. In some centers, Ross procedure is the preferred option particularly in small children. In this procedure the child's pulmonary valve is translocated to the aortic position and a pulmonary homograft implanted. Here, anti-coagulation is avoided but the major disadvantage is that pulmonary homograft dysfunction sets in very soon and recurrent procedures have to be done.

Indications

1. Infants or newborns with critical AS in CCF–require surgery.
2. Children with severe AS (area <0.5 cm^2) or peak systolic gradient between 50-75 mm Hg or those who develop progressive aortic regurgitation. Those with symptoms of angina or syncope and with ECG changes of LVH with strain are candidates for elective valve replacement.
    Mortality-15-20%. Complications-significant AR.

Coarctation of Aorta (CoA)

Coarctation of aorta is typically a discrete stenosis of the proximal thoracic aorta. It occurs in 8-10% of all CHDs and it is more common in males (1.5: 1) and 35% of patients with Turner's syndrome manifest with COA. Coarctation has been identified as the fourth most common lesion requiring surgery in the first year of life.[40]

Environmental influence on development of coarctation has been suggested by a seasonal variation with the incidence of coarctation peaking in the late fall and winter.[41]

Pathology

1. As many as 85% of patients with COA have a bicuspid aortic valve.
2. In symptomatic infants with COA-the descending aorta is supplied blood via ductus arteriosus at birth. Other cardiac defects such as abnormal aortic valve or aortic hypoplasia, VSD (50%), PDA (60%) and mitral valve anomalies are often present which tend to decrease antegrade aortic blood flow *in utero* (Fig. 7.32).
3. Coarctation of aorta is usually a discrete stenosis of the upper thoracic aorta at the point of insertion of the ductus arteriosus.
4. It may be a long segment or tortuous in nature.
5. Less commonly, coarctation occurs in other areas such as ascending aorta or abdominal aorta, where it may be associated with renal artery stenosis.
6. Cystic medial necrosis, consisting of depletion and disarray of medial elastic tissue, occurs common in aorta and may be a histologic substrate for late aneurysm formation.[41]

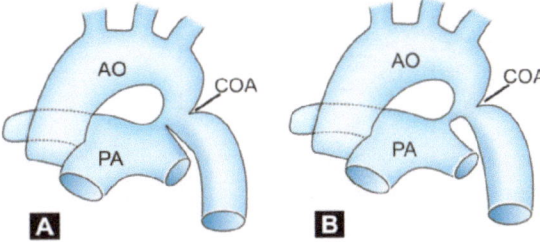

Figs 7.32A and B: (A) Coarctation is at the juxtaductal position so the space is added to the narrowed aorta by the ductus. (B) After ductal obliteration, the added lumen is lost and the aorta becomes severely obstructed, although the severity of the coarctation is unchanged

Hemodynamics

Fetal hemodynamics are readily disturbed by the presence of coarctation of aorta because normally only 10% of the combined ventricular output traverses the aortic isthmus *in utero.* After birth, with closure of the foramen ovale and ductus arteriosus, the entire cardiac output must cross the stenotic aortic segment. Depending on the severity of coarctation and the presence of associated cardiac lesions, these hemodynamic changes may range from mild systolic hypertension to severe congestive heart failure and shock.

Coarctation of aorta increases impedance to left ventricular outflow thereby elevating systolic pressure in the left ventricle, ascending aorta and its branches. If the coarctation is severe or develops rapidly, as in a newborn on ductal closure, left ventricular systolic dysfunction and congestive heart failure may ensue and severe manifestation may set in the first week of life. Immature neonatal myocardium lacks sympathetic innervations and is very poorly compliant and so all the compensatory mechanisms fail. Systolic dysfunction and heart failure in coarctation are confined primarily to early infancy.[42]

Clinical Manifestations (Fig. 7.33)

1. Poor feeding, dyspnea and failure to thrive or signs of acute left ventricular failure may develop in the first 6 weeks of life.
2. Pallor with varying degrees of respiratory distress, oliguria, shock and severe acidosis are common. Differential cyanosis may be present in the presence of added patent ductus arteriosus (R-L Shunt).

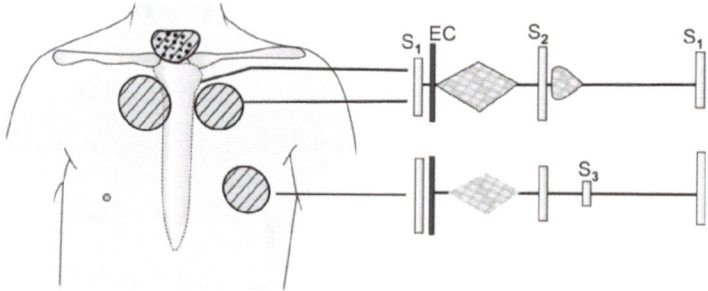

Fig. 7.33: Cardiac findings of coarctation of aorta. A systolic thrill may be present in the suprasternal notch "area shown by dots"

3. Peripheral pulses are weak, and history of claudication may be present. Hypertension may become evident but only after improvement of cardiac functions and a murmur may be heard.
4. Physical examination—hallmark finding.

X-ray Chest (Fig. 7.34)

1. Moderate to severe cardiomegaly and pulmonary vascular markings are increased.
2. In older children and adolescents, normal or mildly enlarged heart.
3. An abnormal contour of aortic arch is common–consists of localized indentation of the aorta at the site of coarctation (reversed 3 sign). Immediately below the 3 sign, a prominent descending aorta may be noted owing to post-stenotic dilation (Fig. 7.35).
4. Rib notching may be found in older patients, but uncommon in those younger than 5 years of age. It is caused by erosion of the inferior surface of posterior ribs by dilated and tortuous intercostals arteries.

Electrocardiography (Fig. 7.36)

Normal or right ward QRS axis and RVH or right bundle branch block (RBBB) are present in most infants with COA rather than LVH. LVH is seen in older children.

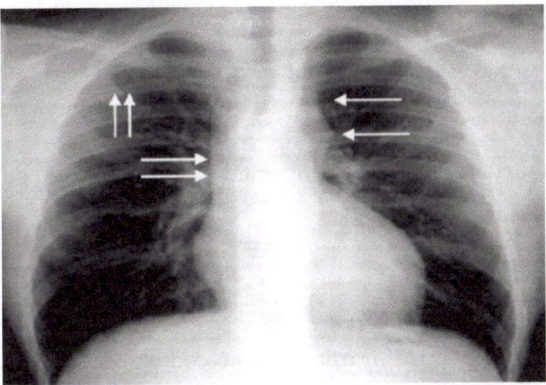

Fig. 7.34: Coarctation of aorta. There are number of features confirming coarctation of aorta. There is the "reverse 3" sign: top arrow represents the aorta just above the coarctation, and the bottom one indicates the dilated aorta just below it (so called post-stenotic dilatation). The ascending aorta is also prominent (double arrows) and the rounded contour of the left heart suggest left ventricular hypertrophy. There is rib notching due to dilatation of the intercostals arteries (double arrows)

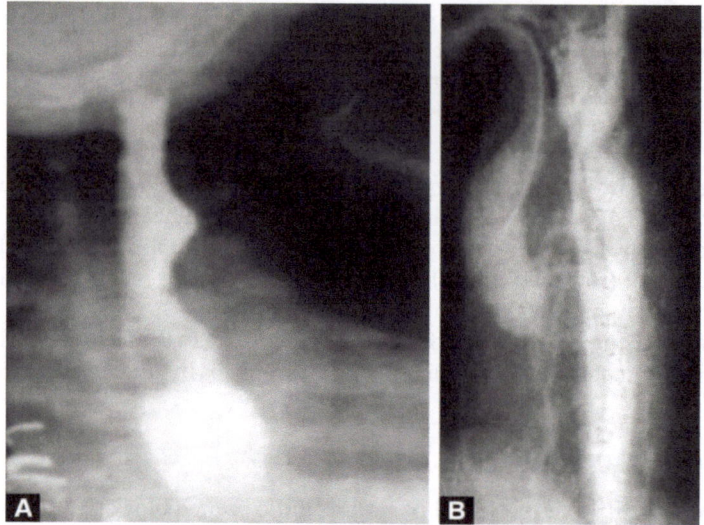

Figs 7.35A and B: Left panel shows barium swallow in PA view showing E sign in coarctation of aorta. Right panel shows aortogram in LAO view showing shelf-like indentation just distal to left subclavian artery caused by coarctation

Physical Examination

Hallmark Finding

1. Arterial pulses below the coarctation are diminished in amplitude and delayed in timing compared to the proximal pulse.
2. Systolic blood pressure is elevated proximal to the coarctation and a systolic pressure gradient is present between the arm and leg.
3. Left ventricular systolic heave.
4. Systolic thrill in supersternal notch.
5. A grade 3/6 ejection systolic murmur arising from coarctation—best heard at upper left sternal border and in left interscapular area posteriorly.

Echocardiography

1. In suprasternal view-a wedge-shaped "shelf" localized narrowing of tissue is imaged in the posterior and lateral aspects of the upper descending aorta, which is distal to left subclavian artery (Fig. 7.37).

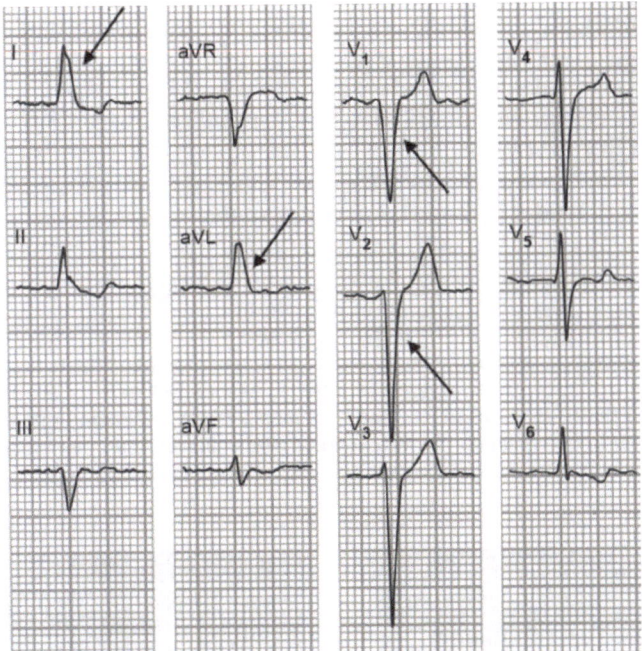

Fig. 7.36: Tracing from a 3 week old infant with coarctation of aorta. Note the marked left ventricular hypertrophy with strain

2. Doppler studies-above and below the coarctation site in conjunction with 2 D echo-gives a proper evaluation (Figs 7.38 and 7.39).

Magnetic Resonance Imaging (Fig. 7.40)

Images in sagittal and parasagittal planes detect coarctation, anatomy of aorta and other associated anomalies, presence or absence of patent ductus arteriosus and collaterals. This investigative modality has a definite place in diagnosis and monitoring follow up after balloon dilatation and to visualize the development of aneurysm if any.

Natural History

1. About 20-30% of all patients with COA develop CCF by 3 months of age. If undetected early death may be precipitated by CCF or renal shut down.

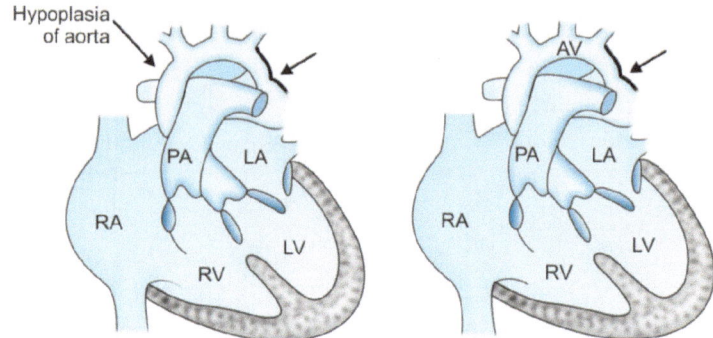

Fig. 7.37: Diagrammatic comparison of the heart and aorta in symptomatic infants and asymptomatic children with coarctation of the aorta. (A) In symptomatic infants, associated defects are frequently found, which include ASD, aortic and mitral valve diseases, and hypoplasia of the ascending and transverse aorta. These abnormalities are shown in heavy lines. (B) In asymptomatic children, the coarctation is usually an isolated lesion, except for bicuspid aortic valve (not shown)

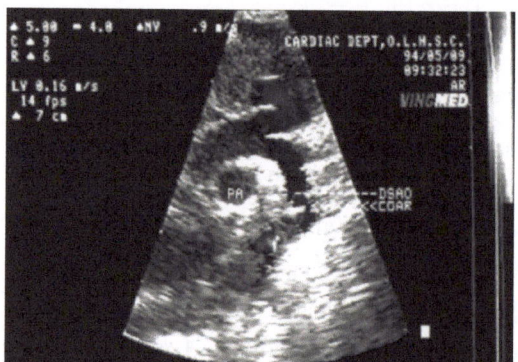

Fig. 7.38: Coarctation of aorta in a suprasternal longitudinal cross section, showing the "shelf like" lesion (arrow), resulting in stenosis of descending aorta. Note that the descending aorta before the lesion is also small and hypoplastic

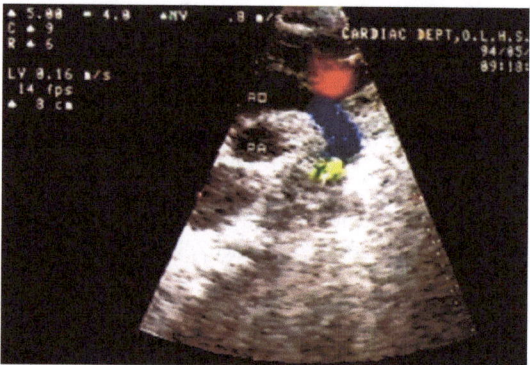

Fig. 7.39: Color flow mapping in the suprasternal window of a patient with coarctation of aorta. Note the change in color to mosaic at the level of the lesion (arrow)

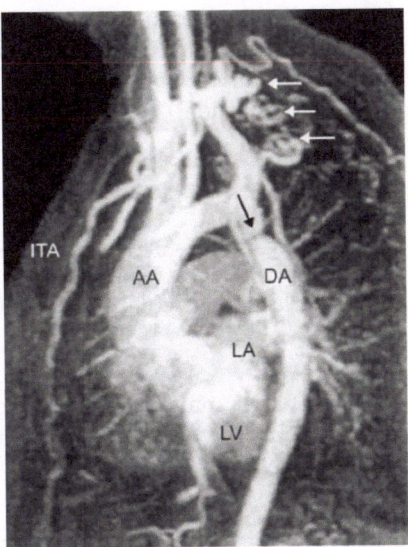

Fig. 7.40: MRI picture of coarctation, black arrow shows coarct segment and white arrows indicate collateral vessels

MANAGEMENT

Medical

1. Prostaglandin E_1 infusion should be started to re-open the ductus arteriosus and establish blood flow to the kidneys in the first week of life.
2. Good dental hygiene and precaution against SBE are important.
3. Decongestive measures-vasodilators (dopamine, dobutamine) diuretics and oxygen have to be started.
4. Hypertensive crisis if it develops should be treated promptly.
5. Balloon angioplasty can be useful procedure in sick infants where surgery is risky but not in newborns. There is a possibility of aneurysm formation with serious late complications.

Surgical

1. Coarctation of aorta with hypertension in the upper extremities or with a large systolic pressure gradient > 20 mm Hg between the arms and legs indicates surgery between 2-4 years of age.[43]

Older children are operated immediately after diagnosis. Late complication, e.g. endocarditis and central nervous system bleeding which rarely occurs if operated early. However surgery before 1 year of age increases risk of re-coarctation.
2. Children with mild COA (<20 mm Hg gradient) may be considered for surgery, if prominent gradient develops with exercise.

Procedure

1. End-to-end anastomosis following resection of coarcted segment is the treatment of choice in children.
2. Occassionaly subclavian artery aortoplasty or circular patch grafts may be performed.

Complications

1. Spinal cord ischemia producing paraplegia may develop after cross clamping of aorta during surgery, which is probably related to limited collateral circulation. Rebound hypertension may occur in the immediate postoperative period.

REFERENCES

1. Fyler DC, Atrial septal defect secundum. In Nadas Pediatric Cardiology, Philadelphia: Hanley & Belfus, 1992;513-24.
2. Sam'anek M. Children with congenital heart disease: Probability of natural survival. Pediatr. Cardiol 1992; 13: 152-58.
3. Holt M, Oram S. Familial heart disease with skeletal malformation. Br. Heart. J. 1960;22L:236-42.
4. Haworth SG. Pulmonary vascular disease in secundum atrial septal defect in childhood. Am J. Cardiol 1983;51:265-72.
5. Shikn DJ, Stejns M, Lintermans JT et al. Influence of age on atrioventricular conduction intervals in children with and without atrial septal defect. J. Electrocardiol. 1982;15:9-14.
6. Murphy JG, Gersh BJ, McGoon MD et al. Long term outcome after surgical repair of isolated atrial septal defect. N. Engl. J. Med. 1990;323:1645-50.
7. Hamilton WT, Dalen Je et al. Atrial septal defect secundum. Clinical profile with physiologic correlates. In. Roberts WC et al. Adult Congenital Heart disease. Philadelphia: FA Dacris Co. 1987;395-407.
8. Sutton MG, Tajik AJ, McGoon DC. Atrial septal defect in patients ages 60 years or older: Operative results and long term postoperative follow up circulation 1982;64:402-09.
9. Steele PM, Fuste V, Colien M et al. Isolated atrial septal defect with pulmonary vascular obstructive disease: Long term follow up and prediction of outcome after surgical correction. Circulation 1987;76:1037-42.
10. King TD, Thompson SL, Steiner C et al. Secundum atrial septal defect: Non-operative closure during cardiac catheterization. JAMA 1976;235:2506-09.

11. Krumsdorf U, Ostermayer S, Billinger K et al. Incidence and clinical course of thrombus formation on atrial septal defect and patent foramen ovale closure devices in 1000 consecutive patients. J.Am.Coll. Cardiol 2004;43:302-09.
12. Nadas AS, Fyler DC. Pediatric Cardiology (3rd ed). Philadelphia. WB Saunders. 1972;348.
13. Tikanya T. Effect of technical development on the apparent incidence of congenital heart disease. Pediatr. Cardiol 1995;16:100-101.
14. Hoffman JLE, Rudolph AM. The natural history of ventricular septal defect in infancy. Am. J. Cardiology 1965;16:634-53.
15. Soto B, Becker AE, Moulaert AJ et al. Classification of ventricular septal defects. Br. Heart J. 1980;43:332-43.
16. Van Hare GF, Soffer LJ, Sivakoff MC et al. Twenty five year experience with ventricular septal defect in infants and children. Am. Heart J. 1987;114:606-14.
17. Ortiz E, Rolemion PJ, Deanfield JE et al. Localization of ventricular septal defect by simultaneous display of superimposed colour Doppler and cross sectional echocardiographic images. AHJ. 1985;54:53-60.
18. Houston AB, Lim MK, Doig WB et al. Doppler assessment of the interventricular pressure drop in patients with ventricular septal defects. Br. Heart J. 1988;60:50-56.
19. Gittenberger–de Grost AC, Van Eastbrugger I, Mondaert AJMG et al. The ductus arteriosus in the preterm infant—Histologic and clinical observations. J. Pediatr. 1980;96:88-93.
20. Rudolph AM, Drorbraugh JE, Auld PAM et al. Studies on the circulation in the neonatal period. The circulation in respiratory distress syndrome. Pediatrics 1961;27:551-66.
21. Fay FS, Cooke PH. Guinea Pig ductus arteriosus. Irreversible Closure after birth. Am. J. Physiol. 1972; 222:841-49.
22. Heymann MA, Rudolph AM. Control of ductus arteriosus. Physical Rev. 1975;55:62-78.
23. Clyman RI, Heymann MAR. Pharmacology of ductus arteriosus. Physical Rev. 1975;55:62-78.
24. McMurphy DM, Heyman MA, Rudolph AM et al. Developmental changes in constriction of the ductus arteriosus. Responses to oxygen and vasoactive substances in the isolated ductus arteriosus of the fetal lamb. Pediatr. Res. 1972;6:231-38.
25. Coceani F, Olley PM. Role of prostaglandins, prostacyclin and thromboxanes in the control of prenatal patency and prenatal closure of the ductus arteriosus. Semin. Perinatol. 1980;4:109-13.
26. Mahomy L, Carnero V, Brett C et al. Prophylactic indomethacin therapy for patent ductus arteriosus in very low birth weight infants. N. Engl. J. Med. 1982;306:506-10.
27. Way GL, Pierce Jr, Wolf RR et al. ST depression suggesting subendocardial ischemia in neonates with respiratory distress syndrome and patent ductus arteriosus. J. Pediatr. 1979;95:609-11.
28. Patel J, Roberto I, Azzopardi D et al. Randomized double blind control trial comparing the effects of Ibuprofen and indomethacin on cerebral haemodynamics on preterm infants with patent ductus arteriosus. Pediatr. Res. 2000;47(1):36-42.
29. Thomas RL, Parker GC, Van Overmeive B et al. Meta analysis of ibuprofen versus indomethacin for closure of patent ductus arteriosus. Eur. J. Pediatrics. 2005;164(3):135-140.
30. Su PH, Chen JY, Su CM et al. Comparison of ibuprofen and indomethacin therapy for patent ductus arteriosus in preterm infants. Pediatr. Int. 2003;45:665-70.

31. Gourmay V, Roze JC, Kuster A et al. Prophylactive Ibuprofen versus placebo in very premature infants. A randomize double blind placebo controlled trial. Lancet 2004:364:1939-44.
32. Brooks JM, Trivedi JN, Patole SK et al. Is surgical ligation of patent ductus arteriosus necessary? The western Australian experience of conservative management. Arch. Dis. Child Fetal Neonatal Ed. 2005; 90(3): F 235-39.
33. Driscoll DJ, Michels VV, Gersony WM et al. Occurrence risk for congenital heart defects in relative of patients with aortic stenosis, pulmonic stenosis or ventricular septal defect. Circulation 1993; 87(suppl.): 1114-20.
34. Roberts WC. The congenitally bicuspid aortic valve. A study of 85 autopsy cases. Am.J.Cardiol 1970; 26: 72-83.
35. Bonowro, Carabello B, DeLeon AC JT. et al. ACC/AHA guidelines for the management of patients with valvular heart disease: A report of the ACC/AHA task force on practice guidelines. J.Am.Coll. Cardiol 1998;32:1486-1588.
36. Frank S, Johnson A, Ross J. Natural history of valvular aortic stenosis. Br. Heart J. 1973;35:41-46.
37. Braunwald E, Goldblatt A, Aygen MM et al. Congenital aortic stenosis. I Clinical and haemodynamic findings in 100 patients. II Surgical and the results of operation circulation 1963:27:426-62.
38. Moller JH, Nakeb A, Edwards JE et al. Infarction of papillary muscles and mitral insufficiency associated with congenital aortic stenosis. Circulation 1966: 34: 87-91.
39. Lnciam GB, Favaro A, Casali G et al. Ross operation in the young: A ten year experience. Ann. Thorac. Surg. 2005; 80: 2271-77.
40. Fyler DC, Buckley LP, Hellenbrand WE et al. Report of the New England regional infant cardiac programme. Pediatrics 1980;65:432-36.
41. Miettinen OS, Reiner ML, Nadas AS. Seasonal incidence of coarctation of aorta. Br. Heart J. 1970:32:103-07.
42. Isner JM, Donaldson RF, Fulton D et al. Cystic medial necrosis in coarctation of aorta: A potential factor contributing to adverse consequences observed after percutaneous balloon angioplasty of coarctation sites circulation 1987;75:689-95.
43. Friedman WF. The intrinsic physiologic properties of the developing heart. In Friedman WE, Lesch M, Sonnenblcik EH. Eds. Neonatal Heart Disease. New York: Grune and Stratton. 1973:21-49.

PART II

Cyanotic: Volume Overload R-L Shunt

Transposition of Great Arteries (TGA)

Transposition of the great arteries (TGA) is a lethal malformation, accounting for 5-7% of all congenital cardiac malformations. Without treatment about 30% die in the first week of life, 50% within first month, 70% within first 6 months and 90% within the first year. The incidence is reported to range from 20.1 to 30.6 per 100,000 live births with a strong 60% male preponderance.

Extracardiac anomalies are less frequent in infants with TGA (< 10%) compared with other congenital heart diseases such as truncus arteriosus (48%), ventricular septal defect (VSD) (34%) and tetralogy of Fallot (31%).[1]

Associated Lesions

Ventricular Septal Defect

The commonest associated anomaly is VSD as in normal hearts

- perimembranous – 33%
- muscular – 30%
- AV canal – 5%
- Outlet – 5%

Perimembranous or muscular VSDs may spontaneously close or become smaller. TGA with a larger VSD and Taussig Bing anomaly (DORV with subpulmonary VSD) are anatomically different but have similar physiology.

Left Ventricular Outflow Obstruction (LVOTO)

The development of LVOTO produces subpulmonary obstruction, which is an important association in patients with TGA. The obstruction may be anatomic or dynamic. It mostly occurs in 20% of patients with TGA with VSD, which progresses to become more severe in 35%.

Other Associated Anomalies

Incidence of PDA is more commonly associated with TGA in 50% of patients at 2 weeks but is usually functionally closed by 1 month. A large PDA is associated with pulmonary vascular disease. Mitral valve abnormalities, e.g. partial or complete cleft of anterior mitral valve are present in 20-30% of cases. Tricuspid valve abnormalities are uncommon.

Anatomy and Pathology (Fig. 7.41)

The common clinical type, (situs solitus of atria) concordant AV (right atrium to right ventricle and left atrium to left ventricle) and discordant ventriculoarterial alignment is widely termed complete TGA. This has come to indicate the transposed great arteries are physiologically "uncorrected", that is the systemic venous blood flows predominantly to the aorta and pulmonary venous blood to pulmonary artery. When the term "corrected" is used, then the systemic venous blood flows to pulmonary artery and pulmonary venous blood to aorta. It should be understood that both physiologically uncorrected and corrected hearts are morphologically complete transposition, e.g. both great arteries are predominantly misplaced across ventricular septum, arise from inappropriate ventricles and thus have discordant ventricular arterial connections (Fig. 7.42).

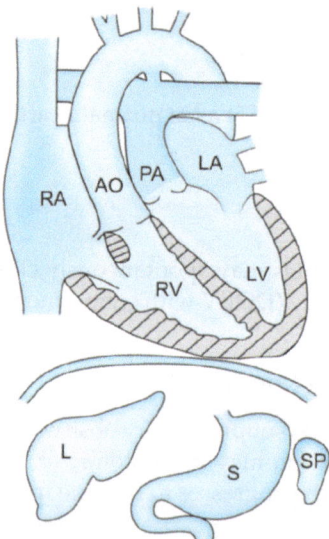

Fig. 7.41: Schematic diagram of complete transposition of great arteries. Aorta (Ao) arises from right ventricle (RV), pulmonary artery (PA) from left ventricle (LV), both great arteries are parallel to each other and connected by a PDA. There is normal position of viscera, atria and ventricles (RA—right atrium, LA—left atrium, L—liver, S—stomch, Sp—spleen)

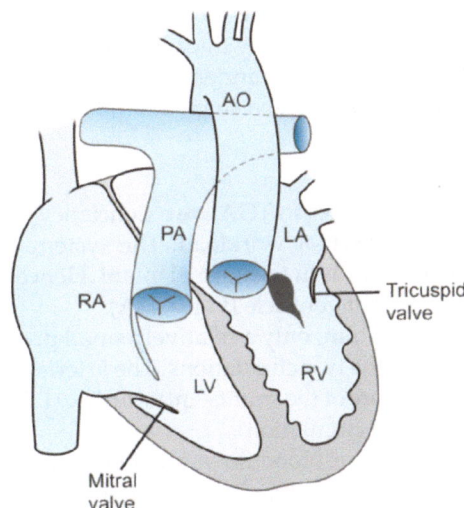

Fig. 7.42: Diagram of congenitally corrected TGA (L TGA). There is an inversion of ventricular chambers with their corresponding atrioventricular valves. The great arteries are transposed, but functional correction results with oxygenated blood going to the aorta. Unfortunately, a high percentage of the patients with L-TGA have associated defects with resulting cyanosis

Van Praagh has favored the following terminology which concerns the TGA. TGA with situs solitus (S) of atria and viscera, usual (D) looping of ventricles and anterior and rightwards (D) aorta. If the transposed aorta at the valve annulus level is positioned to the left of the transposed pulmonary artery, the malformation may be denoted as TGA (S, D, L).[2]

1. The classic complete TGA is called D-transposition, in which the aorta is located anteriorly and to the right of pulmonary artery (PA), and that is why prefix D is used.
2. In D-TGA, the aorta arises anteriorly from R V carrying desaturated blood to the body and PA arises posteriorly from LV carrying oxygenated blood to the lungs. (In normal hearts, aorta arises from LV and lies posterior and lateral to PA which arises from RV). The result of D-TGA is complete separation of systemic and pulmonary circulations, which results in hypoxemic blood circulating through the body and hyperoxemic blood circulating in the pulmonary circuit. Defects that permit mixing of the two circulations (e.g., ASD, VSD or PDA) are necessary for survival.
3. About half of these infants do' not have associated defects other than PFO or a small PDA (simple TGA). VSD is present in 30-40% of patients with D-TGA and may be located anywhere in ventricular septum, where one third of the defects are small. In 5%, there is LVOT obstruction

with intact ventricular septum. In 10% there is a combination of VSD and LVOT obstruction. In TGA, the right ventricular wall is considerably thicker than normal at birth and increases further in thickness with age and LV wall becomes thinner. In infants with TGA the left ventricular cavity is ellipsoid at birth but soon becomes banana shaped.

Physiology

The dominant physiological abnormalities in TGA are a deficiency of oxygen supply to the tissues and an excessive right and left ventricular workload. The systemic and pulmonary circulations function in parallel rather than in series as in the normal infant. Hence the greatest portion of output of each ventricle is re-circulated to that ventricle (Fig. 7.43A).

In TGA with intact ventricular septum, only a relatively small proportion of blood is exchanged by inter circulatory shunts between the two circulations. The arterial oxygen saturations in both the ventricles are dependent on one or more of the shunts–intracardiac (PFO, ASD, VSD) and extracardiac (PDA, broncho-pulmonary collateral circulation).

The effective pulmonary and systemic blood flows and net anatomic right to left and left to right shunts are equal to each other and this volume is the intercirculatory mixing, the flow in TGA on which survival depends (Fig. 7.43B).

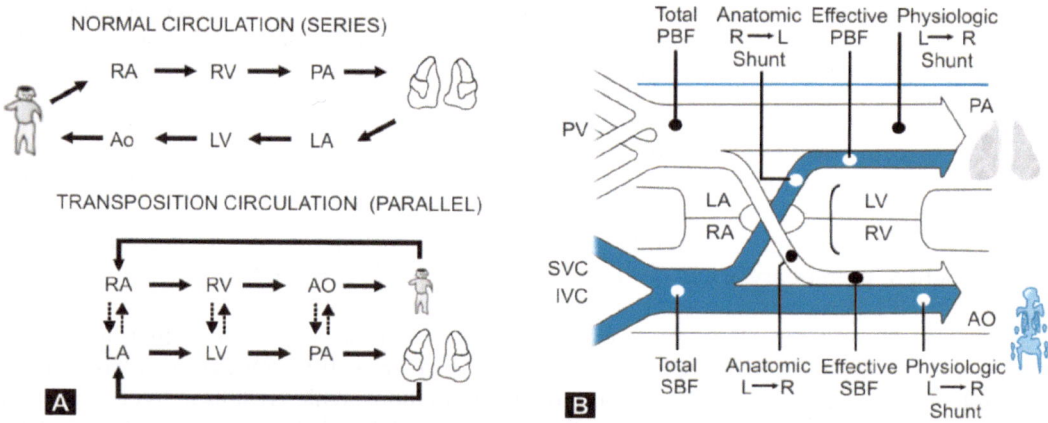

Figs 7.43A and B: The circulation in TGA. A. systemic and pulmonary circulation pathways; In series, with normally related great arteries; In parallel, with TGA. Solid arrows, relatively unoxygenated blood; stippled arrows, oxygenated blood; Dashed arrows–Inter-circulatory shunts. B. Circulation scheme demonstrating flows and shunts in infants with TGA/IVS. Note that the anatomic LR shunt constitutes the effective schematic blood flow (SBF) and anatomic RL shunt, the effective pulmonary blood flow (PBF)

The physiologic left to right shunt represents the volume of the pulmonary venous blood circulating through the lungs without having passed through the body and the physiologic right to left shunt is the volume of systemic venous blood re-entering the systemic circulation without having passed through the lungs.

The extent of inter-circulatory mixing depends on number, size and position of the anatomic communications and on total blood flow through the pulmonary circuit. When the inter-atrial or inter-ventricular shunting sites are of adequate size, the level of arterial oxygen saturation is influenced primarily by the pulmonary to systemic blood flow ratio, with a high pulmonary blood flow resulting in relatively high arterial oxygen saturation. If the pulmonary blood flow is decreased by infundibular or pulmonary stenosis or elevated pulmonary vascular resistance, then there will be a decrease in arterial oxygen saturation, despite adequate anatomic shunting sites. The balances between right and left atrial and ventricular compliances and pulmonary and systemic vascular resistances are important operative factors. Other important aspects are location and size of VSD and influence of LVOTO if present.[3]

A significant role has been postulated for the bronchopulmonary collateral circulation in TGA. Bronchopulmonary anastomotic channels have been visualized angiographically in 73% of infants with TGA and balloon occlusion studies demonstrated that these bronchopulmonary anastomotic channels freely and functionally communicate with pulmonary vascular bed. These communications may play a role in widespread pulmonary vascular disease process observed in TGA. If even at surgery, a significantly large L-R shunt is persisting, then an embolization therapy is warranted.[4]

Clinical Manifestations

Cyanosis, hypoxemia, deterioration of clinical condition or heart failure with early death is the clinical picture of an untreated infant with complete TGA.

The clinical manifestations and course depends on the anatomic and functional factors which influence the clinical picture.

Physiologic–Clinical Classification

1. TGA (IVS or small VSD) with increased PBF and small ICS. A combined marked respiratory and metabolic acidosis along with severe hypoxemia is a hallmark of TGA/IVS with poor mixing.[5]
2. TGA (VSD large) with increased PBF and large ICS.
3. TGA (VSD and LVOTO) with restricted PBF.
4. TGA (VSD and PVOD) with restricted PBF.
   IVS–Intact ventricular septum
   PBF–Pulmonary blood flow.

ICS–inter-circulatory shunting
LVOTO–left ventricular outflow tract obstruction
PVOD–Pulmonary vascular obstructive disease.

1. Prominent cyanosis–Universal finding in complete TGA with ICS. Cyanosis is recognized on first day of life in 92%.[6] Cyanosis is initially mild but progressively becomes deeper. It is more common in males.
2. In an infant–feeding is difficult. Easy fatigability and early heart failure may set in.
3. On examination–healthy newborn with cyanosis.
   Two groups of manifestations are there.
   - Hypoxemia–cyanosis–TGA with ICS
   - Heart failure appears at 2-6 weeks-TGA with VSD
   - Heart sounds-normal

   Murmurs–soft ejection systolic murmur heard at upper left sternal border probably due to increased flow across LVOTO (Fig. 7.44).
4. TGA/IVS with PDA–manifest early with tachypnea and slight cyanosis.

Complications

1. Necrotizing enterocolitis–Mostly seen in infants with TGA and large PDA–where the mesenteric circulation may be at risk because of retrograde diastolic flow in descending aorta and decreased oxygen delivery.
2. Pulmonary vascular obstructive disease (PVOD) is not present in infancy but may appear after successful palliative procedure. In later childhood, because of prolonged PVOD, heart dilates giving rise to severe mitral and pulmonary regurgitation.

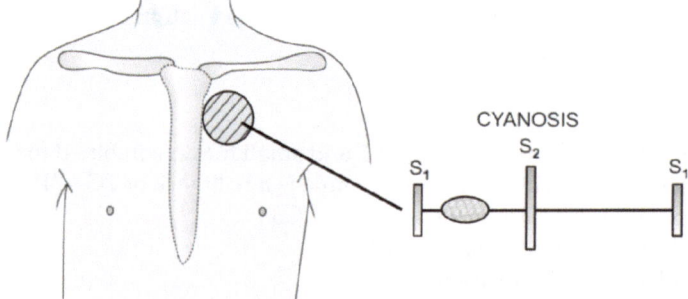

Fig. 7.44: Cardiac findings of transpositions of great arteries. Heart murmur is usually absent, and the S_2 is single in majority of the patients

3. Head circumference of a child with TGA is less than normal[7]–Common presentation is sudden onset of hemiparesis–due to severe anemia and hypoxemia leading on to cerebrovascular accidents in neonate and young infants. In the older child, polycythemia and increased blood viscosity secondary to long standing hypoxemia is the probable cause.
4. Brain abscess–infrequent. If it occurs, it is mostly in surgically uncorrected child beyond 2 years of age.
5. Psychometric assessment–Full scale IQ score for these children as a group is lower than normal population. There is a higher than expected incidence of learning disabilities, speech and language problems and also delayed motor development.

Laboratory Studies

1. Severe arterial hypoxemia (resistant to O_2 inhalation) with or without acidosis is present. A marked combined respiratory and metabolic acidosis along with severe hypoxemia is a hallmark of TGA/IVS with poor mixing.
2. Hypoglycemia and hypocalcemia are occasionally present.

Electrocardiography (Fig. 7.45)

1. RAD (+90° to +200°) with RVH in infants of TGA with ICS–positive T wave in right ventricular leads.
2. CVH may be present in those with associated VSD, PDA–in 60-80%. Q wave in V6 is usually present (70%) in TGA with large VSD but is infrequent when ventricular septum is intact.
3. Dysrythmias are rarely noted in the newborn, but short episodes of bradycardia and functional rhythm may be seen. Atrial flutter may be seen after balloon atrial septostomy.[8]

X-ray Studies (Figs 7.46A and B)

In first few days–heart size is normal.
1. An "egg on side" cardiac silhouette with a narrow neck (purse string appearance) is characteristic. It is associated with increased pulmonary vascularity (plethora). The changes appear after first few weeks of life.[9]

Echocardiography

Two-dimensional echo and color flow Doppler studies usually provide all the anatomic and functional information needed for the management of infants with D-TGA.
1. In parasternal long axis view-the posterior great artery has a sharp angulation before dividing into 2 branches suggesting it to be PA, and proximal portion of great arteries run parallel (Fig. 7.47A).

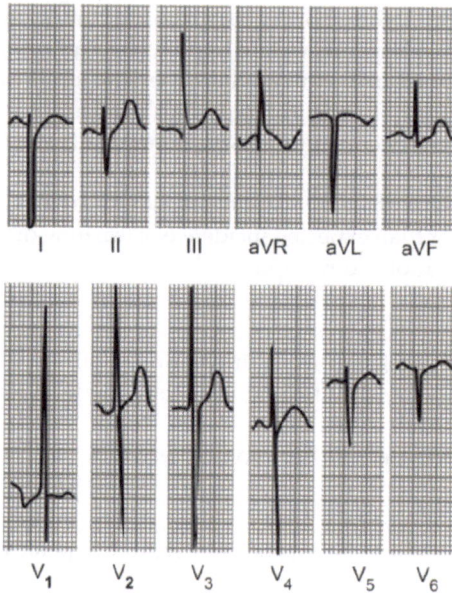

Fig. 7.45: ECG tracing in an infant with complete transposition of great arteries. The QRS axis is +140°. Note the deep S waves in V_5 and V_6 and an upright T wave in V_2 and V_3.

2. In parasternal short axis view–the "circle and sausage" appearance of the normal great arteries is not visible, instead they appear as "double circles". The PA is in center and aorta is anterior and slightly to the right of PA (Fig. 7.47B).
3. Suprasternal and high parasternal views–enable the aorta to be traced, arising from right ventricle to the arch and its branches (Fig. 7.47C).
4. Routine obstetric fetal echocardiography–lead to prenatal diagnosis of TGA.
5. In the apical and subcostal five chamber views, the PA (the artery that bifurcates) arises from LV and aorta from RV.
6. The status of defects, e.g. VSD, LV outflow tract obstruction (dynamic or fixed) or PV stenosis can be evaluated in the view.

Diagnosis

Complete TGA is the most common cyanotic congenital heart disease seen in neonates. The affected babies are usually males, good weight and born of a multiparous mother.

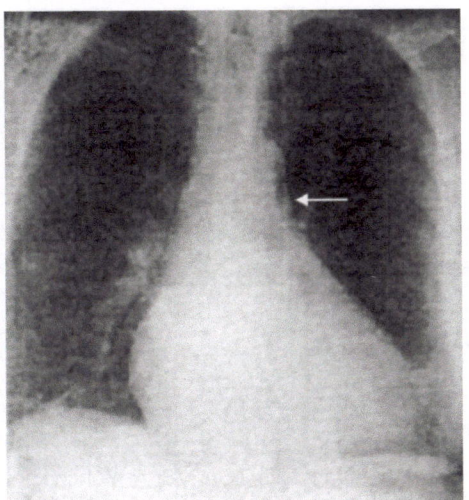 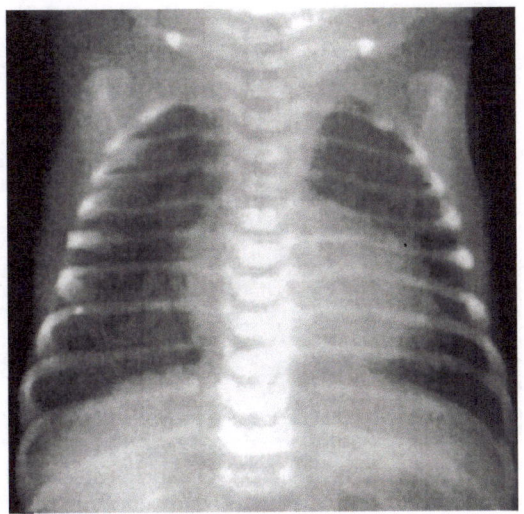

Fig. 7.46A: Globular shaped heart with a narrow superior mediastinum, mild cardiomegaly and increased pulmonary vascular markings in transposition of great arteries

Fig. 7.46B: Chest X-ray of TGA showing 'egg on side' shaped cardiac silhouette with narrow pedicle

1. They usually manifest with either
   - Cyanosis–usually on the first day of life.
   - Congestive heart failure.
2. On examination, second sound is loud and single. A short ejection systolic murmur is audible over the precordium due to LVOTO obstruction (subpulmonary stenosis).
3. X-ray chest–Mild cardiomegaly with "egg on side" appearance of heart with narrow pedicle and also with increased pulmonary vascular markings.
4. ECG–right axis deviation with RVH.

Natural History

1. Progressive hypoxia and acidosis result in death unless the mixing of the systemic and pulmonary blood is brought about by atrial septostomy, but CCF usually develops in 1st week of life.
2. TGA with associated VSD or PDA are the least cyanosed but develop CCF and PVOD by 3-4 months of age-before which corrective surgery is indicated. Without surgery, 90% of patients with TGA die by 6 months of age.

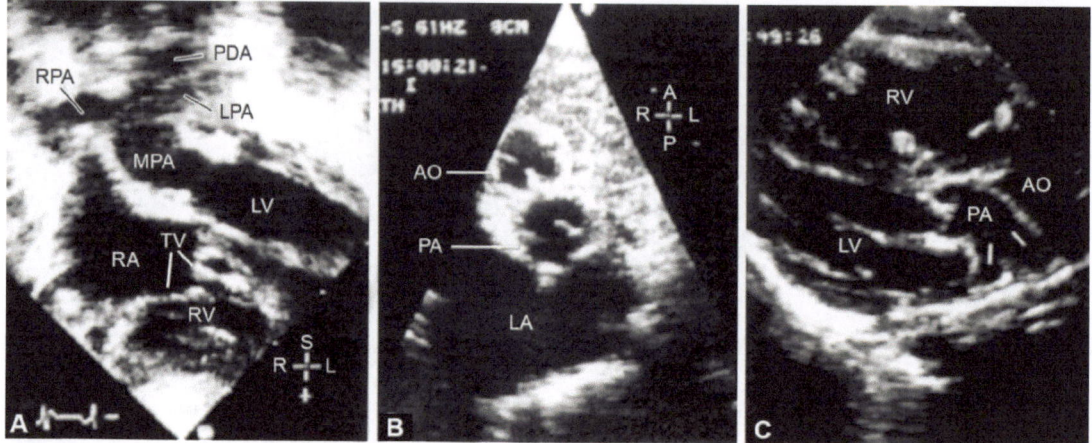

Figs 7.47A to C: Two-dimensional echocardiographic images in an infant with TGA/IVS. A: Subcostal view demonstrates left ventricle (LV) and unobstructed left ventricular outflow tract aligned (connected with normal pulmonary valve, main) MPA, right (RPA), and left (LPA) pulmonary arteries. B: Parasternal short axis view demonstrated slightly/interrelationship of the great arteries consistent with TGA. C: Parasternal long axis view, confirms discordant ventriculoarterial connection; the pulmonary trunk by its abrupt posterior turn shortly distilled to the pulmonary valve and (in other plains of this echo view) the aorta by the origin of brachiocephalic artery

3. In TGA with intact ventricular system, survival is poor due to hypoxia. 17% are alive at 2 months and 4% at 1 year.
4. In presence of ASD–75% survive at 6 months and 65% at 1 year.
5. In presence of VSD–survival is less–40% at 6 months and 30% at 1 year.
6. With VSD and LVOTO–survival is 70% at 1 year and 30% at 5 years.

Management

1. The following measures should be carried out before an emergency cardiac catheterization or a surgical procedure is done.
   a. Arterial blood gases and pH should be obtained and a hyperoxia test should be carried out to confirm cyanotic CHD.
   b. Metabolic acidosis should be corrected and hypocalcemia and/or hypoglycemia should be treated.
   c. Prostaglandin E1 infusion should be started to improve arterial oxygen saturation by re-opening the ductus, which should be continued throughout the procedure.

d. Oxygen should be administered for severe hypoxia, and decongestive measures to be given for evident CCF.
2. Before surgery, cardiac catheterization and a balloon atrial septostomy (Rashkinds' procedure) are often carried out to get a detailed hemodynamic diagnosis for older infants. Blade atrial septostomy may be preferred-where a blade attached to the tip of the catheter which cuts across the inter-atrial septum to produce a shunt.

Surgical
a. Intra-atrial repair operations
   A. *Mustard operation:* A pericardial or prosthetic baffle-which redirects the pulmonary and systemic venous return at atrial level.[10]
   B. *Senning operation:* Modification of Mustard operation. It uses the atrial septal flap and RA free wall to redirect the venous returns.[11]
b. *Rastelli operation:* In patients with additional VSD and severe PS-the redirection of pulmonary and systemic venous blood is carried out at the ventricular level by creating a tunnel and placing a conduit.
c. *Jatene operation:* Arterial switch operation-procedure of choice. The coronary arteries are transplanted to the PA and the proximal parts of the great arteries are anatomosed to the distal ends of the other great arteries, thereby bringing about an anatomic correction. It should be performed before 4 weeks of age. The overall 5 year survival after arterial switch operation-82%.[12]

Total Anomalous Pulmonary Venous Connection (TAPVC)

Total anomalous pulmonary venous connection is that anomaly where the pulmonary veins drain into the systemic veins (TAPVC) or right atrium (TAPVD) rather than the left atrium.

TAPVC accounts for 1% of all CHDs with a male preponderance (4:1).[15] The mechanism of transmission of TAPVC has not been elucidated although a possible association with exposure to lead paint or paint stripping chemicals or pesticides has been established.

Smith et al[16] provided an alternative classification for TAPVC:
1. Supracardiac-without pulmonary venous obstruction.
2. Infracardiac-with pulmonary venous obstruction.
3. An inter-atrial communication (ASD or PFO) is necessary for survival. Also the young age of the patient makes the presence of PDA usual which is not a complicating defect.
4. The left side of the heart is relatively small and there is dilation and hypertrophy of right ventricle and right atrium.

Table 7.2: Transposition of great arteries–surgical options

Anatomy	Surgical option	Comments
TGA/IVS	Physiologic repair	Ususally elective
	Senning/Mustard	Neonatal–1 year
	Anatomic repair (primary)	Neonatal period–before 2 weeks of age.
TGA/IVS with "prolonged" low LV pressure	Physiologic repair Senning/Mustard[13,14]	Elective 1 month–1 year.
	Anatomic repair (delayed)	"Rapid two stage switch"
TGA/VSD	Physiologic repair	Poor long term results
	Senning or Mustard with VSD closure	Poor long term results
	Anatomic repair	Usually neonatal repair
	Arterial switch with VSD closure	PAB–occasionally multiple VSDs
	Interventricular baffler repair	Not all VSDs suitable
TGA/VSD/PS	VSD closure (LV-AO) RV-PA conduit Rastelli[13]	Palliative systemic pulmonary shunt frequently performed Conduit replacement frequently necessary
	VSD closure (LV-AO), anterior translocation of PA with direct connection to RV-"REV" procedure (Lecompte).[14]	Long-term pulmonary regurgitation
TGA/PVOD	Physiologic repair-Palliative	
	Anatomic repair–Palliative	Symptomatic improvement

AO-aorta, IVS–interventricular septum, PA-pulmonary artery, PAB–premature atrial beats, PVOD–peripheral vascular occlusive disease, VSD–ventricular septal defect.

Anatomic Sites of Obstruction to Pulmonary Venous Drainage (Fig. 7.48)

The presence of an obstructive lesion in the anomalous pulmonary venous channel profoundly influences the hemodynamic state and clinical features in a case of TAPVC.

Associated Cardiac Anomalies

Frequently, total anomalous pulmonary venous drainage (TAPVD) occurs as an isolated anomaly in patients with normal visceroatrial situs. It has been reported to be associated with transposition of great arteries, tetralogy of Fallot, single ventricle, truncus arteriosus, tricuspid atresia, hypoplastic left heart syndrome, pulmonary atresia, coarctation of aorta, etc.[17]

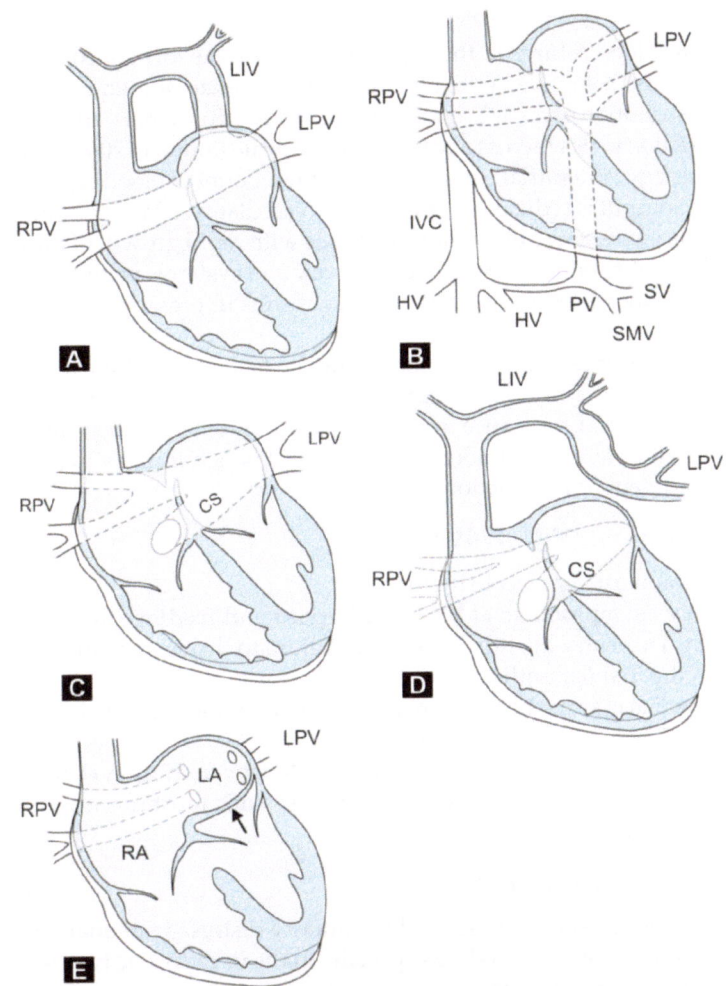

Figs 7.48A to E: Common types of totally anomalous pulmonary venous connection (TAPVC). (A) Supracardiac TAPVC to left innominate vein. The individual pulmonary veins form a horizontal pulmonary venous confluence that connects to the left innominate vein in form of a vertical vein. (B) Infradiaphragmatic TAPVC to the portal vein. (C) TAPVC to coronary sinus. (D) Mixed type TAPVC. (E) Totally anomalous pulmonary venous drainage owing to the malposition of the septum primum

Physiology

In TAPVC, all venous blood returns to the right atrium and some form of communication between right and left sides of the heart is essential for survival. The state of interatrial septum is of prime importance in the distribution of mixed venous blood between pulmonary and systemic circulations. Some degree of restriction to flow across a patent foramen ovale (found in 70-80% of cases) is common.

In presence of restrictive interatrial communication, the amount of blood reaching the left atrium is limited and systemic output is reduced. As pulmonary vascular resistance gradually decreases after birth and as demands for systemic blood flow increases with rapid growth of the infant, pulmonary over circulation is brought about. Since both pulmonary and systemic venous blood return is to the right atrium, therefore increased right atrial pressure results in pressure elevation and congestion in both venous circuits.

On the other hand, presence of a widely patent foramen ovale or ASD allows free communication between the two atria, and distribution of mixed venous blood depends on the relative compliance of the atria and ventricles and resistance imposed by the pulmonary and systemic arterial circuits. The major variable is the state of pulmonary vascular bed which initially depends on presence or absence of pulmonary venous obstruction.

Clinical Manifestations (Fig. 7.49)

TAPVC without pulmonary venous obstruction.
1. Infants are usually asymptomatic at birth. Tachypnea and feeding difficulties appear usually in the first month. This subsequently leads on to failure to thrive, repeated chest infections and cardiac failure in the first 6 months.

    Mild cyanosis which may not be apparent on examination, and the child is usually malnourished with signs of CCF. 75-85% die by 1 year of age.[18]
2. Cardiac findings—Prominent RV impulse is a characteristic finding. A characteristic quadruple rhythm with widely fixed S_2 and grade 3/6 ejection systolic murmur at ULSB. A mid diastolic rumble in always present at LLSB.

With Pulmonary Venous Obstruction

1. *Clinically:* History of marked cyanosis and respiratory distress in neonatal period with failure to thrive. Cyanosis worsens with feeding especially in the infracardiac type when the esophagus compresses the common pulmonary vein.
2. *On examination:* Undernourished newborn with marked cyanosis, tachypnea with marked retraction. Cardiac findings are minimal with a loud and single S_2 and gallop rhythm. A soft ejection systolic murmur in ULSB may be present. Hepatomegaly with pulmonary basal rales are usually present.

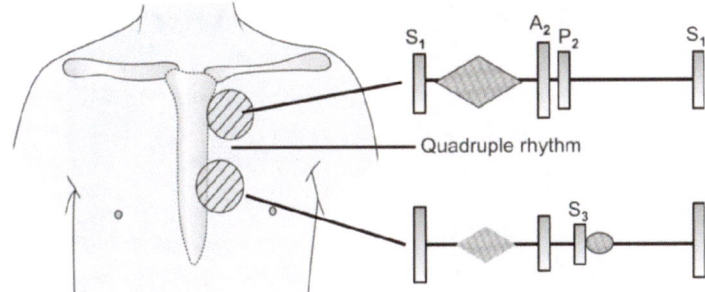

Fig. 7.49: Cardiac findings of total anomalous pulmonary venous return without obstruction to pulmonary venous return

Electrocardiography

1. Tall peaked P wave in lead II or right precordial leads–RAH.
2. RAD with RVH–invariably present with incomplete RBB pattern.

X-ray Studies (Fig. 7.50)

1. Right atrium and RV are enlarged with prominent pulmonary artery segment with increased pulmonary vascular markings.
2. A figure of 8 or "snowman's appearance" of cardiac shadow is seen in patients with TAPVC to left innominte vein, but not before 6 months of age.

Echocardiography (Fig. 7.51)

Common Features

1. A large RV and RA with a relative smaller (hypoplastic) LV and LA and dilated PAs are present.
2. Interatrial communications are usually present: PFO in 70% and ASD secundum in 30% of patients.
3. A large common (common pulmonary venous sinus) may be imaged posterior to the LA in parasternal LA view.
4. M mode echo may show signs of RV volume overload, which slows paradoxical or flat movement of interventricular septum.
5. Doppler studies reveal an increased flow velocity in the PA and continuous flow at the site of pulmonary venous drainage and findings suggestive of pulmonary hypertension.

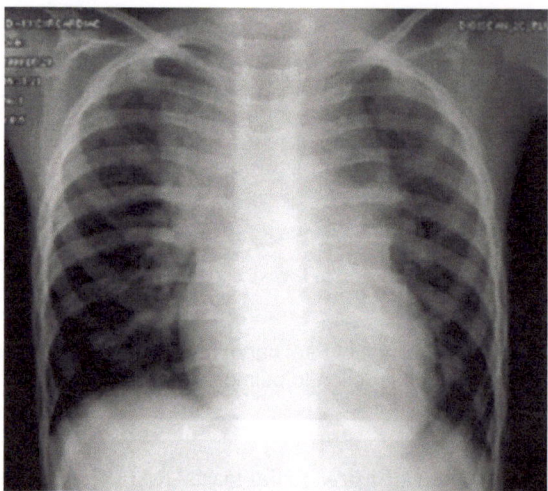

Fig. 7.50: Chest skiagram of TAPVC. Cardiomegaly with increased pulmonary vascularity supracardiac type—"figure of 8" or "Snowman's appearance" configuration

Supracardial Type-Features

The most common site of connection is the left SVC with subsequent drainage to the dilated left innominate vein and right SVC. These abnormal pathways can be seen as images in the suprasternal notch, short axis view, color flow mapping etc. Doppler ultrasound is helpful in defining the direction of flow in left SVC.

Cardiac Type-Features

The most common site of entry is to the coronary sinus, occurring in 15% of cases. A dilated coronary sinus best imaged in parasternal view and apical 4 chamber view may be the first clue to this condition.

Infracardiac Type-Features

A dilated vein descending to the abdominal cavity through the diaphragm. All four pulmonary veins that connect to the confluence can be imaged on subcostal coronal scan.

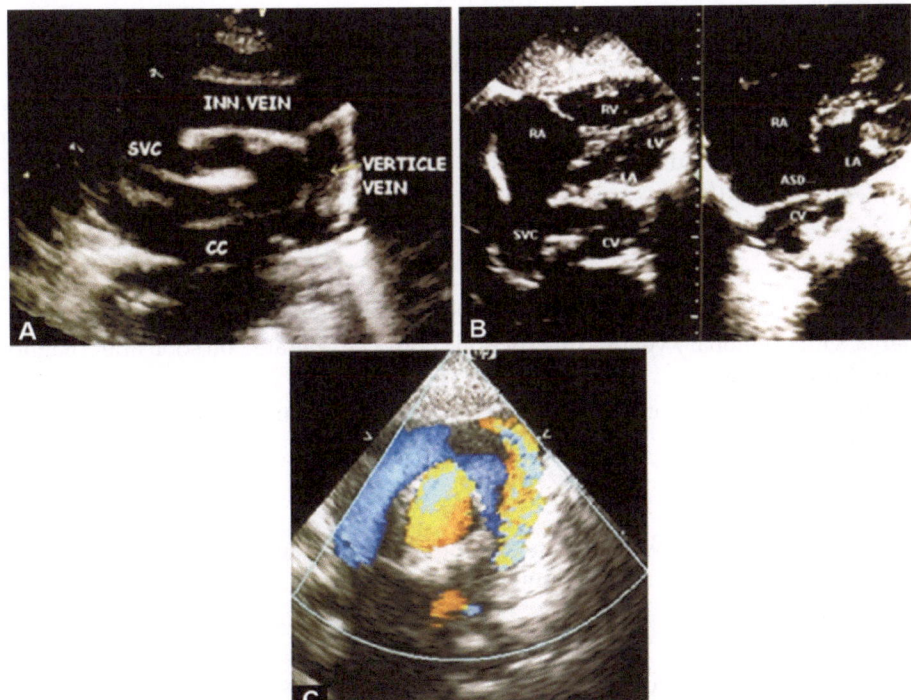

Figs 7.51A to C: Echocardiography of TAPVC. A) suprasternal view showing pulmonary venous confluence (CC) Communicating to left innominate way by left vertical vein, innominate vein joining superior vena cava. B. Subcostal four chamber view in another patient shows pulmonary venous confluence behind the left atrium (LA) which joins superior vena cava, right panel shows a large ASD secundum. C) Color flow mapping in obstructive TAPVC, suprasternal view shows turbulence in left vertical vein. (Courtesy A: Dr. BK Mahala, Narayana Hrudyalaya, Bengaluru, C and D by Dr. SR Anil, Apollo Hospital, Hyderabad)

Mixed Type–Features

Unless all four pulmonary veins are visualized draining into the confluence, mixed type cannot be ruled out. In the most common mixed type, usually upper lobe, of left lung drains to the left SVC and the remaining pulmonary veins in both lungs drain to the coronary sinus.

Natural History

1. CCF occurs in both types of TAPVC and growth retardation with repeated episodes of chest infection also occurs in both.
2. Without surgical repair, two third of the infants without obstruction die before the completion of the first year and the cause of death is usually superimposed pneumonia.
3. Patients with infracardiac type rarely survive beyond 2 months of age.

Surgical

Corrective surgery is necessary for all patients and no palliation exists.

1. All infants with pulmonary venous obstruction should be operated on soon after diagnosis, even in the newborn period.
2. Those infants who have uncontrollable CCF, but without venous obstruction should be operated before 6 months of age.

Procedures

Although the procedures vary with the site of anomalous drainage, all procedures are intended to redirect the pulmonary venous return to the LA.

Mortality

Surgical management is superior to medical management and surgical mortality is 5-10% in the unobstructed variety and 20% in the infracardiac type.

Complications

1. Paroxysms of pulmonary hypertension due to poor compliance of left heart.
2. Postoperative atrial arrhythmias.
3. Obstruction at site of anastomosis, or pulmonary vein stenosis rarely occurs.

MANAGEMENT

Medical

1. Intensive decongestive therapy-digoxin, diuretics, ACE-inhibitors and O_2 inhalation. Metabolic acidosis has to be corrected.

2. Infracardiac type produces pulmonary edema because of venous obstruction-should be put on the ventilator for respiratory support before surgery.
3. If the size of the inter-atrial communication appears to be small, then balloon or blade atrial septostomy should be done to enlarge the communication if surgery is not indicated immediately.

Persistent Truncus Arteriosus

Truncus arteriosus is rare, occurs in fewer than 1 % of all CHDs.[19]

Pathology (Fig. 7.52)

1. Only a single arterial trunk with a truncal valve-gives rise to systemic, pulmonary and coronary circulations. A large perimembranous VSD is usually present and truncal valve may be bicuspid, tricuspid or quadricuspid and is often regurgitant.
2. Maternal diabetes has been implicated as a risk factor and the anomaly has also appeared in dizogotic twins.
3. This anomaly is divided into 4 types.

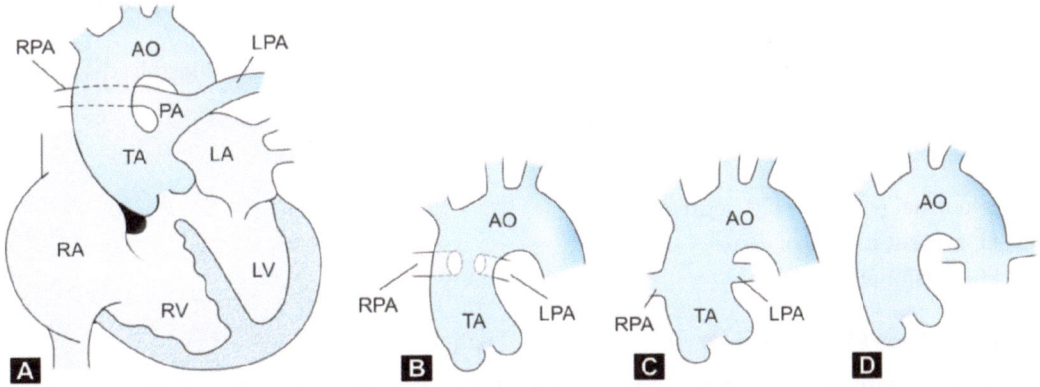

Figs 7.52A to D: Anatomic types of persistent truncus arteriosus (TA) is determined by the branching patterns of pulmonary arteries. A) In type 1, the main pulmonary artery (PA) arises from the truncus and then divides into the right (RPA) and left pulmonary artery (LPA) branches. B) In type 2, the pulmonary arteries arise from the posterior aspect of the truncus. C) In type 3, the pulmonary artery arise from lateral aspects of the truncus. D) In type 4, pseudotruncus arteriosus arteries arising from the descending aorta (AO) supply the lungs

Collete and Edwards Classification[10]

Type I: Short pulmonary trunk originating from truncus arteriosus gives rise to both pulmonary arteries. PBF increases, when both the arteries separate from the truncus arteriosus with no evidence of main pulmonary artery, they may arise close to one another (Type II) or at some distance from one another (Type III).

(Type IV)–Severe form of TOF with pulmonary atresia (pseudotruncus arteriosus) with collaterals supplying the lungs. Types I and II contribute 85% of cases.

4. Coronary artery abnormalities are common and may contribute to high surgical mortality.
5. Evidence of DiGeorge syndrome with hypocalcemia is present in 33% of patients.[21]
6. A right sided aortic arch is seen in 30% of patients and interrupted aortic arch in 10% of cases.

Clinical Manifestations

1. Cyanosis is present at birth. Signs of CCF also appear in the first few weeks after birth, with respiratory distress. These infants die of CCF by 6-12 months. If PVOD supervenes by 6 months, then the child survives till the 3rd decade.
2. On examination-undernourished child in CCF is cyanosed with bounding peripheral pulses. A loud and harsh regurgitant murmur heard along LLSB is suggestive of VSD.
3. If PBF is large, an apical rumble with gallop rhythm and a high pitched early diastolic decrescendo murmur of truncal valve regurgitation may be audible.

Electrocardiography

1. Axis–normal (+ 50 to +120 degrees)
   CVH–present in 70% of cases
   LAH-occasionally present.

X-ray Studies (Fig. 7.53)

Cardiomegaly with increased pulmonary vascularity. A right aortic arch seen in 30% of cases.

Echocardiography (Figs 7.54A and B)

1. A large VSD seen directly under truncal valve.
2. A single large great artery arising from the heart can be identified. An artery branching from the truncus posteriorly is pulmonary artery (Figs 7.55A and B).

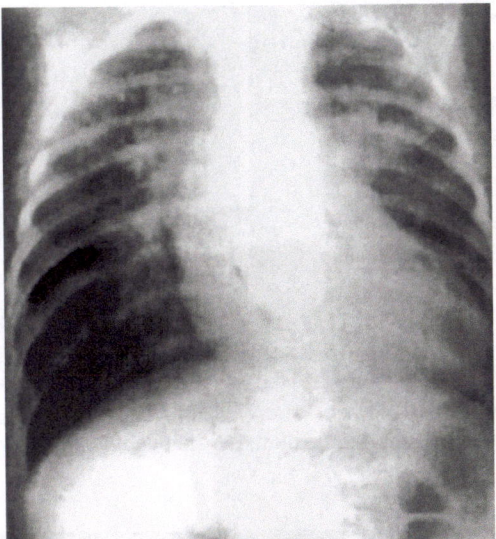

Fig. 7.53: Chest X-ray of truncus arteriosus showing cardiomegaly with LV contour with increased pulmonary vascularity

Natural History

1. Most infants die within 6-12 months depending upon the PBF.
2. Clinical improvement occurs if the infant develops pulmonary vascular obstructive disease (PVOD) by 3-4 months of age. Death occurs by 3rd decade.
3. Truncal valve insufficiency worsens with time.

MANAGEMENT

Medical

1. Vigorous decongestive measures-digoxin, diuretics, ACE-inhibitors with O_2 inhalations.
2. Prophylaxis against SBE should be observed.

Surgical

Palliative Procedure

Pulmonary artery banding may be performed in small infants with large PBF and CCF. The banding can produce distortion of pulmonary arteries and this does not necessary prevent PVODS. This

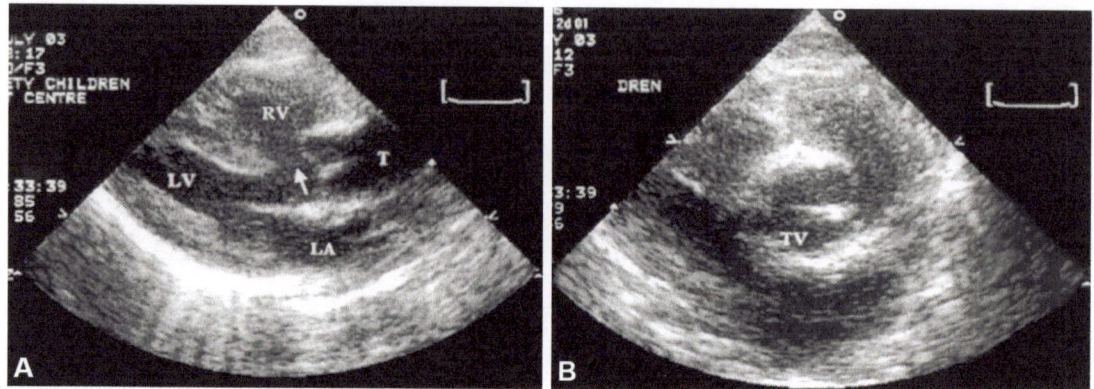

Figs 7.54A and B: Echocardiography of truncus arteriosus: (A) Parasternal long axis view showing a large VSD (arrow) with override of trunk (T) (LA—left atrium, LV—left ventricle, RV—right ventricle). (B) Parasternal short axis view showing thick cusp of truncal valve (TV)

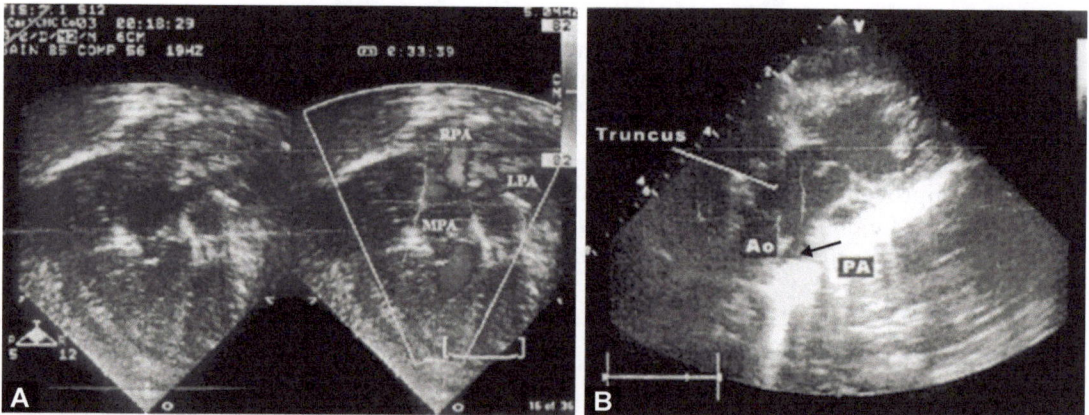

Figs 7.55A and B: Echocardiography of truncus arteriosus: (A) Apical view, main pulmonary artery (MPA) arising from the trunk and dividing to left (LPA) and right pulmonary artery (RPA), left panel shows 2D image, color flow to pulmonary artery is seen in the right panel. (B) Modified subcostal view in another patient showing the pulmonary artery (arrow) arising from the common trunk (Ao—aorta, PA—pulmonary artery)

procedure is associated with high mortality rate (>30%), so it is reserved for only those infants with increased PBF. PA banding is not believed to have any advantage, so primary repair of the defect is recommended.

Definitive Procedure

1. Various modification of Rastelli procedure are performed. The VSD is closed first and later the successive truncal and aortic defects are corrected. Surgical mortality may be between 10-20% and coronary arteries have to be investigated and their interruption has to be avoided. The optional age for this corrective surgery is 3 months (i.e. before the pulmonary vascular obstructive disease begins to develop).
2. Barbero-Marcial operation–Autologous tissue is used to correct type I truncus–again should be performed before 3 months of age.
3. Truncal valve replacement indicated if there is significant truncal valve insufficiency–mortality more than 50%.

CYANOTIC: PRESSURE OVERLOAD RL-SHUNT
Tetralogy of Fallot (TOF)

TOF is the commonest of all cyanotic CHDs seen beyond infancy. TOF is the fifth most common defect overall accounting for 6.8% of all types of CHD. Amongst all patients with TDF, 70.7% had TOF with PS and 20.3% had TOF with pulmonary atresia.

Etiology

The etiology of TOF is heterogenous and includes both environmental and genetic factors, which interact with one another. Several environmental teratogens have been shown specifically to increase the risk of developing TOF with PS, which include maternal phyenylketonuria or trimethadione.[22] Genetic factors are also thought to influence the development of TOF with PS. There are many reports describing families with affected members across generations which support a monogenic or polygenic mode of inheritance or another study which supports the hypothesis that genetic cause of TOF is heterogeneous.[23]

Developmental Considerations

The anatomy seen in TOF is believed to result from incomplete rotation and faulty partitioning of the conotruncus during septation. Malrotation of truncal-bulbar ridges results in malalignment of outlet and trabecular septum and consequent straddling of the aorta over malaligned ventricular septal defect. Van Praagh postulates that the hypoplasia and under development of the pulmonary infundibulum are responsible for infundibular obstruction and malalignment of the outlet septum.[24] A clear mechanistic explanation for abnormal conotruncal development remains uncertain.

Pathology (Fig. 7.56)

The original description of TOF includes the following:
1. Peri-membranous VSD with overriding of aorta.
2. RV outflow tract obstruction-infundibular pulmonic stenosis–in 45-60%.
3. RVH-depending on the severity of PS.
4. Right aortic arch is present in 25% of cases.
5. Pulmonary annulus and MPA are hypoplastic in most patients and obstruction at origin of PA is particularly common.
6. In about 5% of TOF patients, abnormal coronary arteries are also present.

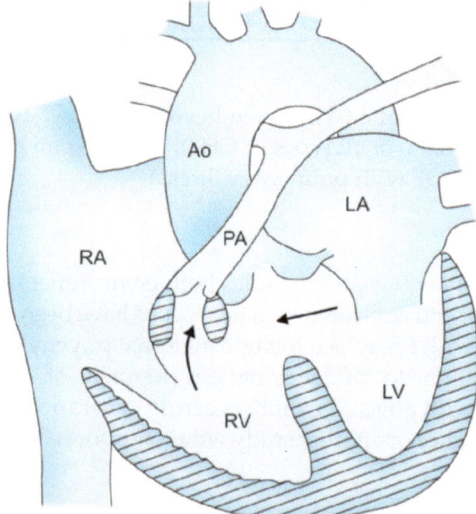

Fig. 7.56: Schematic diagram showing classical features of TOF. 1-RV Infundibular stenosis (thin arrow). 2-Large subaortic VSD (thick arrow) with 3-overriding of aorta (biventricular origin) 4-right ventricular (RV hypertrophy). Pulmonary artery is narrow (PA)

Associated Cardiac Anomalies

The rate of associated cardiac anomalies is very high. Patent foramen ovale and true ASD were found to be present in 83% and left SVC in 11% of hearts with TOF. Anomalous pulmonary venous drainage and Ebsteins anomaly have also been reported in association with TOF.

Pathophysiology and Hemodynamics

The range of physiology seen with TOF is diverse.

Blood Flow

1. The extent and direction of ventricular level shunting will be determined by the cumulative amount of obstructed RVOT.
2. The balance between pulmonary and aortic blood flow will be determined by the difference in impedance between the unobstructed but relatively high resistance systemic vascular bed and the obstructed pulmonary outflow tract.
3. Ventricular septal defect, given its non-restrictive nature, provides the anatomic route of balance between the two circulatory beds.
4. Although the obstruction to pulmonary blood flow in TOF is regarded as being relatively fixed by virtue of the intrinsic anatomy, there is some degree of variation in degree of cyanosis seen in an individual patient.
5. Exercise results in a decrease in arterial saturation secondary to increased R-L shunting which leads on to increase in cyanosis.

The most characteristic and hallmark finding is the subpulmonic stenosis created by the deviation of the outlet or conal septum. All patients with TOF demonstrate anterior and cephalad deviation of this outlet septum and the degree and nature of this deviation determines the severity of subpulmonic obstruction. Moreover deviation of the conal septum can explain the subsequent presence of both ventricular septal defect and overriding of aorta. Because, virtually in all patients, VSD is large and nonrestrictive and right ventricular hypertrophy is secondary to subpulmonic stenosis.

Clinical Manifestation (Fig. 7.57)

1. Most cases of TOF-cyanosis appears 6-8 weeks after birth. Exertional dyspnea, squatting and hypoxic (cyanotic) spells develop later on in life.
2. Acyanotic TOF with a large VSD will present with CCF.
3. Presence of severe cyanosis at birth signifies pulmonary atresia with VSD.
4. Varying degrees of cyanosis, clubbing and tachypnea are present.

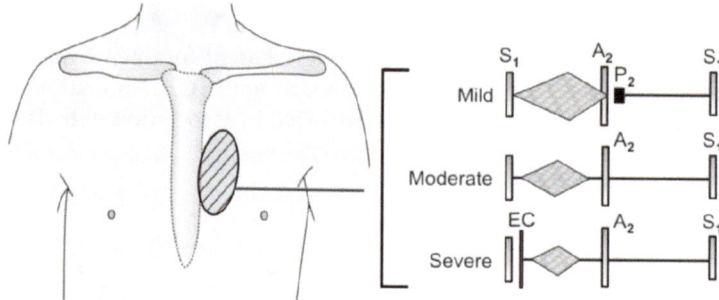

Fig. 7.57: Cardiac findings in tetralogy of Fallot (TOF). A long ejection systolic murmur at the upper end mid sternal border and a loud single S_2 are characteristic auscultatory findings of TOF

5. Physcial examination will reflect the combination of PS, right ventricular hypertension and right to left shunt. There is an accentuated precordial right ventricular impulse.
6. A systolic click originating in aorta is present. S_2 is usually single because aortic component is heard. A loud 3-5/6 ejection systolic murmur is heard at the upper left sternal border. The more severe the PS-softer and shorter is the murmur.
7. Hypercyanotic episodes (cyanotic spells) and squatting.
   - Cyanotic spells (hypoxemic spells) are characterized by a severe and often prolonged decrease in arterial oxygen saturation.
   - Cyanosis is a result of an acute substantial increase in right to left shunting owing to a change in the ratio between pulmonary and systemic vascular impedance.
   - Cyanotic spells are mediated by the dynamic changes in the degree of subpulmonic obstruction clinically correlated by findings of markedly diminished or absent systolic murmur.
   - Mechanism of cyanotic spell–any activity (e.g. exercise, cough, crying or defecation–brings about an increase in catecholamine secretion which stimulates the subpulmonary (infundibular) area, which goes into spasm producing, hypovolemia and acute episode of hypoxia.[25]
   - Spells are characterized by severe cyanosis. Hyperpnea is often present, thought to be in response to acute hypoxia and secondary metabolic acidosis. If prolonged, unconsciousness, convulsions and death may occur.
   - Cyanotic spells were common prior to availability of safe and effective surgery. They occurred more commonly in patients with iron deficiency anemia. In the current era, such an episode

gives, an impetus for surgical intervention and so such life threatening episodes are less common.
- Squatting–is a milder version of hypercyanotic spell. Children assume knee to chest position typically following any activity. This is an instructive gesture to increase systemic vascular resistance thereby improving arterial oxygen saturation.

Electrocardiography (Fig. 7.58)

1. RVH-RAD (+120 – +150 degrees) usually present.
2. RVH is mostly present but with no "strain pattern." RAH occasionally present.

X-ray Studies

Cyanotic TOF (Fig. 7.59)

1. Normal sized heart with decreased pulmonary vascular markings-oligemic lung fields.
2. Typical presentation-concave MPA segment with upturned apex-"boot shaped heart".
3. Right sided aortic arch may be present in 25% of cases.

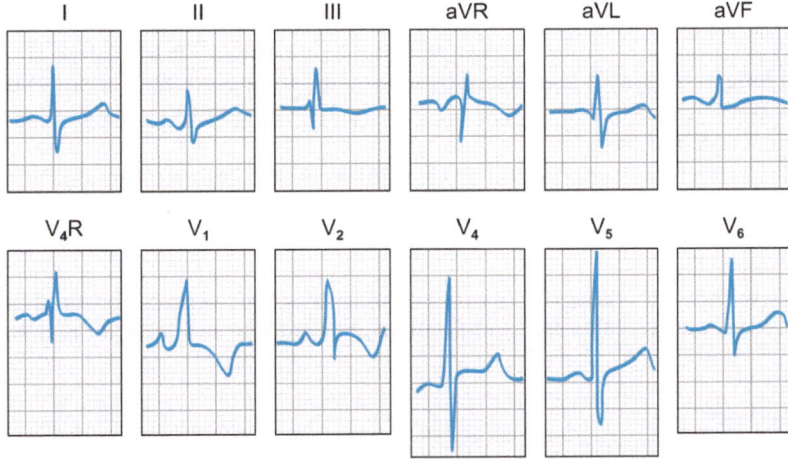

Fig. 7.58: ECGs of patients with TOF with right ventricular hypertrophy. Arrows, RVH in the QRS complex

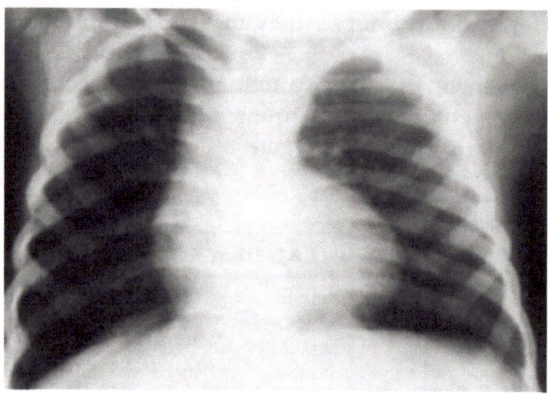

Fig. 7.59: Chest skiagram of TOF. Concave MPA segment with upturned apex-"Boot shaped heart"

Echocardiography

Two-dimensional echo and Doppler studies can make the diagnosis and quantitate the severity of TOF.
1. A large perimembranous infundibular VSD and overriding of the aorta-are visualized in parasternal long axis view. A significant override > 50% suggests double outlet right ventricle.
2. RV outflow tract obstruction with normal pulmonary valve but the branches are smaller than normal (Figs 7.60A and B).
3. Apical four chamber view will provide a clear image of the perimembranous ventricular septal defect and its relationship to the tricuspid and aortic valves.
4. Doppler studies show low velocity R-L or biphasic flow. Pressure gradient across RVOT which can be estimated (Fig. 7.61).
5. Subcostal view shows the integrity of atrial septum, systemic venous and pulmonary anatomy. Aorta and ventricular septal defect and finally right ventricle and infundibular stenosis are also seen.

Natural History

1. Infants who are acyanotic at birth, become cyanosed by 8-12 weeks of life.
2. Hypoxic spells may develop depending upon severity of RVOT, obstruction and thereby growth retardation may develop in future.

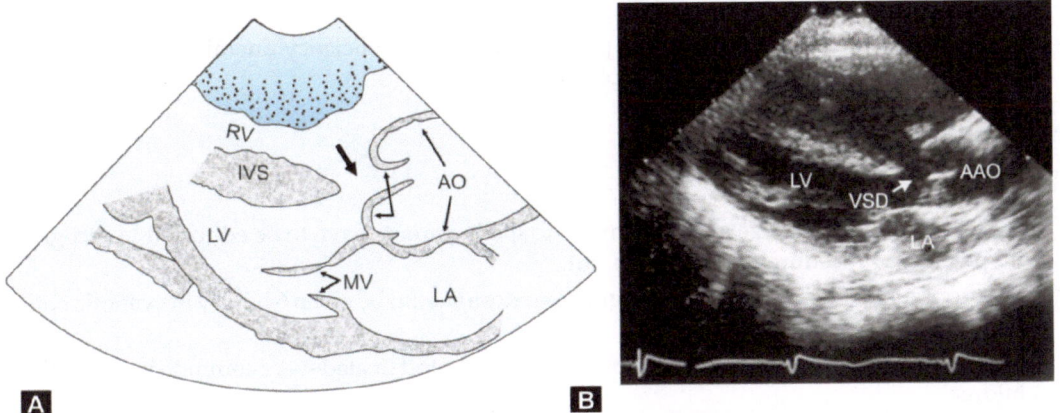

Figs 7.60A and B: Parasternal long axis view in a patient with tetralogy of Fallot. Note a large subaortic ventricular septal defect (arrow) and a relatively large aorta overriding the interventricular septum (IVS)

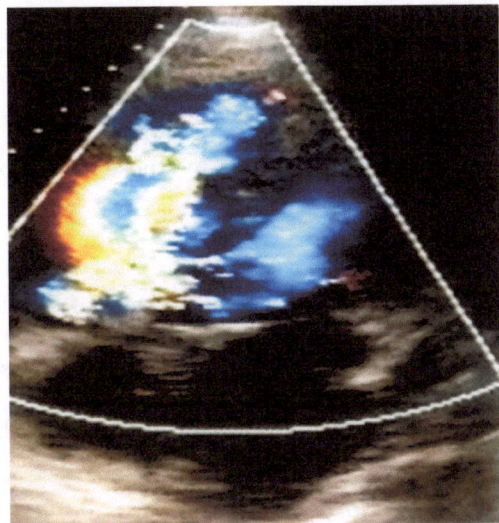

Fig. 7.61: Tetralogy of Fallot–color flow through the ventricular septal defect. "Arrow" on apical four chamber view

3. Brain abscess, cerebrovascular accidents and SBE are common complications.
4. Since central cyanosis predisposes to polycythemia-iron deficiency anemia and coagulopathy should be remembered as potent complications.

Management

Medical

1. Physician should recognize and treat hypoxic spells-parents have to be educated to recognize it and palliative procedures to be carried out.
2. Oral propranolol therapy—0.5 to 1.5 mg/kg per dose should be given 6 hourly in cyanotic patients to prevent cyanotic spells.
3. Relative iron deficiency anemia should be detected early and treated–very common in polycythemic children.

Surgical

Palliative Shunt Procedures

Shunt procedures are performed to increase pulmonary blood flow. Indications are the following especially in the poorer nations where primary repair is difficult.
1. Neonates with TOF and pulmonary atresia.
2. Infants with hypoplastic pulmonary artery annulus and hypoplastic PA.
3. Severely cyanotic infants-younger than 3 months and those who have medically unmanageable cyanotic spells.

The Shunt Procedures

1. Classic Blalock Thomas-Taussig shunt-anastomosis between left subclavian artery and ipsilateral pulmonary artery. Procedure of choice for an infant more than 3 months.
2. Gore-Tex interposition shunt-placed between subclavian artery and ipsilateral PA-ideal for infants less than 3 months.
3. Waterston shunt and Pott's shunt operations have been abandoned because of high percentage of complications.

Currective Surgery-Brock's Procedure

Timing varies depending upon the patient but early surgery is always preferred.

Indications and Timing

1. Symptomatic infants who have favorable anatomy of RV outflow tract and pulmonary artery.
   - Early repair advised, any time after 4 months of age.
2. Mildly cyanotic children who have had shunt surgery-total repair at 1-2 years after shunt operation.

Procedure

Total repair of the defect is carried out under cardiopulmonary bypass and circulatory arrest. For uncomplicated TOF-mortality is between 2-5% during first 2 years.

Complications

1. Bleeding problems-in older polycythemic patients.
2. CCF in presence of anemia-may need decongestive therapy.
3. RBBB in ECG-occurs in 90% of patients
4. Complete heart block-rare.

Tricuspid Atresia (TA)

Tricuspid atresia is defined as complete absence of tricuspid valve with no direct communication between the right atrium and right ventricle. The defect invariably leads to some degree of hypoplasia of right ventricle. Interatrial communication can be a wide patent foramen ovale, may be a secundum atrial septal defect or rarely an ostium primum defect associated with an atrioventricular septal defect. When VSD is present, it is usually perimembranous, but may occur rarely as a part of AV septal defect. Additional cardiovascular anomalies are present in < 20% of patients but less in those with normally related great arteries. Coarctation of aorta is the commonest cardiac abnormality, which occurs in 8% of patients with tricuspid atresia. Tricuspid atresia accounts for 1-3% of all CHDs.[26]

Classification of Tricuspid Atresia[27] (Fig. 7.62)

Type I. Normally related great arteries
   a. Intact ventricular septum with pulmonary atresia.
   b. Small ventricular septal defect and pulmonary stenosis.
   c. Large ventricular septal defect without pulmonary stenosis.

Type II. Transposition of great arteries.
   a. Ventricular septal defect with pulmonary atresia.
   b. Ventricular septal defect with pulmonary stenosis.
   c. Ventricular septal defect without pulmonary stenosis.

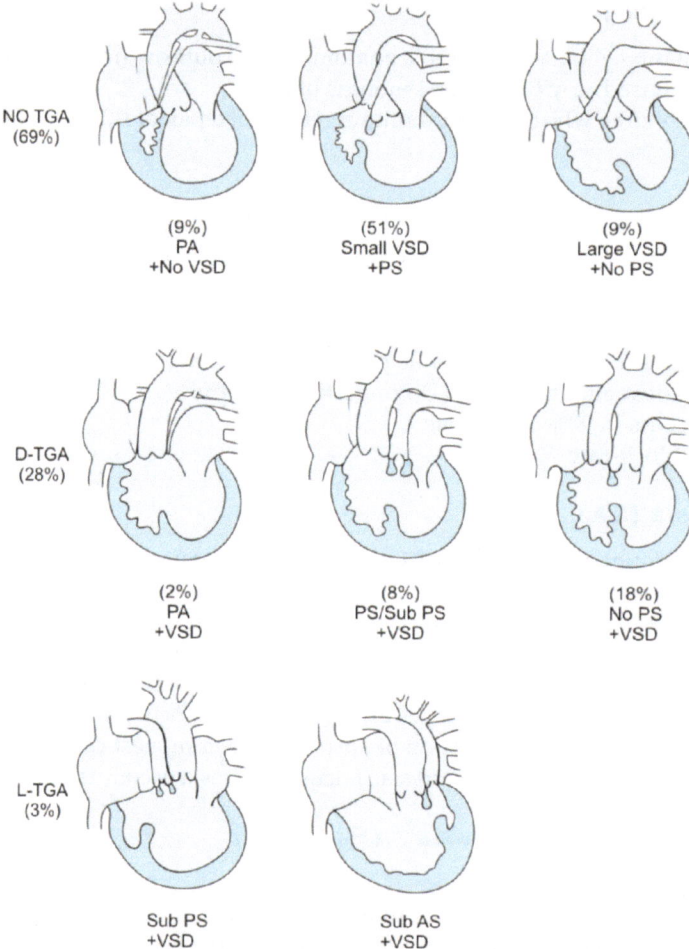

Fig. 7.62: Anatomical classification of tricuspid atresia. In about 70% of cases, the great arteries are normally related and there is a small ventricular septal defect (VSD) with associated hypoplasia of the pulmonary artery (PA). When the great arteries are transposed, the VSD is usually large and PA are large with increased pulmonary blood flow. (Data from Keith JD, Rowe RD, Plad P: Heart disease infancy and childhood, 3rd edition, New York Mcmillan 1978)

Type III. Transposition or malposition of great arteries

Associated complex lesions include truncus arteriosus, subpulomonic PS or AS, coarctation of aorta, AV septal defect.

Clinical Manifestations (Fig. 7.63)

Systemic arterial desaturation is present to some extent in every patient with tricuspid atresia because of complete admixture of systemic and pulmonary vascular return.[28] Cyanosis may not be present at birth but most patients manifest it by 1 week of age.

1. Cyanosis may be in severe form with occasional hypoxic spells. Tachypnoea and poor feeding and incident CCF manifest in infancy as pulmonary resistance decreases.
2. In presence of cyanosis-a grade 2-3/6 regurgitant systolic murmur is usually present with a single S_2 at lower left sternal border. A continuous mumur of PDA is occasionally present.
3. Patients with d-transposition of great arteries usually present with pulmonary overcirculation, pulmonary stenosis is rare. When VSDs present are large, then it is difficult to distinguish these patients from those with normally related great arteries.

Electrocardiography (Fig. 7.64)

1. "Superior" QRS axis (between 0-90°) is characteristic. It appears in most patients without TGA and it presents in 50% of those with TGA.
2. LVH is usually present with RAH or sometimes with combined atrial hypertrophy.

X-ray Chest (Fig. 7.65)

1. Cardiomegaly may be there with enlarged RA and LV. Pulmonary vascularity is decreased in most patients, although it may be increased in patients with TGA.

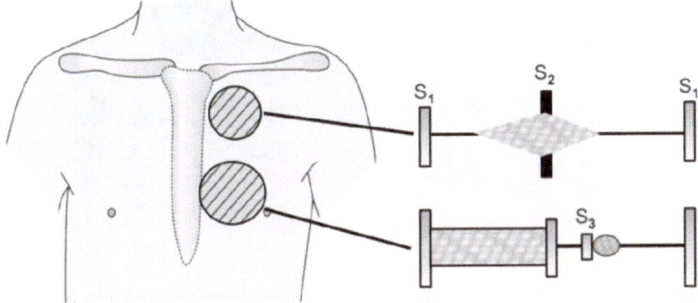

Fig. 7.63: Findings of tricuspid atresia. Associated with patent ductus arteriosus and ventricular septal defect

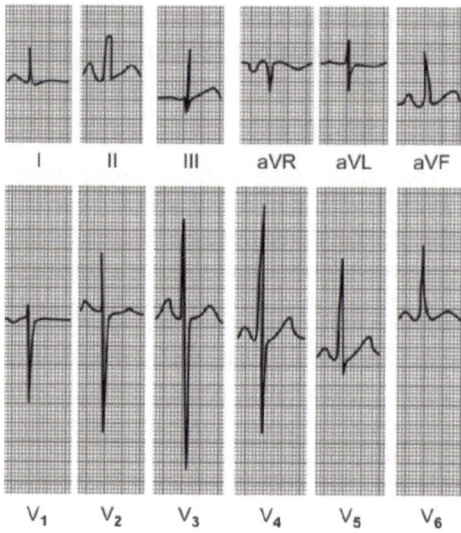

Fig. 7.64: Tracing from an infant with tricuspid atresia showing left anterior hemiblock (– 30°) right atrial hypertrophy and left ventricular hypertrophy

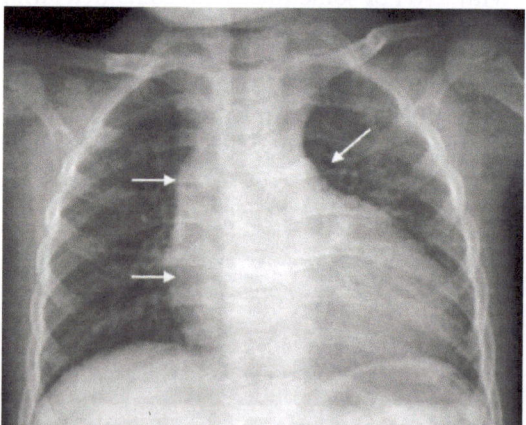

Fig. 7.65: X-ray chest of tricuspid atresia showing prominent right atrium (thin black arrow), concavity over MPA segment (thick white arrow), prominent ascending aorta (thick black arrow) and pulmonary olegemia. (Courtesy: Dr. M Satpathy, Clinical Diag. of Heart disease, Jaypee Med Publishers, 2008)

Echocardiography (Fig. 7.66)

1. Absence of tricuspid orifice, marked hypoplasia of RV and a large LV can be imaged in 4 chamber view. Absence of any communication or flow between RA and RV can be seen.
2. Bulging of atrial septum towards left and size of ASD is usually seen in subcostal view.
3. Size of VSD, presence and severity of PS and presence of TGA should be looked for and other assorted anomalies can be easily visualized.

Complications

1. Repeated chest infection.
2. Hypercyanotic spells.
3. Congestive cardiac failure.
4. Embolic phenomenon including paradoxical embolic episode.
5. Infective endocarditis in older age groups.

Natural History

Survival of patients of tricuspid atresia mainly depends on the type of lesions and on early medical management. In general, prognosis of those patients is worse, when they have in addition high volume transposition of great arteries.
1. Few infants with tricuspid atresia with normally related great arteries survive beyond 6 months without surgical palliation. Some develop CCF because of increased PBF.

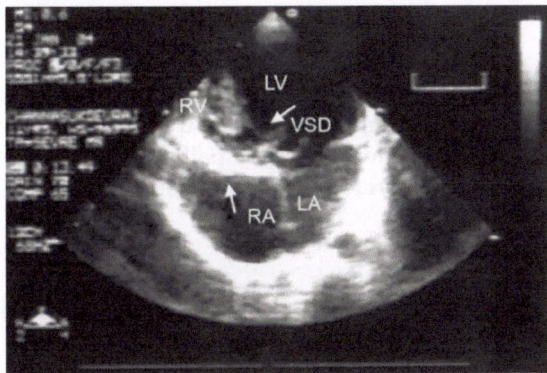

Fig. 7.66: Echocardiogram of tricuspid atresia. Apical four chamber view shows a dense band (large arrow) in place of tricuspid valve, restrictive VSD (small arrow) and underdeveloped right ventricle. (Courtesy: Dr. M Satpathy, Clinical Diag. of Heart disease, Jaypee Med Publishers, 2008)

2. Those who survive for the first 10 years, the chronic volume overload of LV leads on to secondary cardiomyopathy (surgery should be performed before LV dysfunction sets in). These patients are also exposed to risk of infective endocarditis.

Management

Medical

1. Prostaglandin E_1-should be started in cyanosed neonates to maintain patency of ductus.
2. Rashkind procedure (balloon atrial septostomy) may be performed to improve RA-LA shunt.
3. Infants with normally related great arteries and adequate PBF without a VSD do not need any procedure-but should be monitored carefully.
4. If CCF supervenes—decongestive therapy, e.g. digoxin and diureticsa should be given.

Surgical

Palliative

1. Shunt operations
   a. Blalock Taussig shunt—should be performed before 6 months of age.
   b. Bidirectional Glen procedure[29]—Superior cavopulmonary shunt, SVC to right PA shunt (end-to-side)-bidirectional at 6-12 months age group.
2. Pulmonary artery banding—Sometimes necessary to combat CCF can be performed at any age with a mortality of < 5%.

Definitive Surgery

A modified Fontan operation (Choussat procedure)[30] is the definitive procedure for patients with tricuspid atresia. In this operation, systemic venous blood goes directly to the pulmonary artery by bypassing RV, in one or two stages, after one of the palliative shunt operations has already been performed. This procedure has 10 criteria for optimum results.
1. Age 4-15 years
2. Normal sinus rhythm
3. Normal pulmonary venous connections
4. Normal right atrial size
5. Normal systemic venous connections
6. Normal pulmonary artery pressure
7. Low pulmonary vascular resistance

8. Normal LVEF
   9. Adequate sized pulmonary arteries with diameter > 75% of aortic diameter.
   10. Absence of complicating factors from previous surgeries.

Tricuspid atresia represents the best operative risk for such surgery (10% mortality) and the best long term outlook (65% survival 10 years postoperatively).

Ebstein's Anomaly

Congenital lesions of the tricuspid valve resulting in regurgitation are uncommon, the most common of the group is Ebstein's anomaly.[31]

Ebstein's anomaly of tricuspid valve occurs with a prevalence of 0.5% of all types of congenital heart diseases. There is an equal distribution between sexes and associated lesions are not uncommon. In most cases, an interatrial communication is present in the form of either PFO or a true ASD. VSD, pulmonary stenosis or atresia or TOF and coarctation of aorta are rarely associated.

Physiology

Because the degree of anatomic deformity varies greatly, the physiology is also likewise variable.
1. In severe cases of Ebstein's anomaly—central cyanosis is a prominent physical finding which occurs mostly due to R–L shunting at atrial level. During atrial systole, blood flows from true right atrium into atrialized portion of the right ventricle, but during ventricular systole, the blood gets propelled back into true right atrium rather than passing forward into true right ventricle and subsequently into pulmonary artery.
2. In neonatal period—in more severe cases of Ebstein's anomaly, with increased pulmonary vascular resistance, the ability of right ventricle to propel blood forward is compromised. Therefore not enough pressure is generated to open the pulmonary valve, so a functional pulmonary atresia develops and the infant becomes cyanotic and also becomes dependent on patent ductus arteriosus for pulmonary blood flow.[32] Once the pulmonary vascular resistance diminishes, the right ventricle is able to pump forward thereby diminishing RL shunt and diminution of cyanosis occurs.
3. Typically, the cyanosis diminishes in severity over the first few months or years of life and may even disappear entirely only to return later on in life in early adulthood.[33] This happens probably due to worsening of tricuspid valve insufficiency which leads on to further dilation of right atrium and ventricle.
4. In cases with intact atrial septum, cyanosis is absent. Patients present with increased right atrial pressure due to severity of tricuspid regurgitation or stenosis–manifest with–hepatosplenomegaly and jugular pulsations.

Pathology (Fig. 7.67)

1. There is a downward displacement of septal and posterior leaflets of the tricuspid valve into R V cavity, so that a portion of R V is incorporated into RA (atrialized RV) and functional hypoplasia of RV results which is continuous with true right atrium.[34] Tricuspid regurgitation (TR) is present and RA is dilated and hypertrophied.
2. An intra-atrial communication (PFO or ASD) with R-L shunt is present in all.
3. WPW syndrome is frequently associated with the anomaly, and predisposes the patient to tachyarrhythmias.

Clinical Manifestations (Fig. 7.68)

1. Prenatal course of infants born with Ebstein's anomaly is unremarkable. There is no association with maternal age, length of gestation or sex of the fetus.[35] Lithium ingestion in early pregnancy was initially thought as a possible cause, but currently there is some debate as to whether true association exists or not.[36]

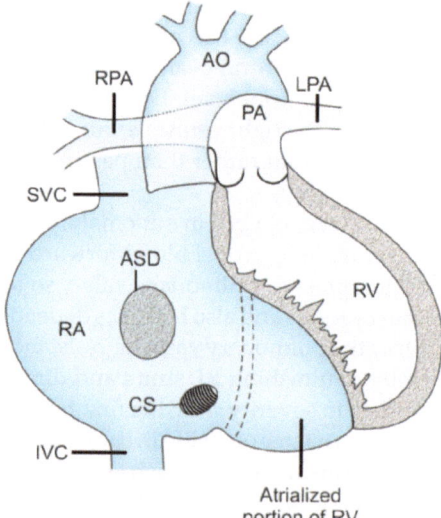

Fig. 7.67: Diagram of Ebstein's anomaly of tricuspid valve. There is a downward displacement of the tricuspid valve, usually the septal and the posterior leaflets into the RV. Part of the RV is incorporated into the RA ("atrialized" portion of the RV). Regurgitation of the tricuspid valve results in RA enlargement. An ASD is usually present. CS, coronary sinus

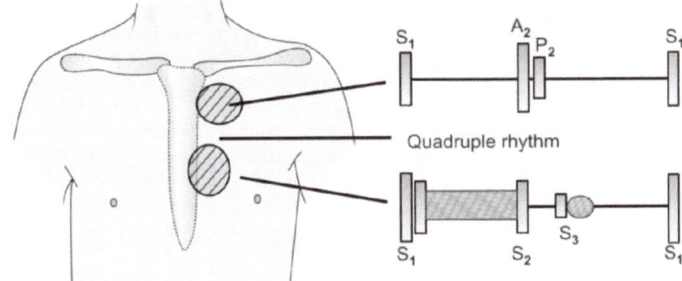

Fig. 7.68: Cardiac findings of Ebstein's anomaly. Quadruple rhythm and a soft regurgitant systolic murmur are characteristic of the defect

2. Mild tricuspid valve deformity–may be symptom free.
3. Severe tricuspid valve deformity–symptoms of congestive cardiac failure and cyanosis may appear early and may be present even *in utero*. As pulmonary vascular resistance decreases, cyanosis improves, may even disappear to reappear later with exertional dyspnea and fatigue.
4. Episodes of supraventricular tachycardia occurs in 20-30% of patients. Exertional dyspnea may be a prominent symptom along with tachycardia especially in older patients, probably as a result of diminished ventricular filling during rapid heart beats.
5. Physical examination
   a. Cyanosis depends on the severity of the lesion
   b. Jugular venous distension with 'a' waves in presence of severe tricuspid regurgitation.
   c. Systolic thrill at lower left sternal border.
   d. Quadruple rhythm
      The rhythm has widely split S_1 (second component being due to closure of tricuspid valve) and S_2 (Usually due to RV conduction delay). Presence of S_3 and S_4 suggest the possibility of Ebstein's anomaly
   - A soft holosystolic, murmur is heard at lower left sternal border which increases on inspiration. Occasionally an ejection murmur of right ventricular outflow tract obstruction may also be present.
   - A mid diastolic rumble may be present–suggestive of true or relative tricuspid stenosis.

Electrocardiographic Features (Fig. 7.69)

1. Right atrial enlargement–prominent feature–typical peaked P waves, may be even notched suggesting combined atrial enlargement.

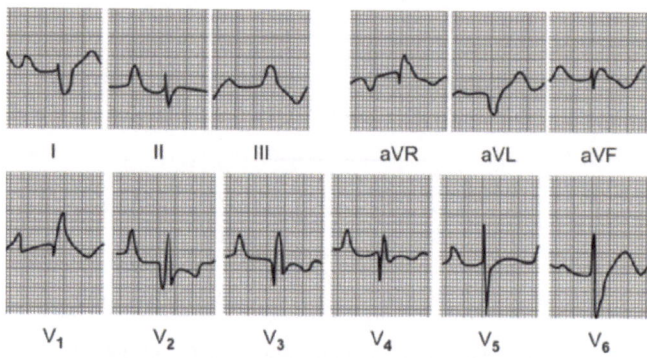

Fig. 7.69: Tracing from a child with Ebstein's anomaly. The tracing shows right atrial hypertrophy, right bundle branch block, and first degree atrioventricular block

2. Right ventricular hypertrophy may be seen though rare.
3. First degree AV block is frequent in 40% of patients. WPW syndrome is present in 20% with occasional episodes of SVT.
4. In older patients because of dilation of RV, atrial flutter or fibrillation may supervene.[37]

X-ray Chest (Figs 7.70A and B)

1. Severe cases–balloon (flask) shaped cardiac contour with a narrow base. If a newborn is born with a huge cardiomegaly, Ebstein's anomaly is the first possibility.
2. Size of right atrium is huge–which in some cases makes up for the entire cardiac silhouette.
3. Pulmonary vascularity is usually diminished when there is cyanosis with right to left shunt.

Echocardiography (Figs 7.71A and B)

2 D echo with color flow Doppler study gives typical morphologic assessment.
1. Apical displacement of septal leaflet of the tricuspid valve is the most diagnostic feature of the anomaly. An elongated somewhat redundant anterior leaflet with a whip-like motion.
2. A large RA, including the atrialized RV and a small functional RV represent the anatomic severity. Evidence of TR, TS and ASD are present (Figs 7.72A and B).

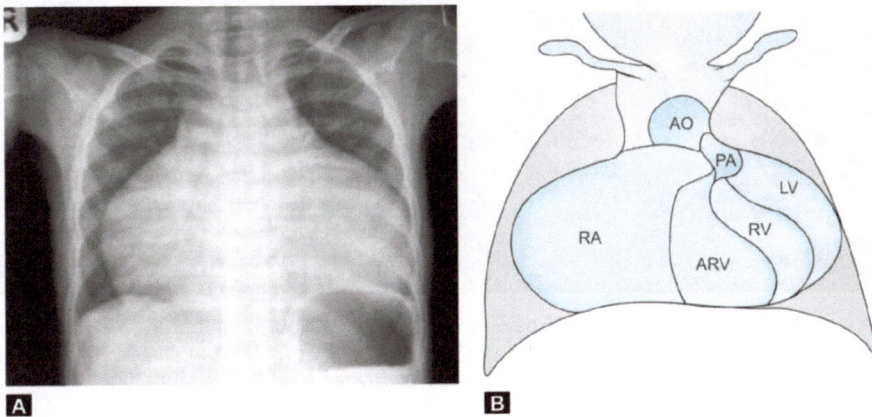

Figs 7.70A and B: Posteroanterior view (A) and diagram (B) of chest X-ray from an infant with severe Ebstein's anomaly. Note extreme cardiomegaly, primarily the right atrium (RA) and diminished pulmonary vascularity

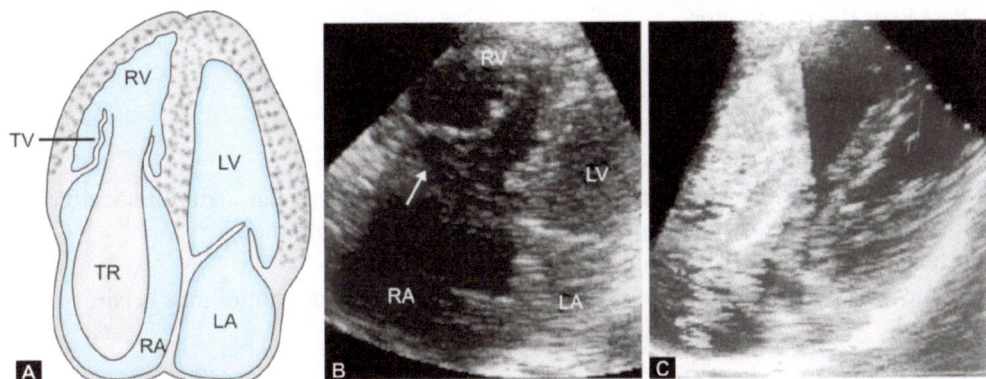

Figs 7.71A and B: (A) Ebstein's anomaly. Apical displacement of tricuspid valve (TV) which is often malformed causing tricuspid stenosis of severe regurgitation as shown. (B) Apical 4-chamber view showing malformation of the tricuspid valve (arrow). (C) Color flow mapping showing severe tricuspid regurgitation

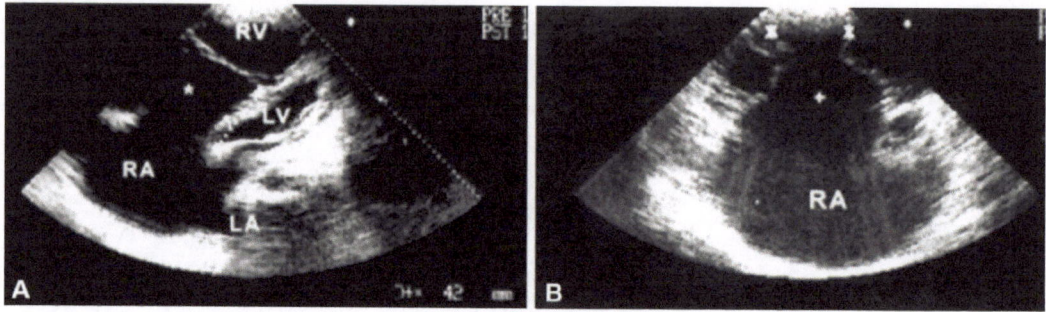

Figs 7.72A and B: Echocardiography of Ebsteins anomaly : (A) Four chamber view shows 42 mm apical displacement of septal leaflet of tricuspid valve, (B) Two chamber view showing dilated RA and atrialized RV. (Courtesy: Dr. M Satpathy, Clinical Diag. of Heart disease, Jaypee Med Publishers, 2008)

3. M-Mode echocardiographic features.
    a. Enlarged right atrium
    b. Increased velocity and amplitude of anterior tricuspid leaflet.
    c. Paradoxical septal motion
    d. Delayed closure of anterior tricuspid valve leaflet.

Complications

1. Heart failure–commonest cause of mortality.
2. Arryhthmia–Supraventricular arrhythmias are common. Ventricular arrhythmia and complete atrioventricular block requiring pacemaker implantation are common.
3. Infective endocarditis–risk throughout life.
4. Systemic arterial desaturation-polycythemia–coagulation abnormalities may occur.

Natural History

1. Cyanosis tends to improve as pulmonary vascular resistance falls during infancy. It appears later on in life.
2. Patients with a less severe anomaly may be asymptomatic.
3. 18% symptomatic infants die in infancy. 30% die before they reach 10 years due to CCF. Median age of death is usually 20 years.

4. Hemodynamic deterioration, with increasing cyanosis, CCF and LV dysfunction develop later on in life.
5. Attacks of SVT with WPW syndrome occur in 15% which may prove fatal.

Management

Medical

1. Varying degrees of activity restriction.
2. In severely cyanotic newborns-intensive treatment with prostaglandin E_1 infusion, inotropic agents and correction of metabolic acidosis necessary before surgery.
3. Episodes of SVT may be treated with adenosine. Betablockers digoxin or verapamil may also be given to prevent episodes of SVT. Radiofrequency ablation techniques have been successful for A V re-entrant mechanisms..
4. Maintenance of good dental hygiene is essential to prevent SBE.
5. If CCF develops, decongestive measures, e.g, digoxin diuretics are indicated.

Surgical

Indications

1. Critically ill neonates who show symptoms within the first week of life (after intensive medical treatment).
2. Severe activity limitation (functional class III or IV).
3. Occurrence of moderate to severe cyanosis, CCF and RVOT obstruction by redundant tricuspid valve.
4. Repeated life threatening arrhythmias with associated WPW syndrome.

Procedures

I. Repair of tricuspid valve and closure of ASD
   a. Danielson technique:[38] Most desirable and best tested technique and used in 60% of patients. It obliterates the atrialized portion of RV and narrows tricuspid orifice which results in a monoleaflet valve (Fig. 7.73).
   b. Carpentier reconstructive surgery:[39] The procedure is the same except that the procedure is in a direction which is at right angles to that used by Danielson. Surgical mortality–15%
2. Tricuspid valve replacement
   - Less desirable approach but may be necessary in 20-30 % of patients.

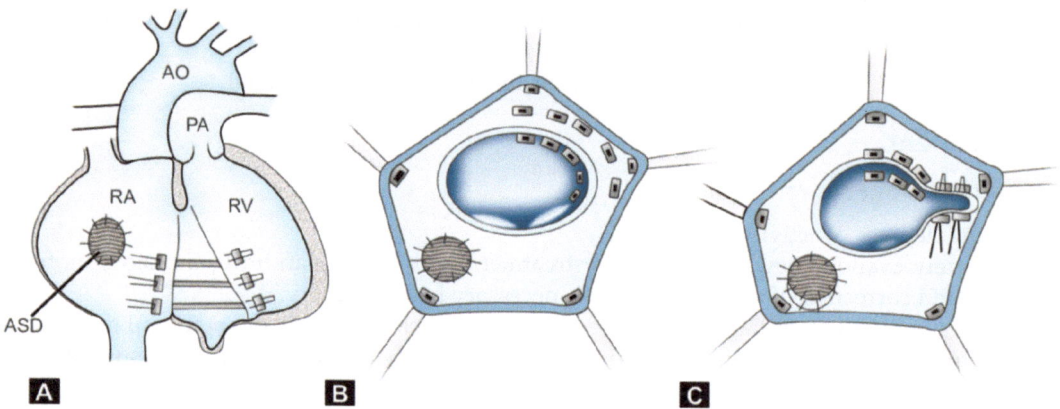

Figs 7.73A to C: Danielson technique for tricuspid valve repair. (A) Series of interrupted mattress switches are placed to obliterate the atrialized portion of the right ventricle (RV). The atrial septal defect (ASD) is closed with a patch. (B) As the switches are tied, the atrialized portion of RV is obliterated, seen through a right atriotomy. (C) Switches are placed to further narrow the tricuspid orifice. The valve is now a monocusp valve (anterior leaflet of tricuspid valve), i.e. mobile and opens widely during diastole

3. Fontan procedure–advocated in patients with severe hypoplasia of functioning RV.
4. For critically ill neonates–
   - Starnes operation—is performed on an urgent basis after intensive medical therapy. The tricuspid valve is closed with a pericardial patch. ASD is enlarged and a systemic to pulmonary artery shunt is created. A fontan type operation is performed later.[40]
5. For patients with recurrent SVT and WPW syndrome, surgical interruption of accessory pathway is recommended.[41] Radio frequency oblation may also be attempted.
6. Finally, in infants and children with severe tricuspid deformity, cardiac transplantation would be the treatment of choice.

Complications

Arrhythmias are the common postoperative complications which include supraventricular arrhythmias and rarely complete heart block.
1. Heart failure–commonest cause of mortality.
2. Arrhythmia–supraventricular arrhythmias are common. Ventricular arrhythmias and complete atrioventricular block requiring pacemaker implantation is common.

3. Infective endocarditis–risk throughout life.
4. Systemic arterial desaturation–polycythemia–coagulation abnormalities may occur.
5. Progressive LV dysfunction if patient survives till adulthood.

REFERENCES

1. Kirklin JW, Barratt-Boyes BG. Complete transposition of great arteries. A long term study. In Kirklin JW, Barratt-Boyes BG, eds. Cardiac surgery, New York. Chuchill Livingstone 1993;1383-1467.
2. Pasquini L, Sanders SP, Parness IA, et al. Caval anatomy in 119 patients with a-loop transposition of great arteries and ventricular septal defect. An echocardiographic and pathological study: J Am Coll Cardiol 1993; 21:1712-21.
3. Anderson RH. Description of origins and epicardial course of the coronary arteries in complete transposition. Cardiol young 1991;1:11-12.
4. Wenovsky G, Bridges ND, Mandell VS, et al. Enlarged bronchial arteries after early repair of transposition of great arteries. J Am Coll Cardiol 1993;21:465-70.
5. Newfeld EA, Paul MH, Muster AJ, et al. Pulmonary vascular disease in complete transpositions of great vessels and intact ventricular septum. Circulation 1979;59:525-30.
6. Levin DL, Paul MH, Muster AJ, et al. D-transposition of great vessels in neonate. A clinical diagnosis Arch Intern Med 1977;137:1421-25.
7. Manzar S, Nair AK, Pai MG, et al. Head size at birth in neonates with transposition of great arteries and hypoplastic left heart syndrome. Saudi Med J 2005;26:453-56.
8. Hayes CJ, Gersomy WM. Arrhythmias after the mustard operation for transposition of great arteries. A long term study. J Am Coll Cardiol 1993;21:465-70.
9. Mathew R, Rosenthal A, Fellows K. Significance of right aortic arch in D-transposition of great arteries. Am Heart J 1974;87:314-17.
10. Mustard WT. Successful two stage correction of transposition of great vessels. Surgery 1964;55:469-72.
11. Senning A. Surgical correction of transposition of great vessels. Surgery 1959;45:966-80.
12. Jatene AD, Foutes VF, Panlista PP, et al. Anatomic correction of transposition of great vessels. J Thorac and cardiovasc Surg 1976;72(3):364-70.
13. Rastelli GC, McGoan DC, Wallace RB. Anatomic correction of transposition of great arteries with ventricular septal defect and subpulmonary stenosis. J thorac Cardiovasc Surg 1969;58:545-52.
14. Lecompte Y, Zannini L, Hazan E, et al. Anatomic correction of transposition of great arteries. J Thorac Cardiovasc Surg 1981;82:629-31.
15. Healy JE Jr. An anatomic survey of anomalous pulmonary veins; Their clinical significance. J thoracic and cardiovasc Surg 1952;23:433-44.
16. Darling RC, Rottiney WB, Craig JM. Total pulmonary venous drainage into the right side of heart: Report of 17 autopsied cases not associated with other cardiovascular anomalies Lab Invest 1957;6:44-64.
17. Smith B, Frye TR, Newton WA Jr. Total anomalous pulmonary venous return: Diagnostic criteria and a new classification Am J Dis Child 1961;101:41-51.

18. Deslisle G, Ando M, Calder AL, et al. Total anomalous autopsied cases with emphasis on diagnosis and surgical consideration. Am Heart J 1976;91:99-122.
19. Burroughs JT, Edwards JE. Total anomalous pulmonary venous connection. Am Heart J 1960;59:913-31.
20. Van Mierop L, Dutsche L. Cardiovascular anomalies in DiGeorge syndrome and importance of neural crest as a possible pathogenetic factor. Am J Cardiol 1986;58:133-37.
21. Collett R, Edwards J. Persistent truncus arteriosus. A classification according to anatomic types. Surg Clin North Am 1949;1245-70.
22. Van Mierop L, Patterson D, Schnaar W. Pathogenesis of persistent truncus arteriosus in light of observations made in a clog embryo with the anomaly. Am J Cardiol 1978;41:755-62.
23. Ferencz C, Loffredo CA, Correa–Villasenor A, et al. Malformation of cardiac outflow tract in genetic and environmental risk factors of major cardiovascular malformations. The Baltimore–Washington Infant study. 1981-1989. Armonk NY. Future Publishing 1997;59-102.
24. Boon AR, Farmer MB, Roberts DF. A family study of Fallots tetralogy. J Med Genet 1972;9:179-92.
25. Rao BN, Anderson RC, Edwards JE. Anatomic variation in tetralogy of Fallot. Am Heart J 1971;81:361-71.
26. Anderson RH, Allwork SP, Ho SY, et al. Surgical anatomy of tetralogy of Fallot. J Thorac cardiovascular Surg 1981;81:887-96.
27. Kothari SS. Mechaisms of cyanotic spells in tetralogy of Fallot–the missing link. Int J Cardiol 1992;37:1-5.
28. Fraser CD Jr, McKenzie ED, Cooley DA. Teralogy of fallot: Surgical management individualized to patient. Am Thorac Surg 2001;71:1556-61.
29. Report of the New England Regional infant cardiac program. Pediatrics 1980;65 (Suppl 2):388-461.
30. Tandon R, Edwards JE. Tricuspid atresia: A re-evaluation and classification. J Thorac Cardiovascular Surg 1974; 67:530-542.
31. Dick M, Fyler DC, Nadas AS. Tricuspid atresia. Clinical course in 101 patients. Am. J. Cardiol 1975; 36: 327-37.
32. Choussat A. Fontan F, Besse P, et al. Selection criteria for Fontan procedure. In. Anderson RH, Shinebourne EA eds. Pediatric cardiology 1977. Edinburgh; Churchill Living stone 1978;559-66.
33. Fyler DC, Buckle LP, Hellenbrand WE, et al. Report of the New England regional infant cardiac program Pediatrics 1980;65:375-461.
34. Newfeld EA, Cole RB, Paul MH. Ebstein's malformation of tricuspid valve in the neonate. Functional and anatomic pulmonary outflow tract obstruction. Am J Cardiol 1967;19:727-31.
35. Schiebler GL, Adams P Jr. Anderson RC, et al. Clinical study of twenty three cases of Ebstein anomaly of the tricuspid valve. Circulation 1959;19:165-87.
36. Kumar AE, Fyler DC, Miettinen OS, et al. Ebstein anomaly: clinical profile and natural history. Am J Cardiol 1971;28:84-95.
37. Zalzstein E, Koren G, Einarson T, et al. A case control study on the association between first trimester exposure to lithium and Ebstein anomaly. Am J Cardiol 1990;65:817-18.
38. Danielson GK, Driscoll DJ, Mair DD, et al. Operative treatment of Ebstein anomaly. J Thorac cardiovascular surgery 1992;104:1195-202.

39. Carpentier A, Chauvad S, Mace L, et al. A new reconstructive operation for Ebstein anomaly of the tricuspid valve. J Thorac Cardiovascular Surg 1988;96:921-101.
40. Starnes VA, Pilbick PT, Bernstein D, et al. Ebstein anomaly appearing in the neonate J Thorac Cardiovascular Surg 1991;101:1082-87.
41. Kugler JD, Gillete PC, Duff DF, et al. Elective mapping and surgical division of the bundle of Kent in a patient with Ebstein anomaly who required tricuspid valve replacement. Am J Cardiol 1978;41:602-05.

CHAPTER 8

Perinatal Cardiology

PART I

Normal Cardiac Findings in the Newborn

Cardiovascular disorders command attention at various times in the perinatal period.

To arrive at a diagnosis of a cardiac disorder in the newborn period, a systematic approach to perinatal cardiology has to be planned out.

Embryology of the Heart

The internal surfaces of the heart and of all the blood vessels are lined by a layer of flattened cells called "endothelium". All components of the heart and blood vessels, i.e. endothelium, muscle and connective tissue are of mesodermal origin. In the early embryonic stage, mesenchyme over the yolk sac, in the connecting stalk and also in the body of the embryo differentiates to form small masses of "angioblastic tissue". This gives rise to endothelium and also to "blood cells". The first blood vessels are derived from endothelium and they proliferate to become interconnected to form a vascular network.

First Phase (Fertilization to Primitive Heart Tube)[2]

The entire cardiovascular system develops from mesoderm. By 18 days of life, the anterolateral plate of mesoderm present over yolk sac, the connecting stalk and the body of the body embryo differentiated to form angioblasts. Angioblasts form the endothelial cell clusters called angiocytes. These spread in a cephalic direction and fuse anteriorly to form a horeshow shaped plexus of small blood vessels.

The heart is first seen in the form of two-endothelial heart tubes (Fig. 8.1A) that soon fuse with one another, in a cranio-caudal direction (Fig. 8.1B). It has an inner endocardium and an outer

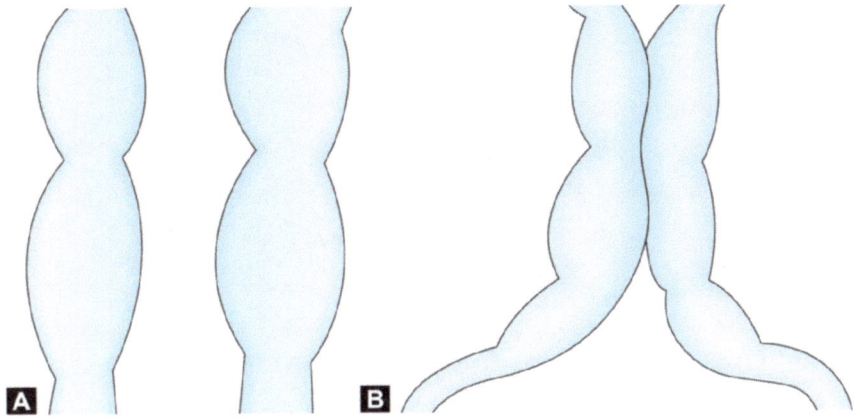

Figs 8.1A and B:[1] Formation of primitive heart tube

myocardium separated by cardiac jelly. Simultaneously the heart tube shows a series of dilatations by 21st–24th day, which from cranial to caudal end are (i) bulbus cordis, (ii) ventricle, (iii) atrium, and (iv) sinus venosus. The ventricle and atrium are connected by a narrow atrioventricular canal (A-V canal). The fusion of the heart tubes in the region of sinus venosus is partial, because it has a central part which communicates with the atrium and of two infused parts called the right and left horns (Fig. 8.1B).

The bulbus cordis represents the arterial end of the heart. It consists of a proximal part called the "conus" (bulbus cordis proper) and a distal part called "truncus arteriosus" (Fig. 8.2). The truncus arteriosus is continuous distally with the aortic sac from which the right and left pharyngeal arches arise. These arteries arch backwards on the lateral side of the foregut to become continuous with the right and left dorsal aortae.

The sinus venosus represents the venous end of the heart.
- One vitelline vein-from yolk sac
- One umbilical vein-from placenta
- One common cardinal vein-from body wall

Fate of Subdivisions of Heart Tubes (Fig. 8.3)

1. *Sinus Venosus*
    a. The body and right horn of sinus venosus are absorbed into the common atrial chamber and form part of the right atrium.

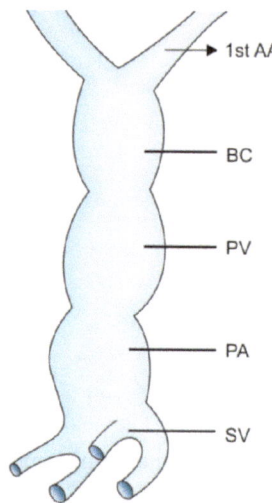

Fig. 8.2:[1] Subdivisions of primary heart tube (AA–aortic arch, BC–Bulbus cordis, PV–Primitive ventricle, PA–Primitive atrium, SV–Sinus venosus

Therefore, the common czardinal vein which forms the terminal part of the superior vena cava and vitelline vein which forms the terminal part of inferior vena cava now open into right atrium.

b. Left horn of the sinus venosus forms part of the coronary sinus which also opens into the right atrium.

Relationship of Pericardial Cavity to Heart Tubes

The endothelial heart tube is derived from the splanchno-pleural mesoderm related to the pericardial cavity (Fig. 8.3). After formation of head fold, this tube lies dorsal to the pericardial cavity and ventral to the foregut (Fig. 8.4). The tube now invaginates the pericardial sac from the dorsal side. As it does, the splanchno-pleuric mesoderm lining the dorsal side of the pericardial cavity proliferates to form a thick layer called the "myoepicardial mantle". When the invagination is complete, the myoepicardial mantle completely surrounds the heart tube. It gives rise to cardiac muscle (myocardium) and also to visceral layer of pericardium (epicardium). The parietal layer of pericardium is derived from somatopleuric mesoderm.

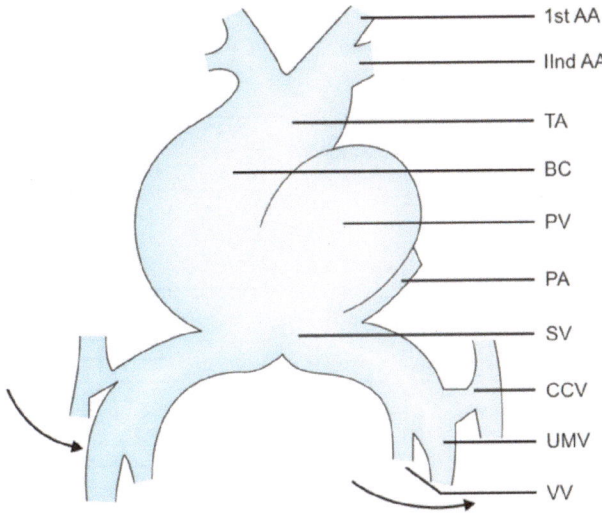

Fig. 8.3: The three paired bilateral venous system (AA – Aortic arch, BC – Bulbus cordis, PV – Primitive ventricle PA – Primitive atrium, TA – Truncus arteriosus, CCV – Common cardinal vein, UMV – Unilateral vein, V V – Vitteline vein. The curved arrows point towards direction of looping

Formation of External Part of the Heart (Fig. 8.4)

The heart tube is for sometime suspended from the dorsal wall of the pericardial cavity by two layers of pericardium that constitute the "dorsal mesocardium". This mesocardium soon disappears and after 23 days post-fertilization, the heart tube lies free in the pericardial sac, suspended by its two ends.

The caudal part of the heart tube, i.e. (atrium and sinus venosus) is embedded within the substance of septum transversum outside the pericardial cavity. The part of the heart tube lying within the pericardial cavity is thus made up of bulbus cordis and ventricle. This part of the tube becomes folded on itself to form a 'V' shaped "bulboventricular loop" and subsequently when the atrium and sinus venosus are freed from septum transversum, they come to lie behind and above the ventricle and the heart tube is now 'S' shaped. At this stage the bulbus cordis (conus) and ventricle are separated by deep bulboventricular sulcus which gradually becomes shallower, so that bulbus cordis and ventricle join to form one chamber which communicates with truncus arteriosus.

The atrial chamber which lies behind the upper part of the ventricle and truncus arteriosus, expands and as it does so, part of it comes to project forward on either side of the truncus. As a result of these changes, the external surface of the heart assumes its definitive shape.

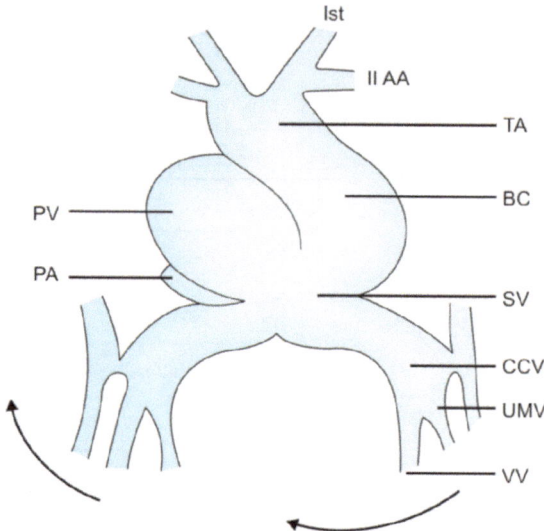

Fig. 8.4:[1] Dorsal view of looping. Arrows are showing towards the direction of looping (AA – Aortic arch, BC – Bulbus cordis, PV – Primitive ventricle, PA – Primitive atrium, TA – Truncus arteriosus, SV – Sinus venous)

Second Phase

27.37 Days of Development

Embryo grows from 5 mm to 17 mm.

The atrial chamber communicates posteriorly with the sinus venosus and antero inferiorly with the ventricle through the atrioventricular canal. It gets divided into two halves when a septum arises from the roof lateral to opening of sinus-venosus-"septum primum" (Fig. 8.5A). This goes downwards and fuses with septum intermedium and upper part breaks down to form foramen secundum.

A second septum develops from the roof of atrium lateral to septum primum-septum secondum which grows downwards and overlaps foramen secundum. The right and left atria now communicate with each other through an oblique valvular opening called "foramen ovale". This foramen ovale persists throughout fetal life (Fig. 8.5).

The right atrium is derived from:
1. Right half of the primitive atrium;
2. Sinus venosus; and
3. Right half of atrioventricular canal.

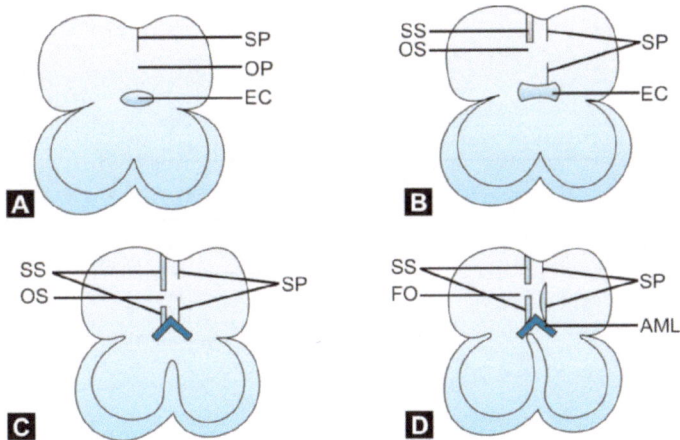

Figs 8.5A to D: Septum formation in the common atrium (SP – Septum primum, OP – Ostium primum, EC – Endocardial cushion, SS – Septum secundum, FO – Foramen ovale, AML Anterior mutual leaflet)

The left atrium similarly is derived from:
1. Left half of the primitive atrial chamber;
2. Left half of atrioventricular canal;
3. Absorbed proximal parts of pulmonary veins.

The conus gives rise to the infundibulum of the right ventricle and to the aortic vestibule of left ventricle.

The ventricles are derived from (Fig. 8.6):
1. Primitive ventricular chamber;
2. Proximal part of bulbus cordis (conus).

- A "spiral septum" appears within the truncus arteriosus, conotruncus and subdivides it into ascending aorta and pulmonary trunk (Figs 8.7A to C).
- The aortic and pulmonary valves are formed at the junction of conus and truncus arteriosus. The mitral and tricuspid valves are formed by the proliferation of connective tissue under the endocardium of the left and right atrioventricular canals.
- Early in development, there are two pairs of lateral dorsal aortae which fuse to form descending aorta. Simultaneously the aortic arches are growing and each arch has a pair of aortic arch arteries. The first, second and fifth arches disappear and third, fourth, fifth and sixth archers form the major cardiac arteries. To summarize, cardiogenesis which starts about 18th day of gestation is

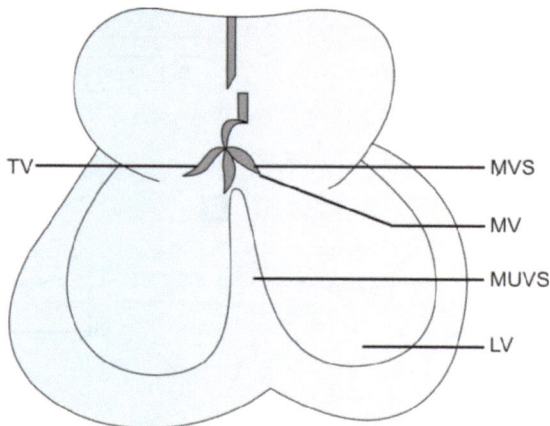

Fig. 8.6: Development of ventricular septum (MV – Mitral valve, LV – Left ventricle, TV – Tricuspid valve, MVS – Membranous ventricular septum, MUVS – Muscular ventricular septum)

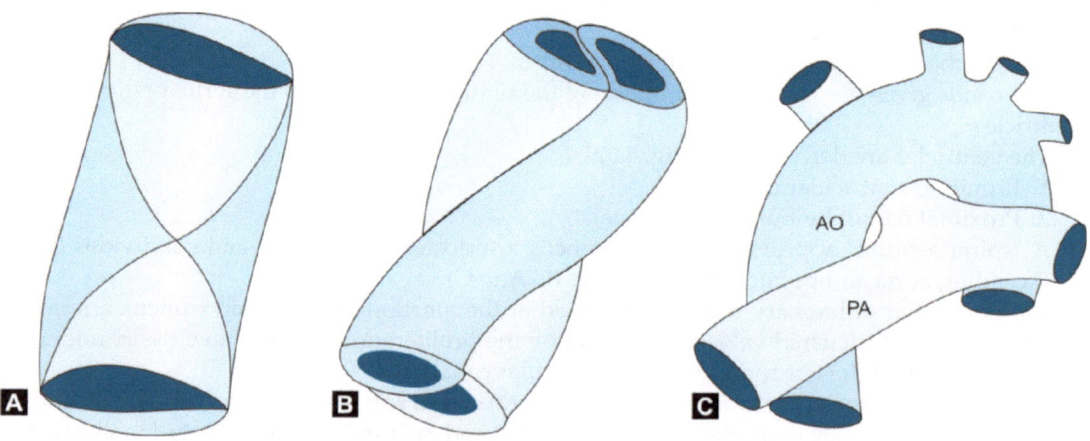

Figs 8.7A to C:[1] Sequential development of pulmonary artery and aorta

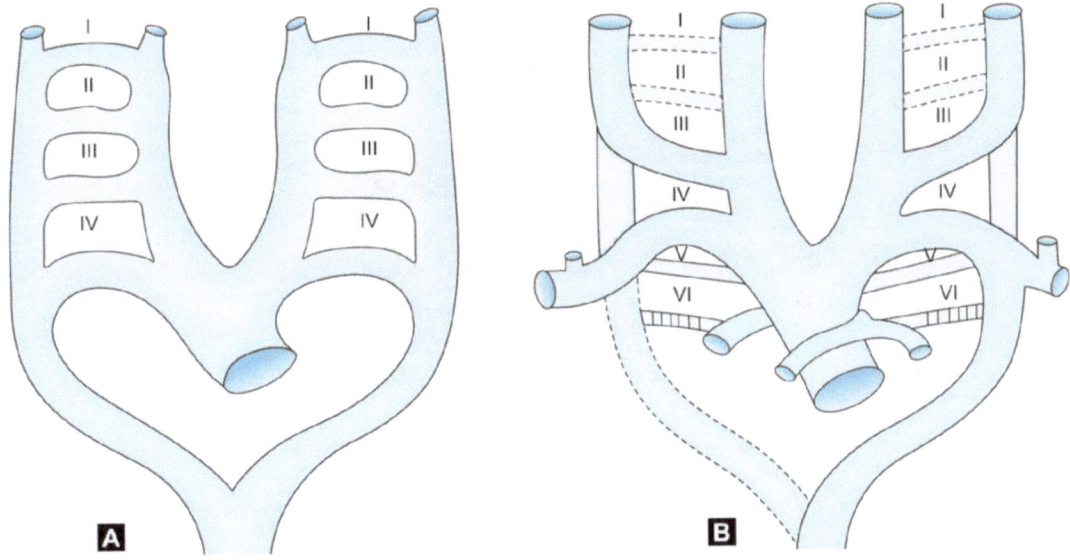

Figs 8.8A and B: Development of aorta and its branches

completed by about 49th day, thereafter maturation process goes on even after birth (Figs 8.8A and B).

Fetal and Perinatal Circulation[3]

Knowledge of fetal and perinatal circulation is an integral part for understanding the pathophysiology and natural history of congenital heart disease (CHD).

Fetal Circulation

Fetal circulation differs from adult circulation in several ways. In adults, gas exchange occurs in lungs while in the fetus, placenta provides the exchange of gases and nutrients.

Course of Fetal Circulation

There are four shunts in fetal circulation: Placenta, ductus venosus, foramen ovale and ductus arteriosus (Fig. 8.9).

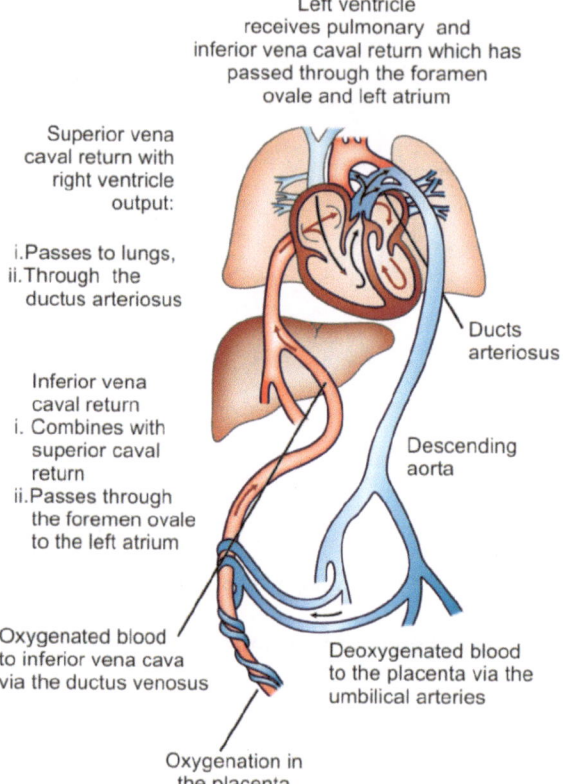

Fig. 8.9: Fetal circulation: arrows indicate the direction of flow. It shows the four sites of shunt – placenta, ductus venosus, foramen ovale and ductus arteriosus

1. The placenta receives the largest amount of combined (right and left) ventricular output (55%) and has the lowest vascular resistance in the fetus.
2. Superior vena cava (SVC) drains the upper part of body including the brain (15% of ventricular output).
   Inferior vena cava (IVC) drains the lower part of body including placenta (10% of ventricular output).
   Since the placenta has oxygenated blood, IVC has 70% and SVC has 40% of the same. The highest PO_2 is found in the umbilical vein (32 mm Hg).

3. Most of the SVC blood goes to RV. One third of the IVC blood with higher O_2 saturation is directed to the left atrium by crista dividens through foramen ovale, whereas the remaining two thirds enters the ventricle and main pulmonary artery (MPA). This means that the brain and coronary circulation receive blood with higher oxygen saturation (PO_2 of 28 mm Hg) than the lower half of body (PO_2 of 24 mm Hg).
4. Less oxygenated blood in the pulmonary artery (PA) flows through the widely open ductus arteriosus to the descending aorta and then to the placenta for oxygenation.

Since the lungs receive only 15% of combined ventricular output, the branches of pulmonary artery are small. This is what gives rise to the pulmonary flow murmur of the newborn. The RV is larger and more dominant than left ventricle (LV). The RV handles 55% of combined ventricular output, whereas the LV handles 45%, in addition; the RV pressure is identical to that of LV and this is reflected in the ECG of newborn which shows dominant RV forces.

Changes at Birth

Within minutes after birth, the gas exchange mechanism has to be transferred from placenta to lungs. With the first breath, the fetal lung expands, it reduces the pulmonary vascular resistance but increases pulmonary blood flow. With the cord being clamped, the placenta is cut off and systemic vascular resistance is increased, thereby increasing aortic pressure.

The primary change is a shift of blood for oxygenation from placenta to the lungs. The placental circulation disappears and the pulmonary circulation is established.
1. Interruption of the umbilical cord results in the following:
    a. An increase in systemic vascular resistance (SVR) as a result of removal of placenta.
    b. Closure of ductus venosus as a result of lack of return of blood from placenta.
2. Lung expansion results in the following:
    a. Reduction in pulmonary vascular resistance (PVR), increase in pulmonary blood flow (PBF) and a fall in PA pressure.
    b. Functional closure of foramen ovale occurs as a result of increased pressure in the LA, in excess of right atrium (RA). The LA pressure increases as a result of increased pulmonary venous return and RA pressure falls as a result of closure of ductus venosus.
    c. Closure of ductus arteriosus (DA) as a result of increased arterial oxygen saturation.

Closure of Ductus Arteriosus

When aortic pressure increases the direction of flow in the ductus is reversed, from aorta to pulmonary artery which is for a short period.

Functional closure of the ductus arteriosus occurs by constriction of the medial smooth muscle in the ductus within 10-15 hours after birth because of increased arterial oxygen tension. It is functionally closed by 72 hours. Anatomic closure of the ductus is completed by 2-3 weeks of age by permanent changes, cellular necrosis of the endothelium and sub-intimal layers of the ductus. Oxygen, prostaglandin E_2 levels and maturity of the newborn are important factors in the closure of the ductus.

Newborn Cardiac Assessment

Newborn infants have right ventricular (RV) dominance with a thick RV wall and elevated pulmonary venous resistance secondary to a thick medial layer of the pulmonary arterioles. The thick pulmonary artery (PA) smooth muscle gradually becomes thinner and by 6-8 weeks of age it resembles that of an adult. Premature infants have less RV dominance and a lower PVR than full term neonates.

PHYSIOLOGICAL PARAMETERS OF CLINICAL IMPORTANCE

Physical Examination

The bedside evaluation of a newborn or a preterm is an absolute necessity.

Normal Physical Findings

The neonatal period is the first month of life where as infancy is up to the end of first year of life.

Full Term Newborn
1. Heart rate-80-180 beats/minute (average-100/minute)
2. Varying degree of acrocyanosis
3. Mild arterial desaturation with arterial PO_2-as low as 60 mm of Hg is quite common-may be due to an intrapulmonary shunt or a transient R-L shunt through patent foramen ovale (PFO) (Fig. 8.10 and Table 8.1).
4. Right ventricle is relatively hyperactive-point of maximum impulse at the left lateral sternal border than the apex.
5. S_2 may be single and ejection click due to pulmonary hypertension may be heard in first few days of life.
6. The newborn may have an innocent heart murmur-gr 2/6 ejection systolic murmur which radiates all over the chest and back. It is due to pulmonary flow and usually disappears after 10-15 days.

Preterm
1. Prevalence and loudness of pulmonary flow murmur are greater in preterms than in full term infants because of thin chest wall.
2. Patent ductus arteriosus (PDA) murmur is more common.
3. The peripheral pulses are of high volume and bounding because of lack of subcutaneous tissue.

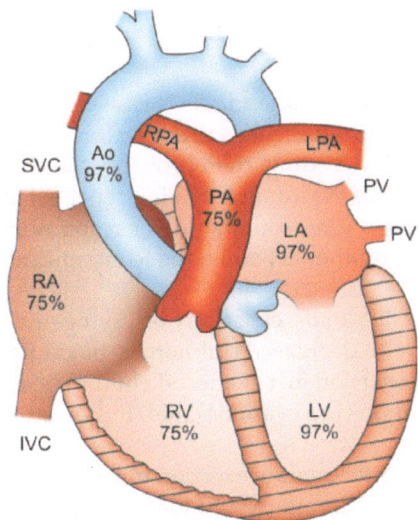

Fig. 8.10: Schematic diagram showing normal oxygen saturation at different levels, oxygen saturation in right side (RA, RV and PA) is approximately 75% and in left side (LA, LV and aorta) is 97% (PV-Pulmonary vein, RPA – right pulmonary artery, LPA – left pulmonary artery, SVC – superior vena cava, IVC – inferior vena cava)

Table 8.1: Normal pressures and oxygen saturation at different sites[2]

	O_2 saturation	Pressure in mm of Hg		O_2 saturation	Pressure in mm of Hg
SVC	70%	–	PV	99%	–
IVC	75%	–	LA	97%	A 3-10
RA	75%	A3-10			V3-12
		V3-10			Mean 3-10
		Mean 2-7	LV	97%	Systole 100-140
RV	75%	Systole 15-30			ED 3-12
		ED 4-12	Aorta	97%	Systole 100-140
PA	75%	Systole 5-30			Dias 60-90
		Dias 4-12			
		Mean 9-18			

ED-end-diastolic, dias-diastolic, SVC-superior vena cava, IVC-inferior vena cava, RA-right atrium, LA-left atrium, RV–right ventricle, LV-left ventricle, FA-pulmonary artery, PV-pulmonary vein

Evidence of Cardiac Abnormalitiy in a Newborn

History

Eliciting reliable history from parents or attendants is essential.
1. *Feeding difficulty:* If the baby is not able to feed properly (breast or bottle feed)–becomes breathless or has excessive sweating during feeding, then probably the child is decompensated.
2. *Repeated respiratory infection:* If the infant is having repeated attacks of breathlessness, cough, restlessness and presence of grunting sounds (lower respiratory tract infection) more than six times per year, indicates high pulmonary flow due to significant left to right shunt.
3. *Other typical histories*
   a. History of discoloration of lips, nails, especially on crying–indicates the possibility of cyanotic congenital heart disease, with decreased pulmonary blood flow probably due to R-L shunt.
   b. History of squatting after exertion in a cyanosed child indicates TOF or TOF like physiology.
   c. History of frequent palpitations in a cyanotic child, Ebsteins anomaly should be the most likely diagnosis.
   d. History of syncope on mild to moderate exertion in an acyanotic child–indicates either severe aortic stenosis (AS), or HOCM, severe pulmonary hypertension or congenitally corrected transposition of great arteries producing bradycardia.
4. *Family history:* A detailed family history–of a child with CHD increases the chance of CHD in subsequent children about ten fold. History of any maternal systemic illness, use of any drug, any infection or exposure to radiation during pregnancy carries significance.

Physical Examination

General Appearance
1. Mongoloid facies – Down's syndrome
   Elfin facies   – William's syndrome
   Moon-like facies – Valvular plmonary stenosis (PS).
2. Presence of polydactyly, fingerized thumb–indicate ASD, VSD.
3. Short neck or low hair line–Noonan's syndrome.

Common clinical syndrome associated with CHD
- Down's syndrome (Trisomy 21)–Endocardial cushion defect, VSD, ASD.
- Turner's syndrome (XO)-Coarctation of aorta.
- Marfan's syndrome–Aortic aneurysm, AR, MVP, dissection of aorta.
- Rubella syndrome–PDA, pulmonary artery branch stenosis.
- Noonan syndrome–PS, ASD with PS.

- DiGeorge syndrome–Aortic arch, conotruncal anomaly.
- Holt Oram syndrome–Familial ASD.
- Ellis-van Creveld syndrome–Single atrium.
- Kartagener's syndrome–Dextrocardia
- William's syndrome–supraventricular AS.
- Laurence Moon Biedl syndrome–TOF.
- Puffiness of face and edema over dorsum of hands and feet–indicate possibility of CHF in infants.
- Poor physical development–in presence of CHD signifies IUGR.
- Birth weight:
  - Larger babies–either born to diabetic mothers or presence of cardiomyopathy or TGA.
- Small babies–low birth weight, premature or weight < 1.5 Kg–have more chances of having congenital heart disease.
- *Color of infant:*
  - Pale, dusky or blue
    Central cyanosis–at palate, tongue, etc. If the color does not improve with O_2 inhalation–suggests a cardiac abnormality.
- *Respiration:* Respiratory distress in newborns and infants is diagnosed by presence of tachypnea, altered depth of breathing, intercostal retraction, flaring of alae nasi, stridor, grunting, etc.

Age	Respiratory–Rate
Newborn	60.
Infants	up to 30
1-4 years	25-28
Adolescents	18-20

- *Arterial pulse:* The peripheral pulses like radial, brachial, femoral, carotid, dorsalis pedis are easily felt in newborns. Pulse varies from 90-160/min in a newborn, average being 125/min. Relatively slow or irregular pulse are common in preterms. Decreased or absent peripheral pulses especially in the lower limbs suggest coarctation of aorta (COA). Weak peripheral pulse suggests low output state or hypoplastic left heart syndrome. Bounding pulse in infants indicate aortic runoff lesions such as PDA, aortic regurgitation or truncus arteriosus.
- Abnormal heart rate (slow or fast) and irregular rhythm–both suggest a cardiac abnormality.
- *Jugular venous pressure (JVP):* JVP is difficult to interpret in newborns and infants because of short neck and tachycardia. If the upper limb veins are visible or become more prominent by raised position the hand from cardiac level, it is presumed that mean venous pressure is increased.
- *Heart murmur:* is usually due to an underlying cardiac disorder. But innocent murmur due to pulmonary flow is more common than pathologic murmurs.

II. Blood Pressure Measurements

Although blood pressure (BP) is not routinely measured in a newborn infant—it has to be measured when a diagnosis of CoA, hypertension or hypotension due to any cause is suspected. It is not possible to measure BP with a conventional sphygmomanometer because "Korotkoff" sounds are very faint and so electronic devices measure blood pressures in newborns and preterms.

In infants, B.P is measured by
1. Flush method–not accurate, so not used anymore.
2. Doppler ultrasound method.
3. Oscilometric (Dinamap) method.

It is recommended that the bladder width of the blood pressure cuff is approximately 50% and the bladder length is approximately 80% of arm circumference midway between the olecranon and acromion. Typically, with such cuffs, the width of the inflatable bag covers two third of the full length of the arm. The equipment necessary to measure blood pressure in children of 3 years of age through adolescence include pediatric cuffs of different sizes.

For premature–newborn–cuff Size 4-8 cm
For infants–6-12 cm
For older children–9-18 cm.

In general, blood pressure obtained by palpation or flush technique is significantly less accurate than auscultation. The systolic pressure is recorded as the first audible Korotkoff sound, with the diastolic pressure correlating best with muffling phases or fourth Korotkoff sound. Every child should have a comparison of upper and lower limb systolic blood pressure. Lower limb systolic pressure is generally 10 mm higher than the upper limb systolic pressure.

Direct Blood Pressure Measurements (Table 8.2)

Many sick full term and premature newborns require intra-arterial recording of BP but normative levels have not been established because of the invasive nature. Blood pressure increases after first few days of life as demonstrated by Doppler ultrasound or oscillometric methods. The full term newborn is declared to be hypertensive when the systolic BP is greater than 90 mm Hg and diastolic

Table 8.2: Direct aortic pressure-normal blood pressure values in first 24 hours[3]

	Full term	Preterm
Systolic	70 ± 10	65 ± 5
Diastolic	41 ± 6	40 ± 4
MAP (Mean arterial pressure)	50 ± 7	48 ± 5

BP is greater than 60 mm Hg. Similarly, in preterm infants, when the systolic BP is more than 80 mm Hg and diastolic more than 50 mm Hg.

Electrocardiography

Normal ECG[4]

The normal ECG of a newborn is different from that of a child or an adult and usually shows the following (Fig. 8.11):

1. Sinus tachycardia-heart rate goes as high as 180.
2. Right axis deviation $+125° - +180°$
3. Small voltage-QRS and T waves
4. RV dominance with tall R waves in V_1, V_2 and V_4R.
5. Benign arrhythmias.
6. Occasional q waves in V_1 (seen in 10% of normal newborns).

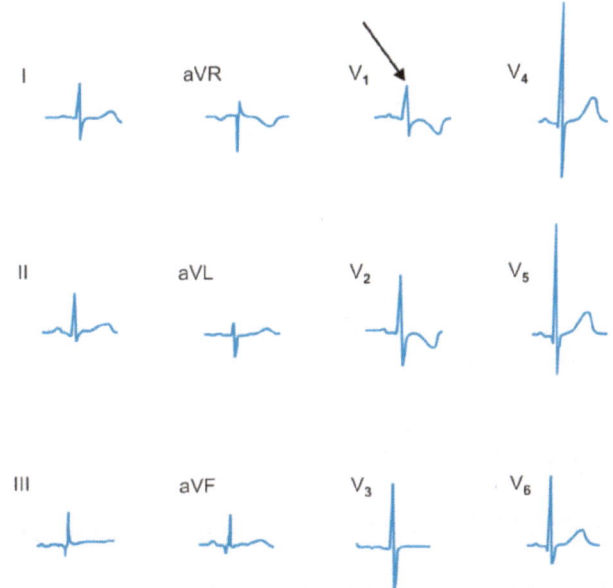

Fig. 8.11:[2] Healthy neonatal ECG. Arrow, normal RV predominance

Abnormal ECG

P wave
1. AP axis is in the right lower quadrant (90°-180°)-suggests atrial situs inversus, asplenia syndrome or incorrectly placed ECG electrodes.
2. A superior P axis-ectopic atrial rhythm or polysplenia syndrome.

QRS axis
1. A QRS axis between 0-150° (left anterior hemiblock)-suggests ECD (endocardial cushion defect) or tricuspid atresia.
2. A QRS axis-less than 30° is abnormal and indicates left axis deviation (LAD) for the patients age. LAD may be seen with LVH.
3. A QRS axis greater than + 180° (– 150° to 180°)-indicates RAD. It may occur with RVH and RBBB.

Left Ventricular Hypertrophy (Fig. 8.12)
1. Relative LAD less than + 60°– suggests LVH.
2. R in V_6 greater than 17 mm in first week.
3. R in V_6 greater than 25 mm in first month.
4. Inverted T in V_6 or T_1 with voltage changes.
5. Adult R/S progression, that is, SV_1 greater than RV_1 (before day 3).

Right Ventricular Hypertrophy (Fig. 8.13)

RVH is difficult to diagnose because of the normal dominance of the RV at this age. However, the following are clues to RVH in the newborn:
1. S waves in lead aVL or V_6 are 12 mm or greater.
2. Pure R waves (no S waves) in V_1 that are greater than 10 mm.
3. R waves in V_1 that are greater than 25 mm or R waves in VR that are greater than 8 mm.
4. Upright T waves seen in V_1 may be also seen in 10% of normal newborns.
5. Upright T waves seen in V_1 after 3 days of age.
6. RAD with QRS axis greater than + 180°.

Atrial hypertrophy (Fig. 8.14)
1. Right atrial hypertrophy (RAH) is revealed by a P. wave amplitude greater than 3 mm in any lead.
2. Left atrial hypertrophy (LAH) is revealed by a P wave duration of 0.08 second or greater (usually with notched P waves in limb leads and biphasic P waves in V_1).

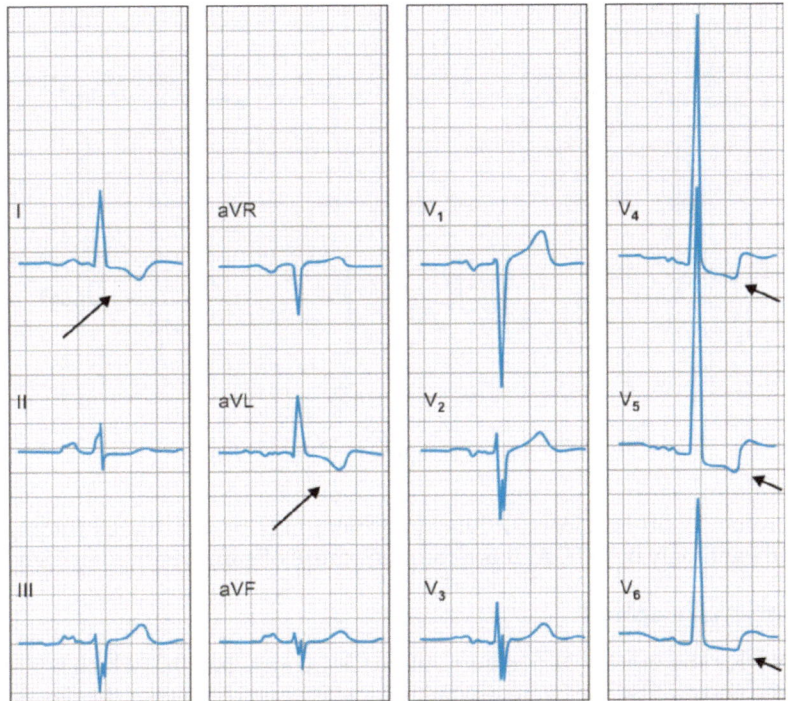

Fig. 8.12:[4] ECGs of patient with left-ventricular hypertrophy. Arrow, ST-segment depression and T-wave inversion

Ventricular Conduction Disturbances

Ventricular conduction disturbances, e.g. RBBB, LBBB, WPW syndrome-QRS duration-0.07 second or more

QRS duration increases with age in normal newborns.
1. RBBB-usually associated with Ebstein's anomaly, COA or ASD.
2. LBBB-very rare in newborns.
3. Intraventricular block (widening of QRS complex)-more significant than RBBB. It is often associated with metabolic abnormalities–hypoxia, acidosis, hyperkalemia, etc.

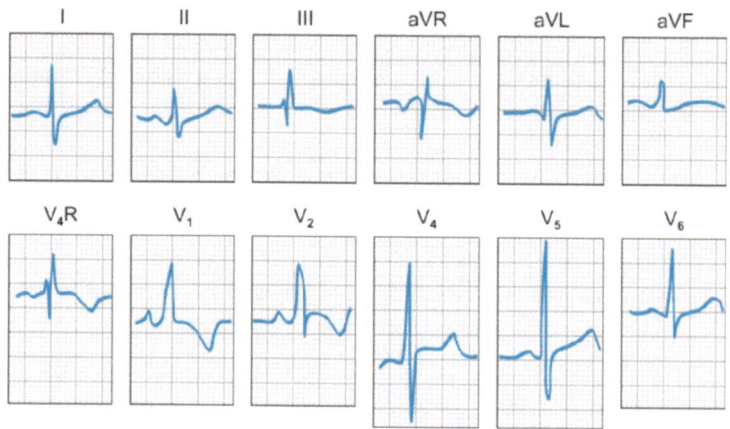

Fig. 8.13:[4] ECGs of patients with right ventricular hypertrophy

4. WPW syndrome (Wolff-Parkinson-White syndrome)-may be an isolated finding or associated with Ebstein's anomaly or L-TGA. It is a frequent cause of supraventricular tachycardia (SVT).

Chest Roentgenography[6]

The cardiothoracic ratio of normal newborn infants is greater than 0.5, which is the normal value in older children and adults. The evaluation of heart size should consider the degree of inspiration judged from level of diaphragm.

Abnormal Chest X-ray[6]

A cardiac problem is suggested by abnormal size, position and silhouette of the heart, by an abnormal shape or position of liver or by increased or decreased pulmonary vascularity.

1. *Heart size:* Cardiomegaly may be seen in the following:
   a. VSD, PDA, TGA, Ebsteins anomaly, HL HS.
   b. Myocarditis or cardiomyopathy.
   c. Pericardial effusion.
   d. Metabolic disturbances-hypoglycemia, hypoxemia and acidosis.
   e. Overhydration or overtransfusion.

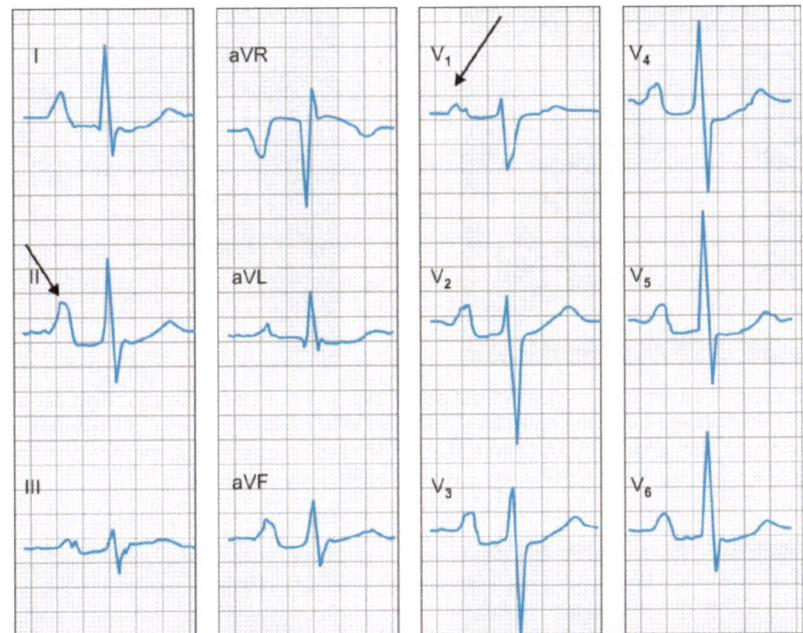

Fig. 8.14:[4] ECG of patients with atrial enlargement. Note the prolonged PR interval (0.28s) in arrows, P-wave changes in right atrial enlargement; and left-atrial enlargement

2. *Abnormal cardiac silhouette*
   a. Boot-shaped heart-seen in tetralogy of Fallot and Tricuspid atresia (Fig. 8.15).
   b. Egg-shaped heart with a narrow waist-TGA (Fig. 8.16).
   c. Large globular heart-Ebstein's anomaly (Fig. 8.17).
   d. Snowman's appearance or "Figure of 8"-TAPVC (Fig. 8.18).
3. *Dextrocardia or mesocardia:* Four common situations in which the heart is located in the right side of chest:
   a. Situs inversus totalis with normal heart (Fig. 8.19).
   b. Hypoplasia of right lung with rightward displacement of a normally formed heart (dextroversion).

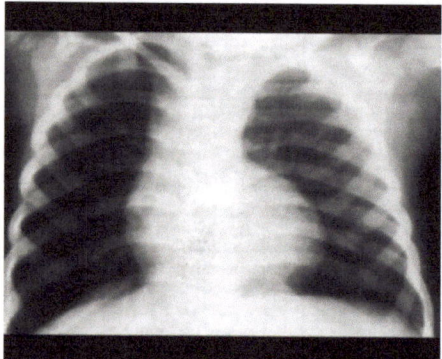

Fig. 8.15: Boot-shaped heart. X-ray chest in patient with tetralogy of Fallot showing normal heart size, RV type apex, presence of pulmonary bay and diminished pulmonary vascular marking. Right aortic arch is also seen

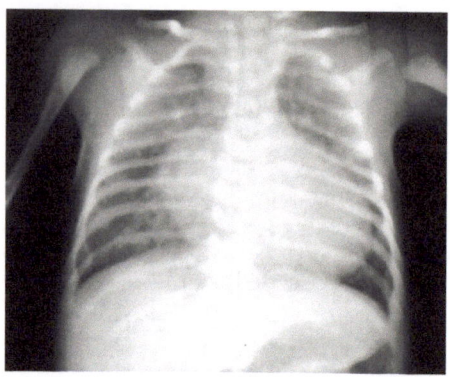

Fig. 8.16: Characteristic 'Egg on side' appearance in d-transposition of great arteries. Note presence of cardiomegaly with narrow pedicle and increased pulmonary markings

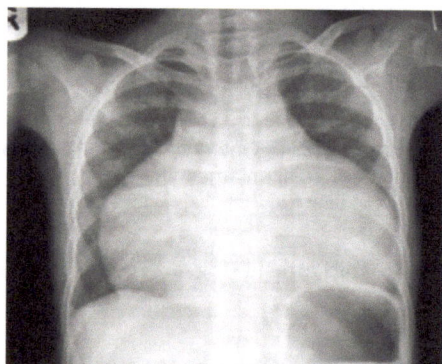

Fig. 8.17: Typical X-ray chest findings in patients with Ebstein's anomaly. Presence of cardiomegaly absent MPA shadow, gross RA enlargement with diminished pulmonary vascular markings

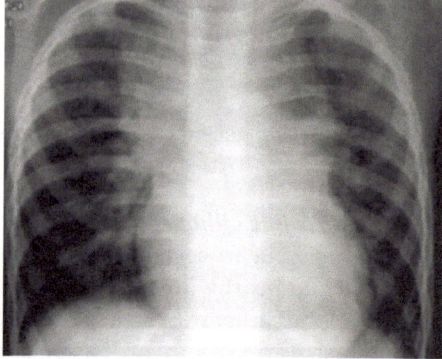

Fig. 8.18: Characteristic 'Snow man appearance' or 'figure of 8' in patient with supracardiac TAPVC draining into left innominate vein through vertical vein. Upper part of figure of 8 is formed by ascending vertical vein, dilated innominate and dilated SVC and the lower part of figure '8' by the cardiac shadow. The pulmonary vasculature is increased

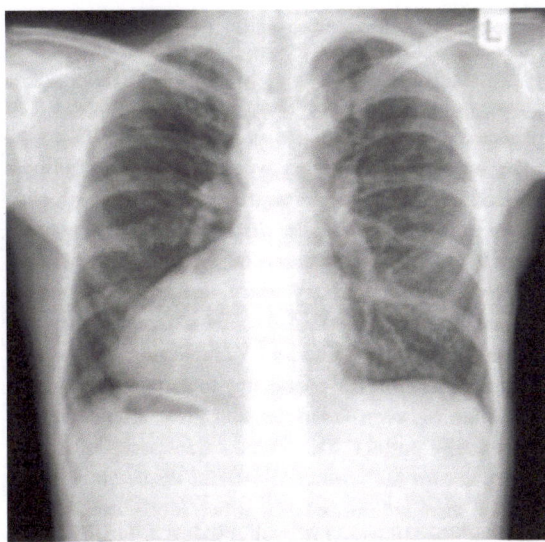

Fig. 8.19: X-ray chest PA view showing situs inversus. Note the presence of stomach bubble on the right side and liver shadow on the left side. The pattern of bronchial bifurcation is also suggestive of situs inversus

    c. Complex cyanotic heart defect including atrial or ventricular inversion.
    d. Asplenia or polysplenia syndrome with midline liver (Fig. 8.20).
4. Pulmonary vascular markings (PVM)
    a. Increased pulmonary vascularity: (Fig. 8.15)
       Cyanotic infant-TGA, truncus arteriosus, single ventricle.
       Acyanotic infant-VSD, PDA, endocardial cushion defect.
    b. Decreased pulmonary vascularity (Fig. 8.16)
       Cyanotic-pulmonary atresia, tricuspid atresia, TOF with pulmonary atresia.
       Heart size is usually normal in these conditions.
       Decreased pulmonary vascularity with marked cardiomegaly–Ebstein's anomaly.
    c. A "ground glass" appearance or a reticulated pattern of lung fields is characteristic of pulmonary venous obstruction and suggests HL HS on TAPVC with obstruction.
5. *Situs of abdominal viscera*
    a. Midline liver-asplenia or polysplenia syndrome with complex cyanotic CHD (Fig. 8.20).

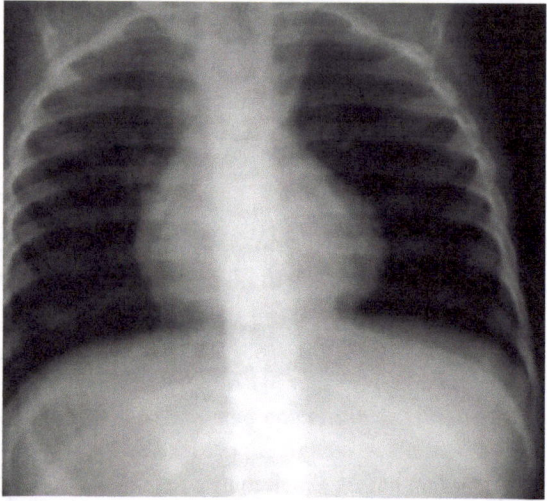

Fig. 8.20: X-ray chest showing large midline liver with dextrocardia. This should immediately alert the physician for presence of complex congenital heart disease associated with isomerism

    b. Left-sided liver (right-sided stomach bubble) with heart on right side of chest-Situs inversus. (Fig. 8.19)
    c. Liver and cardiac apex on same side-suggest complex cardiac defects.

Perinatal Echocardiography (Table 8.3)

The application of high frequency sound waves for cardiac diagnosis in the initial perinatal or newborn period has revolutionized the diagnostic process and promoted the early and prompt intervention necessary for survival of many with serious cardiac defects. Safe, accurate, non-interventional fetal diagnosis can be made in the second trimester of pregnancy and they can be verified by repeat Echo/Doppler study in the immediate newborn period. Surgical treatment of severe cardiac defects can be undertaken without cardiac catheterization in most instances. Echocardiography has multiple modes of examination which include M-mode, Two-dimensional and Doppler echocardiography. Two-dimensional echo examinations are performed by directing the plane of the transducer beam along a number of cross-sectional planes through the heart and great vessels by four transducer

Table 8.3: Echocardiography–Indications[5]

I. Familial
   a. Family history of CAD in first degree relative
   b. Family history of chromosomal related disorders.
      - Down's syndrome
      - Edward's syndrome
      - Turner's syndrome
      - Patau's syndrome
      - Noonan's syndrome
      - Tuberous sclerosis
II. Maternal
   - H/o exposure to teratogens
      A. X–rays
      B. Infections–Rubella-PDA
         – Coxsackie B
         – Toxoplasmosis
      C. Drugs–Alcohol-ASD
         – Lithium–Ebstein's anomaly
         – Phenytoin sodium, valproate, carbamazepine
         – Warfarin
         – Hypervitaminosis D–Supravalvular AS
   - Metabolic disorders
      A. Diabetes mellitus–HOCM
      B. SLE–Complete heart block.
      C. Hyperthyroidism–Fetal tachyarrhythmia
      D. Phenyl Ketonuria
III. Fetal
   A. Extracardiac anomalies
      i. Anatomic–exomphalous, diaphragmatic hernia.
      ii. Chromosomal–Trisomy 13-15, 18 or 21 detected–Amniocentesis
   B. Fetal arrhythmias
      Fixed bradycardia
      Irregular rhythm
      Tachycardia (>180/bpm) in absence of amnionitis.
   C. Intrauterinc growth retardation
   D. Non immune hydrops fetalis–abnormal fetal situs.

locations-parasternal, apical, subcostal and suprasternal notch positions. The parasternal long axis view is the most basic view and shows the left ventricular inflow and outflow tracts.

Indications for Two-dimensional Echo Examinations

1. Routinely screen newborns and small infants who appear to have cardiac defects or dysfunction.
2. To rule out cyanotic congenital heart disease (CHD) in newborns with findings of persistent fetal circulation.
3. PDA has to be suspected in a newborn with ventricular dysfunction or in a premature infant who is on a ventilator.
4. To confirm diagnosis in infants and children with findings of certain cardiac defects.
5. To confirm or rule out cardiac abnormality suggested on clinical examination, X-ray chest, ECG, etc.
6. To monitor and see the effect of drugs, e.g. indomethacin therapy in PDA, LV dysfunction in CCF etc.

Benefits of Fetal Echocardiography

Fetal Echocardiography[5]

Congenital heart disease (CHD) is the most common severe congenital abnormality which may amount to approximately 50 to 75,000 children being born with a major CHD every year. Prenatal diagnosis of congenital heart disease also results in referral of mothers with affected fetuses to a tertiary care center where an affected newborn can be looked after in an integrated manner.

Detection of congenital heart disease before delivery is clinically important due to the potential life threatening implication at birth. Early detection of cardiac anomalies offers the possibility of termination of pregnancy, delivery and immediate postnatal care in the same institution.

Fetal echocardiography has definite benefits as stated below:

1. A normal fetal scan is very reassuring for a family with a previous child affected with a congenital heart disease.
2. Parental counseling and education allowing the potential parents to be better prepared psychologically at the time of delivery. If a serious defect is detected, e.g. hypoplastic left heart syndrome, parents can be given a choice of termination of pregnancy.
3. The pregnant mother is transported and the baby delivered in a center well equipped with neonatal cardiac care, thus allowing a smooth transition from pre to post natal life. Timely institution of prostaglandin infusion for ductus dependant lesions helps in avoiding acidosis and hypoxia.

4. Management of arrhythmia *in utero* can be life saving and if features of hydrops are present, an early delivery can be undertaken if drug therapy is not effective.
5. Fetal echocardiography will play a major role in future to guide in utero treatment in some cardiac defects which are amenable to surgery and intervention.

Optimal Timing of Screening

Transvaginal examination of fetal heart is possible as early as 9-10 week of gestation. However transabdominal optimum echo pictures are generally possible by 16 weeks onwards. Thus the ideal time for fetal echocardiography is at about 18-22 weeks, because at this age almost all details of cardiac structures are possible to evaluate. A relook at mid second trimester of gestation may be necessary even if an earlier first trimester scan was normal, as some of the congenital heart defects can develop later e.g. hypoplasia of a ventricle secondary to inflow or outflow obstruction.

ACKNOWLEDGEMENTS

All the diagrams on Embryology have been taken from "Human Embryology"[1] by Dr. Inderbir Singh.

PART II

Recognition of Cardiac Disorders in the Fetus and Newborn Period

Most pediatric cardiologists face problems in diagnosing cardiac disorders in the following situations:
- Antepartum-myocardial dysfunction, arrhythmia or a congenital heart defect which has been detected by fetal echocardiogram.
- Early neonatal life-presence of cyanosis, respiratory distress and suspicion of patent ductus arteriosus in preterms.
- Late neonatal life–presence of a murmur, presence of signs of congestive cardiac failure. The following topics relating to fetal and neonatal period will be discussed in some detail.
    1. Fetal
    2. Preterm neonate
    3. Transient myocardial ischemia
    4. Presence of heart murmur in a newborn
    5. Cyanotic neonate
    6. Congestive cardiac failure
    7. Arrhythmias.

Fetal

Recognition of a Cardiac Abnormality[7]

Cardiovascular system is the first major system to function in the embryo and the heart starts to function in the beginning of fourth week. Until recently fetal heart rate monitoring was the only means to identify a fetus with a possible cardiac problem. Even now, only about 10% of congenital heart diseases (CHD) are detected prenatally. Fetal echocardiography allows precise and clear anatomic definition of the fetal heart by 16 weeks of gestation with motion mode (M-mode), and two dimensional scanning. Color Doppler studies can determine cardiac abnormalities even as early as 10 weeks. Finding a normal complement of chambers, valves, septae and normal continuity (mitral aortic, septal-aortic) helps to rule out the presence of congenital malformation of the heart and they have been instrumental in diagnosing over 20 types of cardiac abnormalities in the fetus (Table 8.4).

Many complex congenital malformations require prostaglandin E_1 to maintain ductal patency after birth to supply either pulmonary blood flow in (pulmonary atresia) or systemic perfusion in (interrupted aortic arch). If ductal dependent complex CHDs (TGA with PS, pulmonary atresia) are diagnosed prenatally, then appropriate obstetric plans are made for availability of prostaglandin E_1 which can be administered soon after birth to avoid ductal closure, or even termination of pregnancy.

Table 8.4: Cardiac abnormalities detected by fetal echocardiography

Structural abnormalities	
A. Cyanotic	
• Transposition of great vessels	• Truncus arteriosus
• Pulmonary atresia	• Double outlet right ventricle
• Tetralogy of Fallot	• Single ventricle
• Tricuspid atresia	• Atrioventricular canal defect (Complete)
B. Acyanotic	
• Coarctation of aorta	
• Ventricular septal defect	• Hypoplastic left heart syndrome
• Atrial septal defect	• Aortic stenosis
(Ostium secundum), (Ostium primum)	• Absence of pulmonary valve

Fetal echocardiography has also been useful in detecting fetal arrhythmias and heart failure *in utero* as well as to monitor antiarrhythmic and decongestive therapy *in utero*. It also provides valuable information regarding cardiac function and effect of gestational age on growth of cardiac structures, which is helpful in family counseling.

Echocardiographic Assessment of Fetal Cardiovascular Abnormality

Performance: M-mode echocardiographic studies of human fetus provide insight into the relative size and pressure of fetal ventricles. The timing of mechanical events during various phases of cardiac cycle as reflected by wall motion and motion of cardiac valves may be used to analyze the cardiac rhythm.[10] Two dimensional imaging may provide insight into relative chamber and blood vessel volume and pressure. The addition of colour flow Doppler adds further information regarding the function of atria, ventricular and semilunar valve and flow important fetal flow pathways such as ductus venosus, foramen ovale and ductus arteriosus. Pulsed Doppler flow analysis has been used to estimate regional blood flow distribution within the human fetus during the third trimester of pregnancy.

The risk of fetal echocardiography is considered minimal and Doppler studies are also considered safe. Pulsed wave Doppler delivers more energy than color Doppler and continuous wave Doppler delivers the least energy of all.

During certain medical therapeutic measures for the mother, fetal echocardiography has an important role in monitoring the health of the fetus, specifically, when indomethacin is used for preterm labor or polyhydramnios which has been shown to cause multiple abnormalities in the fetus. Constriction of ductus arteriosus or tricuspid regurgitation has been found in up to 10% of fetuses of mothers receiving indomethacin. The effect appears to be greatest in fetuses greater than 34 weeks of gestation. Pulsed Doppler evaluation can quantify the constriction and also the flow through the ductus and therapy can be adjusted if significant gradient across the ductus is found. Pulmonary hypertension has resulted from surgical constriction of fetal lamb ductus and thereby the risk of postnatal pulmonary hypertension may mandate early labor if ductal constriction is present.

The common occurrence of both an abnormal foramen ovale and flow through the ductus arteriosus in fetal transposition of great arteries (TGA) may be explained by the pathophysiology of TGA. In normal fetal circulation, more highly oxygenated blood from the placenta crosses the foramen ovale, resulting in oxygen saturation in the left ventricle of 10% higher than that in the right ventricle. In the fetus with normally related great arteries, this blood is pumped to the ascending aorta. In fetuses with TGA, this more highly oxygenated blood in the left ventricle is pumped to the pulmonary artery, and subsequently returns to the left ventricle through pulmonary veins and makes the oxygen saturation in the left ventricle even higher than in the normal heart. It is speculated that increased oxygen content in the pulmonary artery may lead to ductal constriction and decreased pulmonary vascular resistance.

Intrauterine Interventions[9]

The future is bright for a fetus detected with certain congenital heart lesions with poor fetal or neonatal outcome as fetal cardiac surgery is on the horizon.

The primary aim of prenatal intervention in congenital heart disease is to reverse the pathological process and to preserve cardiac structure and function, thereby preventing postnatal disease. A secondary aim of prenatal intervention is to modify the severity of the disease to enhance postnatal surgical outcome. Balloon dilatation of aortic or pulmonary valve has been performed in late gestation in human fetuses with failing heart but the technical success of such fetal valvuloplasty is currently poor and the indications for fetal interventions are limited. If antegrade flow could be established earlier in gestation, perhaps normal or near normal left or right heart growth and function can be ensured.

Neonatal Alert in Fetus with Duct Dependent Lesion

This first step of prime importance in all duct dependent lesions, diagnosed antenatally, such as critical left heart obstructive lesion, transposition of great arteries and pulmonary atresia is fetal transport with a planned delivery at a site where neonatology, pediatric cardiology and congenital heart surgery services are readily available. Planning allows for prostaglandin infusion and mechanical ventilation to be available if needed.

What is it that Parents want to know?

The value of prenatal diagnosis can best be assessed in light of what parents expect from these studies. A detailed prenatal diagnosis has an impact on prenatal counseling and on the process of obtaining informed consent from parents whose fetuses have complex congenital heart disease.

The counseling process consists of a detailed description of anatomic abnormalities in the fetus. The details of neonatal care, involving timing, location and mode of delivery, details of medical support including potential need for prostaglandin E infusion for the maintenance of ductal patency and the potential need for reparative or palliative surgery in the neonatal period are discussed. The parents are given the chance to meet the doctors involved in looking after the infants at different stages, e.g. neonatologist, pediatric surgeon or cardiac surgeon, etc.

The parents are mainly interested in learning about the prospects of survival and they are mostly related to associated anomalies, genetic syndrome or underlying anatomy. The prospects for cardiac and neurodevelopmental outcome are discussed and the parents are encouraged to ask the questions and have their doubts cleared.

II. Preterm Neonate

Only about 7% of combined ventricular output passes into the lungs in the fetus with 85% of the right ventricular output crossing the arterial duct into the descending aorta. Patency of the arterial duct is maintained by the circulating and locally produced prostaglandins *in utero*. As gestation progresses, the duct becomes more sensitive to the constrictive effect of oxygen. At birth, with the onset of spontaneous respiration, the low resistance placenta is removed, thus increasing systemic vascular resistance. Expansion of lungs elicits an immediate decrease in the pulmonary vascular resitance due to vasodilatation of pulmonary vascular bed. The shift of systemic and pulmonary vascular resistances causes a reversal of flow of ductus arteriosus from right to left to predominantly left to right. In theory this leads to increase in pulmonary blood flow and decrease in venous return, thereby there is an increase in left atrial pressure exceeding the right atrial pressure which ultimately leads on to closure of foramen ovale. The pulmonary vascular resistance continues to fall in first 48 hours and in a normal newborn, the ductus closes functionally within the first few days.[8]

The increase in pulmonary arterial oxygen closes the duct and as left atrial pressure rises, the foramen ovale also closes. In preterm infants, because of hypoxemia and acidosis and also with higher levels of circulating prostaglandins, the duct does not close, leading on to further respiratory distress.

Cardiovascular Sequelae of Prematurity

Patent ductus arteriosus	- Present in 50% preterms
Persistent pulmonary hypertension (PPHN)	- Associated with asphyxia RDS
Pneumopericardium	- On positive pressure ventilation
Aortic thrombosis	- From umbilical artery catheterization
Infective endocarditis	- Associated with sepsis
Right heart failure	- Associated with severe RDS.

Patent Ductus Arteriosus

Persistent patency of the ductus after birth can be desirable or undesirable.

It is undesirable for the ductus to remain patent as an isolated anomaly. Conversely, it is desirable for the ductus to remain patent, if it is associated with certain forms of cyanotic congenital heart disease that fall into 3 general categories:

1. Ductus serves as the only source of pulmonary artenal blood flow, e.g. pulmonary atresia with intact ventricular septum.
2. Ductus is the only source of systemic arterial blood flow, e.g. aortic atresia or complete interruption of aortic arch.
3. Ductus constitutes the only means of bidirectional mixing, e.g. transposition of great arteries with intact atrial and ventricular septa. These circulations have been called" ductal dependent".

Pathophysiology of Ductus Arteriosus Patency

The ductus arteriosus represents a persistence of the terminal portion of the left pulmonary or sixth branchial arch. The ductus is more muscular than the pulmonary artery and aorta which are elastic, and it also has a loose structure with increased amount of acid mucopolysaccharide in the muscular media. During fetal life it is well developed by 6th week of gestation, forms a bridge between pulmonary artery and dorsal aorta and it serves to divert blood away from the fluid filled lungs towards the descending aorta and placenta.

After birth, when the full term newborn starts breathing, the oxygen concentration increases; which brings about longitudinal and circumferential vasoconstriction, but the biochemical basis of elevated oxygen concentration bringing about vasoconstriction has never been proven. A cytochrome P450 hemoprotein which is located in plasma membrane of vascular smooth muscles cells, appears to act as a receptor for the oxygen induced events in the ductus. Oxygen brings about membrane depolarization which is responsible for increase in smooth muscle intracellular calcium and formation of potent vasoconstrictor endothelin-l. The ductus also produces several vasodilators which oppose the vasoconstricting effects of oxygen. The increase in oxygen concentration releases the prostaglandin and nitric oxide which are potent vasodilators. Therefore, closure of ductus at birth occurs through a process that alters the balance between dilating and constricting factors.

Oxygen has a greater constrictor effect in the mature ductus arteriosus which is due to a developmental alteration in the sensitivity of the vessel to locally produced vasodilators. Isolated ductus arteriosus, in preterms, is much more sensitive to the dilating action of PGE_2 and nitric oxide than the near term ones. In addition to being much more sensitive to vasodilators, the ductus in extreme premature (27-28 weeks gestation) fetus also has decreased contractile capacity. These factors probably account for the persistence of ductus arteriosus in premature infants. Inhibitors of prostaglandin production such as indomethacin, ibuprofen and mefenamic acid have proved to be effective in closing ductus. Elevated cortisol concentrations in fetus have been found to decrease the sensitivity of ductus to PGE_2 and so prenatal administration of glucocorticoids reduces the incidence of ductus arteriosus in preterms. It is also suggested that preterm infants have low concentration of thyroid hormone leading on to decreased consumption of oxygen which leads on to increased incidence of PDA. In the full term newborns, the ductal closure is complete within 1 to 3 months.

Ductal closure is dependent on initial ductal constriction, which is associated with developing hypoxia, which mediated a series of events that leads to disruption of the internal elastic lamina and endothelial cell. Smooth muscle cells, proliferate, forming internal mounds that impinge on the ductal lumen ultimately leading on to anatomic closure. In preterm infants, hypoxia may not occur and so constriction does not take place. Thus in preterms < 30 weeks gestation, a symptomatic patient ductus arteriosus remains as a reality.

The incidence of PDA in premature infants is inversely related to gestational age. In a recent multicenter trial of indomethacin prophylaxis in premature infants weighing < 1000 gm, the incidence of PDA in placebo group was 50%. In premature infants with PDA, diagnosis should be done before treatment is initiated. Studies in extremely premature infants with a hemodynamically significant PDA it was observed that, although the total left ventricular output was increased, flow was decreased in the abdominal aorta and its branches, though there was no change in the flow in anterior cerebral arteries.[10]

Very low birth weight infants with PDA have been found to have increased flow in the ascending aorta and decreased flow in the descending aorta with an associated metabolic acidosis. Such alterations in cardiac output distribution have been implicated in the high incidence of intracranial hemorrhage and necrotising enterocolitis. The continuous distension of pulmonary vessels during diastole may be important in production of pulmonary vascular disease and bronchopulmonary dysplasia.

Clinical Manifestations

1. *History*
   a. A preterm newborn-with hyaline membrane disease-not able to wean the infant off the ventilator and later on increase the ventilator settings and oxygen requirements.
   b. Intermittent apneic spells and episodes of bradycardia.
   c. Congestive heart failure occurs in 15% of premature infants with birth weight less than 1750 gm and in 40 to 50% in those with birth weight less than 1500 gm.
2. *Physical examination*
   a. Hyperdynamic precordium.
   b. Bounding peripheral pulses, with tachycardia.
   c. Classic continuous (machinery) murmur in the infraclavicular area-diagnostic. The murmur may be systolic in those infants on ventilators.
3. *Investigations*
   a. Chest X-ray-cardiomegaly with evidence of pulmonary plethora. Presence of hyaline membrane disease-may be difficult to assess.
   b. ECG-usually normal. Occasionally may show LVH.
   c. Echocardiography
   Two-dimensional echo-anatomic information, about diameter, length and shape of ductus (Fig. 8.21)
      i. *Doppler-Ductal shunt patterns:* A continuous positive flow indicates a pure left to right shunt with the PA, pressure lower than aortic pressure (Fig. 8.21). In pure right to left shunts, flow

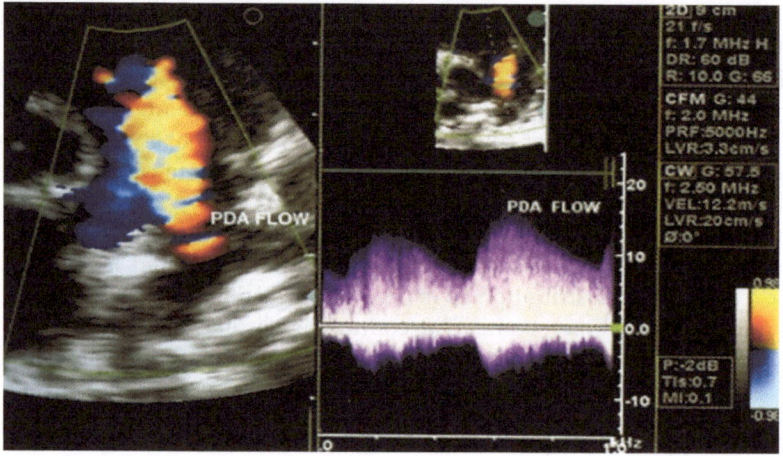

Fig. 8.21: Echocardiography of PDA, left panel showing color flow from descending aorta to pulmonary artery along its left margin and right panel showing continous turbulence obtained from the same site

is continuously negative away from the PA, indicating that the PA pressure is suprasystemic. A bidirectional shunting pattern (early negative flow in systole followed by late positive flow in diastole) is found in infants with a PDA with severe PA hypertension.

ii. *Pressure in the pulmonary artery (PA):* A high ductal flow velocity indicates a low PA pressure and a low flow velocity indicates a high PA pressure.
iii. *Perfusion status:* Increased flow velocity in the left PA suggests a large L-R shunt through the ductus. High PA pressures and a lower flow velocity indicate poor perfusion of lungs- bad prognostic sign during first 24-48 hours. Pulmonary artery and descending aorta flow patterns indicated by left atrial: aortic ratio being increased above 1.3 : 1.

Management

For symptomatic infants, either pharmacologic or surgical closure of the ductus is indicated. A small PDA that does not cause symptoms should be followed medically for 6 months without surgical ligation because of the possibility of spontaneous closure of the ductus.

Medical

1. Fluid restriction-120 ml/kg/day.
2. Diuretics-1 mg/kg, given 2-3 times a day-low success rate.

3. Oral iron-to improve hematocrit: Higher hematocrits diminish excessive shunting through the PDA and help ensure systemic oxygen delivery when perfusion is limited.
4. Oxygen inhalation and maintenance of neutral thermal environment reduces the demand on left ventricular output.
5. Pharmacological

Indomethacin

In most intensive care nurseries, indomethacin has replaced surgery as the preferred therapy for a persistent PDA.

In infants (weight more than 1250 gm and older than 7 days)-0.2 mg/kg of lyophilized indomethacin given I/V over 20-30 minutes as an initial dose. It can be repeated after 12 and 36 hours in the same dose in a similar manner.

In infants less than 1250 gm-0.1 mg/kg for the second and third dose only (unless they are older than 7 days).

A single loading dose of indomethacin (0.2 mg/kg) without subsequent maintenance doses can be effective in preventing clinical symptoms associated with PDA when given within first 24 hours.

In infants < 27 to 28 weeks gestation it is optimal to document closure at around 1 week of life and if the ductus is not closed ligation should be performed preferably.

Contraindications to use of Indomethacin

1. Poor renal function–if urine output is less than 1 ml/kg/hour or serum creatinine is more than 1.7 mg/dL.
2. Low platelets and bleeding disorders-indomethacin impairs platelet function for 7-9 days. It should not be given if the platelet count is less than 50,000/c.mm
   Indomethacin is not given when there is frank renal or gastrointestinal bleeding but can be given in presence of intracranial bleeding.
3. Necrotizing enterocolitis-presence of ductus arteriosus brings about bowel ischemia producing necrotising enterocolitis and indomethacin further reduces the bowel blood flow.
4. Sepsis-impairs blood cell motility.
5. Hyperbilirubinemia.

Surgical

If indomethacin is contraindicated or if the infant is full term and/or beyond 7 days, then surgery is indicated.

III. Transient Myocardial Ischemia

Prevalence: Since myocardial ischemia is rarely recognized, the true incidence is unknown.

Pathogenesis

1. Prenatal and perinatal asphyxia leading on to hypoxic pulmonary vasoconstriction which in turn brings about subendocardial necrosis in the papillary muscles and other areas of ventricles in the newborns. This usually results from the imbalance of the oxygen supply and demand.
2. These newborns usually have pulmonary hypertension, bidirectional shunts at atrial ductal levels and tricuspid regurgitation. Echo demonstrates varying degrees of LV dysfunction.

Clinical Manifestations Depend on Severity of LV Dysfunction

1. Full term newborns with moderate to severe asphyxia (Apgar Score <5 at 1 minute)-develop tachypnea with mild cyanosis.
2. The patient may also have systolic murmur of TR or MR, congestive cardiac failure with gallop rhythm develops in 1/3 of cases and the patient rarely goes into shock.
3. Severe CHF with cardiogenic shock-due to severe myocardial dysfunction.
4. ECG-generalized flat T waves with minor ST segment depression which may be seen in normal newborns also. Abnormal Q waves suggestive of anterior or inferior infarction may be seen in the limb and precordial leads.
5. Chest X-ray-Cardiomegaly of varying degrees with pulmonary venous congestion.
6. Echocardiogram-Varying degrees of myocardial dysfunction, enlarged LA and LV with decreased contractility of the posterior wall of LV and mitral regurgitation. All the abnormalities improve in 1 to 2 weeks time
7. Laboratory tests:
   a. PO_2 and pH-mildly reduced
   b. Hypoglycemia-commonly seen
   c. Serum creatinine-elevated
   d. Myocardial perfusion scan-diffuse impairment of thallium uptake-which is normal in cases of myocarditis.

Management

1. Mild cases
   Supportive measures   - O_2 administration

2. Severe cases
   - Correction of acidosis
   - Treatment of hypoglycemia
   - Ventilatory support
   Short acting inotropes
   - Dopamine
3. Fluid restriction and diuretics

Prognosis

1. Mild transient myocardial ischemia-usually recovers unless it is very severe.
2. In severe cases also-acidosis usually resolves and ECG abnormalities also resolve within a few months.

IV. Heart Murmurs

Innocent Murmurs

As in older children and infants, not all murmurs are organic. Full term newborn infants are monitored since birth, and 50% of them are found to have innocent systolic murmurs anytime in the first week of life and in preterms, they are even higher.

Four common innocent murmurs are:

1. *Pulmonary flow murmur:* Most common heart murmur and even more common in prematures. It is a soft systolic murmur best heard at the upper left sternal border (ULSB) transmits to both sides and last for almost 6 months. It is because of increased velocity of blood flow between main pulmonary artery and its branches, also referred to as peripheral pulmonary stenosis murmur.
2. *Transient systolic murmur of PDA:* Audible in ULSB and left infraclavicular area on the first day and usually disappears shortly thereafter. It is soft, grade 2/6 and is usually systolic. It is believed to originate from a closing ductus arteriosus.
3. *Transient systolic murmur of TR:* Indistinguishable from that of VSD. It is a regurgitant murmur heard at LLSB. It disappears however in a day or two. In newborns with fetal distress leading on to birth asphyxia, which produces PVR (pulmonary vascular resistance) and produces tricuspid regurgitation and it disappears when PVR falls.
4. *Vibratory innocent murmur:* Counterpart of Still's murmur in older children. It is an ejection systolic murmur best audible at the LLSB or near the apex and has a low frequency vibratory quality, sometimes it may be difficult to differentiate from that of VSD.

Pathologic Heart Murmurs

Most pathologic murmurs should be audible during the first month of life, with the exception of ASD. However, the time of appearance of a heart murmur depends on the nature of the defect.

1. Heart murmurs of stenotic lesions (e.g., AS, PS, COA) are audible immediately after birth and persist because, they are not affected by level of PVR.
2. Heart murmurs of LR shunt lesions that depend on the reduction of PVR (dependent shunt) may appear later. The murmur of small VSD is audible immediately after birth whereas that of a large VSD may not be audible until 1-2 weeks of age.
3. The continuous mumur of a large PDA does not appear till 2-3 weeks and a crescendo systolic murmur is heard in the infraclavicular area.
4. The murmur of ASD appears late in infancy with insidious onset. It becomes loud after a year or two. A newborn or a small infant with large ASD may not have a heart murmur.

The most important point assessing an asymptomatic neonate with a murmur is to be sure that there is no duct dependent structural heart disease because such infants will collapse when the duct closes. Presence of duct will be confirmed by the echocardiography.

V. Cyanosis in the Newborn

Most newborns with cyanotic heart disease are cyanotic at birth. Cyanosis may be peripheral, and central.

Peripheral Cyanosis

Clinical cyanosis associated with normal arterial oxygen saturation but with sluggish circulation.

Central Cyanosis-Clinical Approach

Early detection of cyanosis in a newborn is crucial. Clinically, the lips, finger and toe nails, mucous membrane, conjunctiva, etc. would be cyanosed in central cyanosis. The tongue is a good place to look for cyanosis because it is not-affected by color or even the circulation is not sluggish in this area. Cyanosis is recognized when the arterial oxygen saturation is 85% or lower but in newborn, cyanosis is evident even when O_2 saturation is 90%. It may be present in a variety of conditions (Table 8.5).

Often history and physical examination allow differentiation between the causes of cyanosis, but in practice the need to differentiate between a cardiac and respiratory disorder is the commonly encountered situation. If doubt exists, then a number of simple tests usually suffice as shown in Table 8.6.

Hyperoxia (Nitrogen Washout) Test

This test should not be performed in infants where even short periods of hyperoxia may be a risk factor for retinopathy. In fact the blood gas analysis may provide the same result without formally conducting the test. This test was basically described to distinguish between respiratory and cardiac

Table 8.5: Neonatal central cyanosis

Respiratory disease	Preterm infants, who are likely to have respiratory distress
	Often improved by increasing oxygen concentration
Cardiac disease	Most are term infants
	May be otherwise well
	May have other cardiovascular signs
	Unlikely to improve by oxygen
Persistent pulmonary hypertension (PPHN)	May have been asphyxiated
	Associated with respiratory and less commonly cardiac disease. Cyanosis variable
Methemoglobinemia	Very rare. May have family history or maternal exposure to oxidizing agents. Asymptomatic
Cerebral disease	Mediated via respiratory or pulmonary vascular derangement
Hypoglycemia	
Hypocalcemia	

Table 8.6: Tests to distinguish between causes of cyanosis

	Cardiac	Respiratory
Chest X-ray	May be normal	Rarely normal
	May have abnormal heart size or shape	Often diagnostic
	Vascular markings may be abnormal	
	Lung changes can be non-specific	
	(obstructed TAPVC may resemble hyaline membrane)	
ECG	May be normal	Usually normal
	Occasionally helpful	
Arterial blood gas	Oxygen low	Oxygen low
	Carbon dioxide normal/low	Carbon dioxide normal/high
Hyperoxia test	Usually fail	Often pass

cause when echocardiography was not available and cardiac catheterization would be necessary to distinguish between the two. The baby is placed in an inspired oxygen concentration of 85% or more for over 10 minutes, the arterial PO_2 usually rises beyond 100 mm Hg in an underlying respiratory disorder, although some mixing cardiac conditions, e.g. TAPVC and double inlet ventricles will also achieve this. Failure of hyperoxia test makes cyanotic CHD more likely although infants with severe respiratory disease and PPHN will also fail.

Cyanotic Congenital Heart Disease

There are three groups of cyanotic congenital heart disease (Table 8.7).

Treatment

Following parameters have to be clarified to plan the treatment:
1. Assess if the cyanosed infant has any other congenital abnormality.
2. If possibility of serious infection is present, then antibiotics have to be started after culture has been taken.
3. Parents have to be informed about the seriousness of the infant's condition and option for surgery has to be informed.
4. Decide whether prostaglandins are required.

Prostaglandin E-series: Indicated in those cyanosed infants, where ductus arteriosus has to be kept patent, which will increase lung blood flow even without balloon atrial septostomy.

Indications

1. Very blue infants (PAO_2 saturation < 70%).
2. Acidotic infants.
3. Those who are getting bluer (duct has closed) and unresponsive to oxygen.
4. Those who are in shock.

Prostaglandins will usually improve oxygenation and prevent deterioration in those with obstruction to blood flow through the right heart and in transpositions. They are vasodilators of ductal tissues and maintain patency for several days.

Table 8.7: Classification of cyanotic congenital heart disease

Category	Examples	Comments
Right to left shunts	Tricuspid atresia Pulmonary atresia with intact ventricular septum Critical pulmonary stenosis.	Cyanosis recognised in early newborn period-gets worse as duct shuts
Common mixing	Tetralogy of Fallot Total anomalous pulmonary venous drainage Double inlet left ventricle	Cyanosis usually appears after 6-8 weeks Often only mildly cyanosed Degree of cyanosis depends on degree of pulmonary stenosis
Transpositions		Degree of cyanosis depends on number/size of shunt lesions and not on presence of pulmonary stenosis

Prostaglandin E-2 types
  E_1-parenteral
  E_2-oral but can be given parenterally also.
  Dosage regimen given below is for prostaglandin E_1 but similar intravenous doses can be used for prostaglandin E_2 also.

Parenteral: Prostaglandin E_1-0.05-0.1 µg/kg/min (5 ng/kg/min)-may be increased in instalments of 0.05 µg/kg/min (if no side effects are encountered) to 0.4 µg to achieve therapeutic effect. Subsequently reduce to 0.025 µg/kg/min in stages. But such an increase is rarely necessary. The drip should not be flushed-it may cause apnea. Oral/nasogastric dose-25 µg/kg/hour is given hourly initially. The dose might have to be doubled.

*Side effects-*Apnea, jitteriness. convulsions, fever and flushing, diarrhea, hypertension.
  Serious side effects from gastric administration are uncommon.
  Apnoea is a serious side effect, has to be kept in mind while starting a parenteral line.

Persistent Pulmonary Hypertension of Newborn (PPHN)

Persistent pulmonary hypertension of newborn may result from one of the three causes:
1. Underdevelopment of lung–congenital diaphragmatic hernia[11]
2. Mal-adaptation of the pulmonary vascular bed to extrauterine life–postnatal stress.
3. Mal-development of pulmonary vascular bed–alveolar capillary dysplasia[11]

Prevalence

PPHN occurs in approximately 1 in 1500 live births.

Etiology

1. Decreased cross-sectional area of pulmonary vascular bed–underdevelopment of lung.
   – Congenital diaphragmatic hernia
   – Primary pulmonary hypoplasia
2. Pulmonary vasoconstriction-in presence of normal vascular bed
   – Alveolar hypoxia (meconium aspiration, hyaline membrane disease hypoventilation)
   – Birth asphyxia
   – Circulatory shock-LV dysfunction
   – Infections-group A β-hemolytic streptococcal infection
   – Polycythemia (hyperviscosity syndrome)
   – Hypoglycemia and hypocalcemia

3. Increased pulmonary vascular smooth muscle hypertrophy (medial layer)
   - Caused by-chronic intrauterine asphyxia
   - Maternal use of prostaglandin synthesis inhibitors (aspirin, indomethacin)-early ductal closure.

Pathophysiology

1. PPHN is a continuation of pulmonary hypertension, which causes varying degrees of cyanosis from R-L shunt through a PDA or PFO. No CHD present.
2. In general pulmonary hypertension caused by the second group is easy to control in comparison to the first and third group where it is impossible to reverse.
3. Varying degrees of myocardial dysfunction often occur in association with PPHN, manifested by global decrease in contractility and TR. These abnormalities are caused by global ischemia and aggravated by hypoglycemia and hypocalcemia.
4. Current thinking suggests–vasodilating newborn pulmonary circulation which may be the result of increased production of NO, and regression of potassium channels.[12] Studies by Belik et al[13], also suggested that the mechanical properties of fetal pulmonary vascular smooth muscle cells differ from those of a normal newborn.

Clinical Manifestations

1. Cyanosis and respiratory distress, 6-12 hours after birth-in full terms or preterms. History of asphyxia/meconium aspiration present.
2. Cyanosed newborn, tachypnoic and grunting.
3. Prominent RV impulse with single and loud P_2.
   - Gallop rhythm (LV dysfunction) with soft pansystolic murmur (TR).
   - Hypotension in severe cases of myocardial dysfunction.
4. Arterial desaturation (umbilical artery) in severe cases.
5. ECG-usually normal for age. T-wave abnormalities may suggest myocardial dysfunction.
6. Chest X-ray-varying degrees of cardiomegaly
7. Echo and Doppler studies-no cyanotic CHD is found
   - PDA with R-L or bidirectional shunt may be present.
   - RV is dilated with flattened interventricular septum.
   - RA pressures are increased with R-L shunt through PFO.
   - Evidence of dysfunction may be present
8. Cardiac catheterization-not indicated.

Treatment

Principles of treatment are:
1. To lower PVR and PA pressure through oxygen administration, induction of respiratory alkalosis and use of pulmonary vasodilators.
2. Correct myocardial dysfunction
3. Stabilize the patient and treat associated conditions.

1. *General supportive measures:*
   a. Vital signs and oxygen saturation are carefully monitored.
   b. Hypoglycemia. hypocalcemia (ionized calcium < 3.5 m Eq/L) and hypomagnesemia (magnesium <1.2 mg/100 ml)
   c. Polycythemia is treated
   d. Body temperature maintained between 36.50-37.20°C.
2. *Oxygen*: To maintain PO_2 of 100 mm Hg. 100% oxygen is administered initially by an oxygen hood, and if it is not successful, then intubation with positive airway pressure at 2-10 cm of water would be helpful.
3. *Mechanical ventilation:* Used to improve oxygenation and to produce metabolic alkalosis if the previous measures are not successful.
4. *Tolazoline (Priscoline):* Loading dose-0.5-1.0 mg/kg by slow IV infusion, followed by 2-4 mg/kg/hour. Tolazoline is not specific pulmonary vasodilator but two thirds of patients respond with an increase in systemic oxygenation. Since it lowers systemic vascular resistance (SVR)-hypotension is a side effect one should be aware of and BP monitoring has to be done during infusion. Other side effects include gastrointestinal bleeding, decreased platelet count and decreased urine output.
5. *Nitric oxide inhalation:* Promising therapy for severe PPHN. Prolonged low dose nitric oxide therapy brings about sustained improvement in oxygenation leading on to recovery. Inhaled nitric oxide brings about selective pulmonary vasodilatation without causing systemic hypotension. Its predilection for pulmonary circulation is due to rapid binding of nitric oxide to hemoglobin. The vasodilator effects of nitric oxide are mediated by cGMP.[14]
6. *Phosphodiesterase inhibitors*: Effects of cGMP are limited to rapid degradation of phosphordiesterases.[15] Phosphodiecterase type 5 inhibitors prevent the breakdown of cGMP and may potentiate vasodilatation with inhaled nitric oxide (iNO). Sildenafil is an oral phosphodiesterace type 5 inhibitor that has been proven safe and may have greater acute hemodynamic effects than inhaled nitric oxide and may further reduce pulmonary vascular resistance.[15] Sildenafil has been tried in varying doses from 20-80 mg given 3 times a day in adults and has been found to be successful in exercise capacity and other functions. Randomized clinical trials evaluating sildenafil in children with PAH are in progress.[16]

7. High frequency oscillatory ventilator-found to be effective in patients with severe PPHN. About 40% can escape extracorporeal membrane oxygenation.
8. Extracorporeal membrane oxygenation (ECMO)-has been shown to be effective in the management of selected patients with severe PPHN.
9. Myocardial dysfunction-can be managed by following measures:
   a. Dopamine used along with tolazoline (dose 10 µg/kg/min) by I/V infusion to improve cardiac output
   b. Dobutamine may be added if signs of CHF are present (dose 5-8 µg/kg/minute by I/V infusion)
   c. Correction of acidosis, hypoglycemia and hypocalcemia.
   d. Diuretics and digoxin may be added at a later stage.

Prognosis

1. Prognosis is good for neonates with mild PPHN.
2. For those requiring maximum ventilator setting for a prolonged time, chances of survival is small-and those who survive, develop bronchopulmonary dysplasia and other complications.
3. Neurodevelopmental abnormalities may manifest. About 50% develop hearing loss, abnormal EEG in 80% and cerebral infarction (45%) probably related to degree of alkalosis, duration of ventilator support and use of furosemide and aminoglycosides.

IV. Heart Failure in the Newborn

Congestive cardiac failure (CCF) is a fairly common manifestation of CHD and other non-cardiac causes as listed below:

Cardiac Causes

1. *Congenital heart disease*
   - At birth — Hypoplastic left heart syndrome (HLHS)
     Severe TR or PR
     Large systemic A V-fistula
   - First week — TGA
     Large PDA in preterms
   - 1-4 weeks — Critical AS or PS
     Coarctation of aorta
2. *Primary myocardial disease:* Myocarditis, myocardial ischemia (asphyxia cardiomyopathy)
3. *Arrhythmias:* PSVT, atrial flutter/fibrillation, congenital heart block.

Non-cardiac Causes

- Birth Asphyxia—myocardial ischemia
- Metabolic—hypoglycemia. hypocalcemia
- Severe anemia, neonatal sepsis.
  There are certain lesions-where cyanosis and heart failure co-exist.
  1. TGA-with large VSD and/or PDA with coarctation of aorta
  2. Truncus arteriosus
  3. Double inlet ventricle
  4. Tricuspid atresia-with coarctation and/or TGA with large VSD
  5. Hypoplastic left heart syndrome
  6. Total anomalous pulmonary venous connection.

Clinical Features

Common manifestations are:
1. Poor feeding, breathlessness, grunting, clammy extremities and worried expression–easy fatigability.
2. Unexplained weight gain inspite of poor feeding–probably due to collection of fluid.
3. Failure to thrive-in later neonatal period.
4. On examination - Tachycardia, respiratory distress, cold sweat
   Hepatomegaly
   Facial edema-rarely seen
   Gallop rhythm

Ross Classification

Can qualify the degree of heart failure in an infant.

Mild - Feed - < 3.5 oz
       Resp. rate - > 50/minutes
       Abnormal respiratory pattern, diastolic filling sounds, hepatomegaly

Moderate - Feed - < 30 z/feed
         - Time taken for feed - 40 minutes
         - Resp. rate - 60/minutes
         Diastolic filling sounds moderate hepatomegaly.

Severe - Heart rate - > 170/minutes
       - Decreased perfusion, severe hepatomegaly

Management

Investigations

- X-ray chest — Cardiomegaly
- ECG — Helpful in diagnosing selective chamber hypertrophy and rhythm disturbances.
- Echocardiogram — Assessing ventricular function and visualizing cardiac defects.
- Serum electrolytes and ABG monitoring — Important in cyanotic condition.

Acute Management Principles

1. Ensure that ventilation and oxygenations are adequate and avoid hyperoxia (which may increase left to right shunting).
2. Prostaglandin infusion-duct dependent systemic/pulmonary circulation could be present.
3. Diuretics-furosemide (1 mg/kg/IV) give symptomatic relief.
4. Avoid hypoglycemia.
5. Treat anemia, sepsis, electrolyte imbalance.
6. Inotropes-Digoxin, captopril, etc.

Chronic Management

1. Adequate calorie intake - essential nasogastric feeding 150 ml/kg–Calorie dense formula– 0.8 K/ml 2 hourly.
   Avoid sodium supplements if possible by controlling hyponatremia with altered diuretic dose.
2. Diuretics
   - Furosemide (1 mg/kg 8-12 hrly) with potassium supplements.
   - Spironolactone (1 mg/kg 8-12 hourly).
3. Digoxin
   - 4-5 µg/kg 12 hourly and adjust according to blood levels 6 hours post dose.
4. ACE-Inhibitor
   - Captopril-1 mg/kg 8 hourly and increase dose to 1.5-2 mg/kg in 3 divided doses. Side effects-hyperkalemia, rise in creatinine, neutropenia, liver function derangement.
5. Others
   - Prostaglandins reopen or maintain patterns of ductus.
   - Peritoneal dialysis–In low output states which impaired renal function.

Arrhythmias

Arrhythmias though rare, are not uncommon in full term and preterm newborns. Maternal diabetes, toxemia, and other postnatal conditions, e.g. asphyxia, hypothermia, metabolic and electrolyte imbalance all contribute to rhythm disturbances.

Full term Newborns

1. Heart rate - The normal resting heart rate-110-150 beats/min.
   - During sleep or any activity-ranges between 80-190 beats/min
2. Benign arrhythmias–Premature atrial contraction (PAC) is the commonest arrhythmia occurring in 10-35% of all normal infants.
3. Non-sinus rhythm   - 35%
   Junctional rhythm   - 25%
   Premature ventricular contraction (PVC) - 1-13%
   SVT   - 4%

Preterm and Low Birth Weight Newborns

- Bradyarrhythmias are seen more frequently in preterms. Sudden sinus bradycardia (< 90/min) is observed in about 90% of preterms.
- Sinus arrhythmias-100%

Selected Arrhythmias in the Newborn

Supraventricular Tachycardia (SVT) (Fig. 8.22)

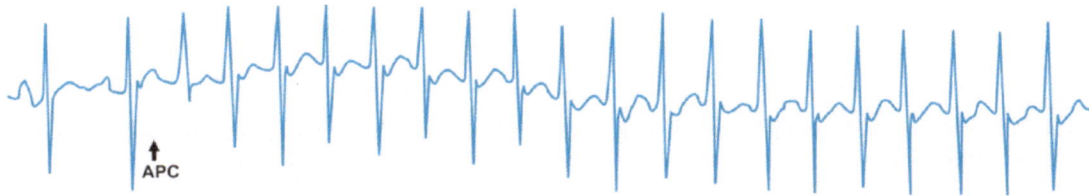

Fig. 8.22: Onset of a supraventricular tachycardia recorded on 24 h tape. Note the atrial premature contraction (APC), which initiated the re-entry circuit. The QRS complexes are of narrow morphology and the P waves can be seen buried in T waves

Classification

3 types - Reciprocating A V tachycardia-most frequent.
    Non reciprocating A V tachycardia.
    Nodal tachycardia.

1. Clinically - Rapid heart rate-200-300 beats/min, usually start and end abruptly.
    - WPW syndrome–responsible for 50% of SVT
2. Short episodes of SVT - Asymptomatic.
3. Sustained SVT - Restless, tachypnoic, feeding difficulties.
    - Develop signs of CCF and collapse in 24-48 hours.
4. Fetal SVT - Severe CCF - death.

Associated structural heart disease-Ebstein's anomaly, tricuspid atresia and cardiac tumors.

Treatment

1. Adenosine - Treatment of choice.
    Rapid I/V bolus-50 µg/kg every 2 minutes.
    Going up to maximum of 250 µg/kg when in CCF.
2. If adenosine fails - DC Cardioversion followed by digitalization and diuretics.
3. SVT of short duration - Digoxin.
4. Vagal stimulation - Ice bag applied over face or eye ball pressure–breaks SVT in some newborns.
5. Fetal SVT - Digitalize the mother–I/V 8-12 µg/kg over 24 hours followed by maintenance 0.5-0.75 mg/kg.
    Fetal/maternal digoxin levels are ratio of 0.6 : 1.

Disturbances of Atrioventricular Conduction (Figs 8.23A and B)

A disturbance in conduction from the normal sinus impulse to the ventricular response is assigned to one of the 3 causes, depending upon the severity of conduction disturbance.

First Degree A-V Block

The P-R interval is prolonged (>0.12 sec in newborn) usually in CHDs.

Endocardial cushion defect (ECD), ASDs, Ebstein's anomaly, digitalis toxicity and metabolic disturbances. No treatment is indicated.

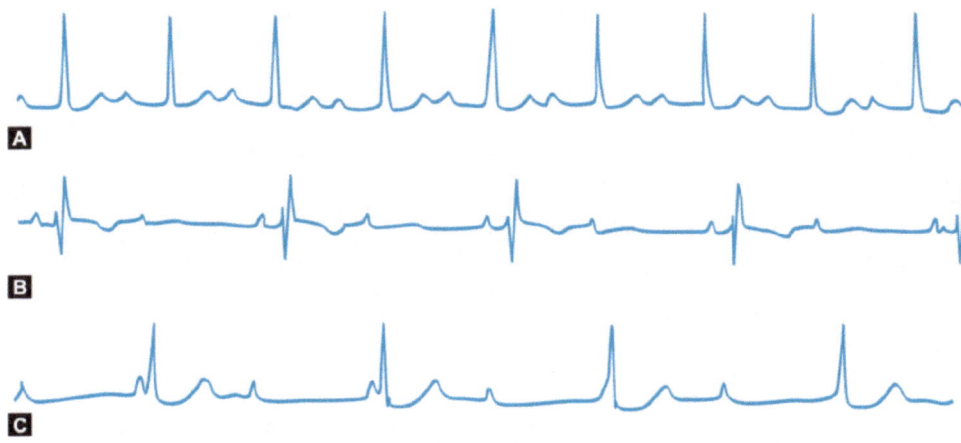

Figs 8.23A to C: ECGs demonstrating the different kinds of heart block. (A) First-degree heart block with a prolonged P-R Interval of 320 ms. (B) Second-degree heart block with 2: 1 conduction. (C) Complete heart block with an atrial rate of 80 beats/min and a ventricular escape rhythm of 39 beats min

Second Degree A-V Block

Three types-Mobitz I and II and higher grade AV block.

These conditions are associated with myocarditis, cardiomyopathy, certain CHDs, postoperative state and digitalis toxicity. Treatment should be to treat the underlying cause. Prophylactic pacemaker therapy may be indicated in Mobitz II and high grade second degree AV block.

Third Degree A-V Block (Complete Heart Block)

In complete heart block, P rate is normal (for newborn) QRS is slower than P rate. QRS duration is normal, because the block is above bifurcation of bundle of His. Maternal lupus erythematosus, or other collagen diseases are frequently associated with congenital complete heart block-and 30% may be associated with underlying CHD manifesting with CCF.

These newborns have 5-10% chances of sudden death-pacemakers have to be implanted.

REFERENCES

1. Inderbir Singh. Cardiovascular system in Human embryology (5th edition) 1993.
2. Vijayalakshmi, Eds M. Satpathy, BR Mishra. Bedside diagnosis and classification of congenital heart diseases–clinical diagnosis of congenital heart disease–First Edition. Jaypee Medical Publishers 2008;14-26.

3. Samal AK, Mishra BR. Foetal and Neonatal circulation–First Ed; Eds. M. Satpathy, BR Mishra. Jaypee Medical Publishers 2008;11-13.
4. Wagner Galen S, Lein TH. Abnormal wave morphology–chamber enlargement–in Marriott's Practical Electrocardiography–10th Ed. Galen S. Wagner–Lippincott, Williams and Wilkins 2001;71-90.
5. Saxena A, Soni NR. Fetal Echocardiography: Where are we?–Indian J. Pediatr 2005;72:603-08.
6. Savitri Shrivastava. X-ray chest for evaluation of Pediatric Heart Diseases–IAP speciality series on Pediatric Cardiology–ed. RK Kumar, SS Prabhu, MZ Ahamed–Jaypee Brothers Medical Publishers 2008;1:11-20.
7. Shakuntala Prabhu, Sumitra Venkatesh. Fetal cardiology–IAP speciality series on Pediatric cardiology eds. RK Kumar, SS Prabhu, MZ Ahamed. Jaypee Brothers Medical Publishers 2008;1:216-24.
8. Charles S, Kleinman, Julie Glickstein, Roxanna Shaw. Fetal Echocardiography and Fetal cardiology. In Moss and Adam's Heart Disease in Infants, children and adolescents including foetus and young adults–7th ed. Lippincott, Williams and Wilkins 2008;592-614.
9. Schmidt B, Roberts RS, Fanaroff A, et al. Indomethacin prophylaxis, patent ductus arteriosus and risk of bronchopulmonary dysplasia: Further analysis from the Trial of indomethacin Prophylaxis in Preterms (TIPP). J. Pediatr 2006;148:730-34.
10. Shimada S, Kasai T, Konishi M, et al. Effects of patent ductus arteriosus on left ventricular output and organ blood flows in preterm infants with respiratory distress syndrome treated surfactant. J Pediatr 1994;125:270-77.
11. Kitagawa M, Hislop A, Boyden EA, et al. Lung hypoplasia in congenital diaphragmatic hernia. A quantitative study of airway, artery and alveolar development. J Surg 1971;58:342-46.
12. Chang JK, Moore P, Fineman JR, et al. K+ channel pulmonary vasodilatation in fetal lambs; Role of endothelium derived intric oxide. J Appl Physiology 1992;73:188-94.
13. Belik J, Halayk A, Rao K, et al. Pulmonary vascular smooth muscle: Biochemical and mechanical changes. J. Appl Physiol 1991;71:1129-35.
14. Palmer RM, Ferrige AG, Moucada S. Nitric oxide release accounts for the physiological activity of endothelium derived relaxing factor. Nature 1987;327:525-26.
15. Beavo JA, Reifsnyder DH. Primary sequence of cyclic nucleotide phosphodiesterase enzymes and the design of selective inhibitors. Trends Pharmacol Sci 1990;11(4):150-55.
16. Michelakis E, Tymchak W, Lien D, et al. Oral sildenafil is an effective and specific pulmonary vasodilator in patients with pulmonary arterial hypertension: Comparison with inhaled nitric oxide. Circulation 2002;105:2398-03.

CHAPTER 9

Rheumatic Fever: Recent Advances

Rheumatic fever (RF) is generally classified as a connective tissue or collagen vascular disorder. Acute rheumatic fever occurs as a result of complex interaction between Group A streptococcus (GAS), a susceptible host and the environment. Its anatomical hallmark is damage to collagen fibrils and to the ground substance of the connective tissue. The rheumatic process is expressed as abnormal immune response leading to an inflammatory reaction that involves multiple organs: especially the heart, joints and the central nervous system. The major importance of acute RF is it's ability to bring about fibrosis of heart valves, leading to crippling hemodynamics of chronic heart disease.

Epidemiology

Acute rheumatic fever (RF) continues to be a major public health problem in the developing countries, where it is the most common cause of acquired cardiac disease in children and young adults.[1] Worldwide it is estimated that > 470,000 cases of RF occur annually in patients of all ages, most cases occur in the developing countries where the reported incidence is as high as 200-300/100,000.[2] Community based surveillance suggests that the true incidence in some areas may be high as 500/100, 000 (Table 9.1).[3]

Although individuals of any age can be affected, acute RF is mainly an acquired disease of children (5-15 years) and young adults world-wide. The two most important predisposing factors are poverty and overcrowding.[4] The higher incidence of severe carditis in the young and earlier

Table 9.1: Rheumatic fever in school children[7] (1997)

Country	Prevalence/1000
Japan	0.7
USA	0.6
Asia (Other)	0.4-21.0
Africa	0.3-15.0
South America	1-17.0

development of chronic valvular heart disease in the developing countries are because of result of recurrences of acute rheumatic fever leading to rapid deterioration of cardiac function which needs early cardiac surgery. This also reflects on the failure of medical care delivery system in developing countries to provide secondary prophylaxis for rheumatic children. In contrast, it's incidence which has been declining in the western countries (United States and Western Europe) has been attributed to the wider use of antibiotics especially after initiation of penicillin in the treatment of streptococcal pharyngitis, improved economic standards and decreased crowding in homes and schools, as well as increased awareness and availability of health care.[5] Changes in the streptococcal strains and decreased virulence may also have contributed to the decline in RF seen in the developed countries.[6] The prevention of rheumatic fever in the developing countries is the same now as it was during the second world war in the developed countries.

Pathogenesis

Group A streptococcal (GAS) infection of the pharynx and not the skin precedes the onset of rheumatic fever. Because of the latent period of 6-8 weeks between the streptococcal infection and the onset of clinical manifestations, rheumatic fever is generally regarded as an immune mediated reaction.

Environment

Despite epidemiologic link between GAS pharyngitis and RF other factors clearly influence the incidences of RF. In developing countries overcrowding, poverty, poor nutrition, poor hygiene and poor access to health care are common and contribute to rapid spread (respiratory droplets) and increased virulence of GAS.[8]

Agent

An untreated GAS tonsillopharyngitis is the antecedent event that precipitates rheumatic fever and it does not follow streptococcal skin infection which leads on to post-streptococcal glomerulonephritis. Proper antimicrobial treatment of, streptococcal pharyngitis with eradication of the organism virtually eliminates the risk of rheumatic fever. In situations conducive to epidemics (military population, overcrowding) as many as 3% of acute streptococcal sore throats may be followed by rheumatic fever.[9] Approximately 0.3% (non-epidemic) to 3% (during streptococcal epidemics) of individuals who have not had RF will develop the illness following an untreated symptomatic or asymptomatic streptococcal pharyngitis and recent reports suggest that even asymptomatic pharyngitis may lead on to RF in up to two third of the cases.[10]

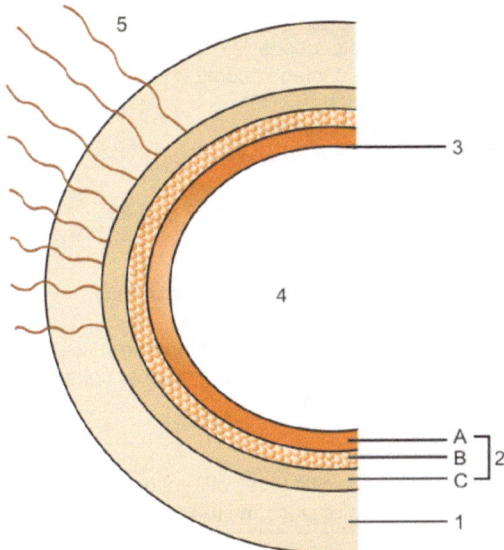

Fig. 9.1:[11] Antigenic structure of streptococcus: (1) Capsule (hyaluronic acid), (2) A- Peptidoglycan (cell wall rigidity), B- Carbohydrate (group specific), C- Lipoteichoic acid fimbriae, (3) Cytoplasmic membrane (4) Cytoplasm (5) Pili covered with lipoteichoic acid[11]

The major factors that are related to the risk of rheumatic fever are the magnitude of the immune response to the antecedent streptococcal pharyngitis and persistence of the organism during convalescence. The strain virulence of streptococcal organism influences the likelihood of development of RF.

The concept that RF is associated with infections due to virulent encapsulated (mucoid) strains capable of inducing strong type of specific immune responses to M protein and other streptococcal antigens (Fig. 9.1). It has been strengthened by the observations made during the outbreak of acute RFs during 1980's in the United States (Table 9.2). The M. protein is thought to be a major virulence factor because it affects the ability of host cells to undergo phagocytosis. Epitopes of M protein molecule cross react antigenically with human heart and brain tissue.[11] There are reports from community that heavily encapsulated (mucoid) strains give rise to increase in number of RF cases.[12] Decrease in RF cases in developed countries is partly due to a change in GAS strains (altered expressions M.Proteins).

Table 9.2: Pathogenesis of rheumatic fever

Group 12 A Streptococcus
Tonsillopharyngeal infection only
Intensity of infection
- Brisk antibody response
- Persistence of the organism

Rheumatogenic strains
- M types 1,3,5,6,14,18,19,24,27 and 29

Non-rheumatogenic strains
- 2,4,12,22 and 28

M proteins-distinct structural characteristics
- Long terminal antigenic domain
- Epitomes that are shared with human heart tissue
- Heavily encapsulated forming mucoid colonies
- Resist phagocytosis

Susceptible host
Genetic predisposition
- Presence of specific β cell alloantigen
- High incidence of class, II HLA antigens

The Host

Children between the ages of 5-15 years are the most commonly affected. RF is uncommon before 5 years, almost never occurs before 2 years and is uncommon beyond the age of 35 years.[13] Children with RF before 5 years manifest with only arthritis and rarely present with chorea and when present, cardiac involvement is more severe and persistent RHD is common.[14] With exception that chorea is more common in girls, there is no definite gender predisposition.[15]

Although only a small proportion of individuals with untreated first attack of streptococcal pharyngitis may develop RF (3%), incidence of the same disease following streptococcal pharyngitis in those who have had a previous attack of RF is more (50%). Familial predisposition to the disease has also been reported[16] and a higher concordance rate between identical twins (18.77%) than in fraternal twins (2.5%).[17] Higher rates of RF and RHD have also been reported in certain ethnic groups, specifically Maoris and Pacific islanders in New Zealand, Samoans in Samoa and Hawaii and aboriginal people in Antartica.[18] These observations strongly suggest a genetic basis for susceptibility to RF. A specific β cell alloantigen identified by monoclonal antibodies has been described in almost all patients (99%) of RF but only in 14% of controls.[6] Furthermore, susceptibility to RF has been linked with HLA-DR, 1, 2, 3 and 4 haplotypes in various ethnic groups.

Pathogenesis

Rheumatic fever occurs as a result of complex interaction between GAS organism, host and environment. Although the relationship to a preceding streptococcal pharyngitis is established and well accepted, the pathogenesis of RF is incompletely understood. Current evidence suggests that pharyngitis is caused by a rheumatogenic strain of GAS in a susceptible individual. This results in streptococcal antigenic component that mimics normal human tissue antigen, leading to abnormal humoral and cellular immune responses. Several times evidence led to and support the concept of RF occurring after GAS pharyngitis:
1. Documented relationship between GAS pharyngitis epidemics and RF.[19]
2. Immunologic evidence of a preceding streptococcal infection via rising antibody titres.[20]
3. Adequate treatment of GAS pharyngitis can prevent RF.[21]
4. Antibiotic prophylaxis can prevent RF recurrences.[22]
5. Mass prophylaxis with penicillin terminated RF epidemics in military and civilian population.[23]

Most of clinical manifestations occur approximately 10 days to 5 weeks (average 18 days) following GAS pharyngitis in a susceptible host. Importance of host susceptibility in the pathogenesis of RF is important because abnormal immune response to GAS infection is genetically controlled. Recently a alloantigen detected by monoclonal antibody (D8/17) has been reported to occur in >99% of patients with RF compared with only 14% in general population.[24] This β lymphocyte alloantigen has not yet been confirmed and has to be studied further.[25]

Pathology

The basic pathology of acute rheumatic fever is an exudative and proliferative inflammatory response affecting the connective tissue and basement membrane (type IV collagen) in several organs principally the heart, joints, brain, skin and subcutaneous tissues. A generalized vasculitis affecting small blood vessels is also noted.

The basic structural change in collagen is fibrinoid degeneration. The pathologic changes in rheumatic carditis are primarily perivascular and interstitial without evidence of myocyte necrosis. Two phases have been described: The exudative phase occurs in the first 2-3 weeks after the disease onset and is characterized by interstitial edema, cellular infiltration (T cells, B cells, macrophages), fragmentation of collagen and scattered deposition of fibrinoid (eosinophilic granular material. During the second proliferative or granulomatous phase, which lasts for months to years,[26] the Aschoff nodule considered pathognomonic and morphologic hallmark of RF and RHD, may be found in the endocardium, subendocardium or myocardial interstitiom.[27]

Aschoff body is an aggregate of large cells with polymorphous nuclei and basophilic cytoplasm arranged as a rosette around a vascular core of fibrinoid, and the aggregate is usually perivascular.

These nodules are seen only in the heart in the acute phase, mostly either in the interventricular septum, wall of the left ventricle or left atrial appendage. They may persist for many years even in patients with no evidence of recent or active inflammation. Recent studies suggest that cells in Aschoff bodies located underneath and activated valvular endothelium play an important role in antigen presentation to infiltrative T cells, which have been recognized as critical in the evolution of RHD.[28]

Immunopathogenesis

Although our understanding of the pathogenesis of RF and RHD is incomplete, the importance of the host immune response to a preceding GAS infection is clear.

Current evidence supports the following:
1. GAS pharyngitis in a genetically susceptible host leads to breakdown products and streptococcal antigens that are cross reactive with heart proteins (molecular mimicry).[28]
2. The immune response that occurs in response to the infection leads to cross reactive and cytokine production.[29]
3. The antibodies injure the valvular endothelium leading to vascular adhesion molecule related infiltration of T cells, cells and macrophages leading to further inflammation and damage.[30]
4. Cellular infiltration contributes to formation of Aschoff bodies.
5. Activated lymphocytes and macrophages from Aschoff bodies express large amounts of HLA class II molecules on their surface and may play an important role in antigen presentation to T cells that have been recognized as important effectors of chronic rheumatic valvular disease.[27]
6. Infiltrative T cells are cross reactive with streptococcal M protein and cardiac myosin and laminin, a valve protein; CD4+ T cells have been recognized as major effectors of this process leading to chronic RHD.[31]
7. Cytokines (in particular interleukin-4) appear to be important in persistence and progression of rheumatic valvular lesions in a susceptible host.[32]

Heart

Grossly, the pericardial surface may have white fibrinous shaggy exudates: all cases show lymphocytic and mononuclear infiltration of pericardium. Aschoff nodules may be present in the pericardium.

The endocardium is most commonly affected. Myocarditis may also occur as a part of pancarditis but the mural endocardium (valves-valvulitis) is usually affected particularly on the left side, e.g. mitral valvulitis with edema and cellular infiltration of the leaflets and chordae tendinae. Small 1-2 mm friable verrucous vegetations occur on atrial surface of mitral valve or on ventricular side of aortic valve.

The verrucae seen at the edges of the leaflets are usually small and attached firmly to the surface. The acute pathological changes, e.g., edema, presence of verrucae on leaflets and probably papillary muscle dysfunction result in incomplete closure of the valve in the acute stage and subsequently fibrosis results in thickening and deformity of the leaflets and finally, shortening of chordae tendinae results in valve stenosis and or incompetence.

Clinical Features

Acute rheumatic fever is diagnosed by the use of revised Jones criteria. These criteria were first put forward by Dr.T.Duckett Jones in 1944, and after repeated modifications, was updated again in 1992. The criteria are three groups of important clinical and laboratory findings (Table 9.3).

As already discussed after the initial episode of group A (β-hemolytic streptococcal pharyngitis, a latent period of 6-8 weeks follows after which the clinical syndrome of acute rheumatic fever evolves, characterized by the major manifestations).

- Polyarthritis
- Carditis
- Chorea
- Erythema marginatum
- Subcutaneous nodules

These features may occur singly or in combination.

The minor criteria are fever, arthralgia, elevated acute phase reactants and a prolonged PR interval on electrocardiogram.

Apart from these, vague manifestations of malaise, easy fatigability, pallor and history of epistaxis and abdominal pain may be present.

Family history of rheumatic fever may also be present.

The latest update allows the diagnosis of RF to be made in patients with isolated chorea, indolent carditis (detected months after acute illness) or prior history of RF or RHD.[33]

Major Manifestations

Arthritis

The latency period between GAS infection and most manifestation of RF ranges from 10 days to 5 weeks (latency for chorea is 1-6 months).

Arthritis occurs in about 80% of patients and is characteristically migratory and not deforming. The joints commonly affected in order of prevalence are knee, ankle, wrist, elbow, hip and shoulder. The joint pains start suddenly, extreme in intensity by 12-24 hours and all the signs of inflammation e.g., (swelling, tenderness, redness and heat) also appear. The joint though mildly swollen, is exquisitely

Table 9.3: Diagnosis of acute rheumatic fever-guidelines (Jones criteria 1992 updated)

Major manifestations	Minor manifestations
Carditis	
Polyarthritis	Fever
Chorea	Arthralgia
Erythema marginatum	Elevated acute phase reactants
Subcutaneous nodules	Erythrocyte sedimentation rate (ESR)
	C-reactive protein
	Prolonged P-R interval

Plus

Supporting evidence of antecedent group A β-hemolytic streptococcus infection
- Has sore throat
- Positive throat culture or rapid streptococcal antigen test-less reliable because they do not distinguish between recent or chronic stroptococcal infection
- Rising or elevated streptococcal antibody titer

If supported by evidence of preceding group A streptococcal infection, presence of two major manifestations or one major and two minor manifestations indicate a high probability of acute rheumatic fever.

Criteria for diagnosis of:	
Primary episode of RF	2 major or 1 major plus 2 minor plus evidence of preceding strep infection
RF recurrence in a patient without RHD	2 minor plus evidence of preceding strep infection
RF recurrence in a patient with RHD Chorea or indolent carditis	No criteria or evidence preceding strept infection needed.

tender with limitation of active and passive movements. The pain and swelling usually subside in the next few days.

Once the affected joint starts improving, the second joint starts getting involved and migratory polyarthritis lasts for about 3-6 weeks. Multiple joint involvement at the same time is unusual and smaller joints of the hands and feet may be rarely affected. Arthritis responds dramatically to aspirin, which can be used as a therapeutic test. If significant improvement does not take place within 48-72 hours inspite of administration of therapeutic serum salicylate, the diagnosis of acute rheumatic fever should be questioned.

Carditis

Rheumatic carditis is usually a pancarditis involving endocardium, myocardium and pericardium in varying degrees. Clinically rheumatic carditis is also associated with murmur of valvulitis of mitral or aortic regurgitation, and it is the only manifestation of rheumatic fever which leads to permanent disability. Carditis is noted in atleast 30-70% of patients with acute RF. Approximately 80% of patients who develop carditis do so within the first 2 weeks of the RF illness. If there is no cardiac involvement in the first 2 weeks, the likelihood of subsequent cardiac involvement during the acute phase is low.[34] If the cardiac involvement is mild, patients may show complete resolution of cardiac findings, but patients with moderate to severe carditis are more likely to experience evolving RHD.[35] In the acute stage, carditis may lead to death or to severe morbidity caused by congestive cardiac failure and subsequently leads to chronic valvular heart disease. However, carditis may often be asymptomatic and is detected only when the patient manifests with joint pains or congestive cardiac failure.

Endocarditis: Mitral regurgitation (MR) the dominant cardiac abnormality in patients with RF, occurs in approximately 95% of cases with acute rheumatic carditis. Mitral regurgitation occurs because of a combination of annular dilatation and chordal elongation that results in abnormal coaptation and in some prolapse of anterior mitral leaflet. Rarely the mitral valve chordae rupture which makes the leaflet prolapsed producing mitral regurgitation (Fig. 9.2).

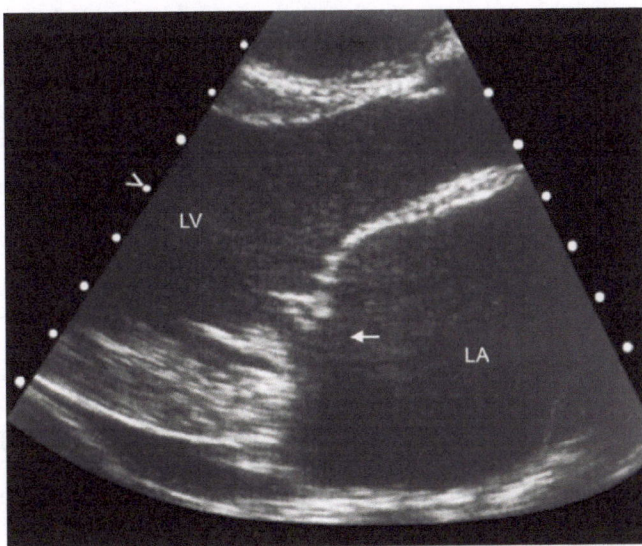

Fig. 9.2: Acute rheumatic carditis. Two-dimensional echocardiographic parasternal long-axis image showing prolapse of the tip of the anterior leaflet, resulting in a regurgitant orifice (arrow) and left heart dilation. Note also the small pericardial effusion. LA, left atrium, LV, left ventricle. With courtsey—Fillen HD, Dairen DJ, Shada RE

Most patients with mild mitral regurgitation are asymptomatic. Those with moderate to severe MR, usually present with features of left heart failure, including paroxysmal nocturnal dyspnea, cough, hemoptysis and ultimately pulmonary edema. Children younger than 5 years of age with RF and carditis may present insidiously with fever, lethargy, vague pains, fatigue. Presentation of RF with carditis with heart failure is more common in older children.[36] On examination, tachycardia is the earliest sign of carditis. A high pitched holo systolic murmur of MR is best heard at the apex usually radiating to axilla and back. It is best heard at end expiration in left decubitus position. In addition low pitched mid diastolic apical murmur may be heard due to increase diastolic flow across the mitral valve (Carey Coomb's murmur)[37] which is never heard in isolation.

Aortic regurgitation (AR) occurs in approximately 20-25% of patients with carditis usually with MR. Isolated AR occurs in 5% of patients with acute rheumatic carditis. Some have reported leaflet prolapse to be one of the mechanisms of this acute valvular dysfunction.[38] Patients with mild AR are asymptomatic and those with moderate to severe AR result in heart failure, leading to a combination of low cardiac output and pulmonary edema. Patients with acute severe aortic regurgitation are tachycardiac and tachypneic, unlike the findings of chronic aortic regurgitation. On auscultation, the decrescendo diastolic murmur is softer, lower pitched and shorter than the murmur heard with chronic regurgitation and this murmur may be easily missed because of tachycardia in the acute phase. A short ejection systolic murmur is heard over the LVOT because of increased flow. A low pitched mid to late diastolic rumble with pre-systolic accentuation is heard in the mitral area – called "Austin Flint murmur". Acute rheumatic aortic regurgitation is less likely in comparison to mitral regurgitation to disappear with resolution of the acute inflammatory phase of the illness.

Echocardiography: The diagnosis of rheumatic carditis is usually based on the presence of significant murmurs, which may not be picked. Thus it is important to emphasize that heart failure does not occur in acute or chronic RHD in the absence of significant valvular dysfunction. It is well established that Doppler echo is more sensitive in picking up minor degrees of valvular regurgitation than clinical examination. On the other hand, in normal cases also, mild regurgitation may be picked up especially across mitral and aortic valves on Doppler echo.

Myocarditis-may accompany endocarditis and is detected by cardiomegaly and congestive cardiac failure (CCF), in the presence of a significant murmur. Heart failure usually starts as left ventricular failure which manifests as tachypnea, breathlessness and acute pulmonary oedema. Although acute rheumatic carditis has long been considered a pancarditis and clinically are related to valvular pathology and regurgitation rather than myocarditis and myocardial dysfunction.[39] Furthermore there may be evidence of subtle abnormalities of contractility, left ventricular ejection, fraction remains normal.[40]

Pericarditis-does not occur alone in RF, it is always a part of pancarditis. It can be diagnosed by the presence of pericardial friction rub or by the demonstration of fluid in the pericardial cavity on echocardiography. Pericarditis occurs in approximately 4-11% of patients with acute rheumatic carditis.[41] When it occurs, it is invariably associated with significant left sided valvular disease. Clinically the patients may have the typical positional chest pain and shoulder pain seen with pericarditis and echocardiography confirms the presence of pericarditis.

Chorea (Sydenham's Chorea)

Chorea can occur alone (pure chorea) or in association with carditis: it affects only 10% of patients with acute RF. It usually occurs in girls between 8-12 years of age. The latent period between streptococcal infection and onset of chorea is long (2-6 months) with normal ESR and ASO titre. The two components of sydenham's chorea are emotional liability and choreiform movements. The symptoms usually last for 3-4 months and sometimes may even last for 1 year. Chorea occurs because of neuropathologic changes and inflammation in basal ganglia, cerebral cortex and cerebellum.[42]

In a patient with chorea, examination may reveal the following points:
1. Pronator sign-child tends to pronate the hands when extending the arms above the head.
2. On squeezing the patient's hand-"milking sign" irregular contractions of the fingers may be felt.
3. Spooning sign-hyperextension of the fingers when asked to extend the hand and forearm.
4. Tongue-when projected looks like a "bag of worms".
5. Knee jerks-classically pendular.

Movements are abrupt and erratic, fidgetiness facial grimaces, halting or explosive speech, irritability, poor attention span and deterioration in scholastic performace.

Although combination of chorea and carditis is common occurring in 47% of patients with RF in a recent series[43] cardiac involvement is relatively mild and heart failure uncommon. However rheumatic cardiac involvement in these patients may evolve and may progress over time and some presenting with chronic RHD years after acute RF illness.

Erythema Marginatum

It is a classical manifestation of RF but is not seen in India. It usually occurs in 5% of patients with RF and appears early and sometimes associated with carditis.

Erythema marginatum appears as large bright pink macule or papule which spreads quickly to give a serpiginous edge with a fading centre. Face is usually spared and the rash is characteristically seen on the trunk and limbs. The rash is painless, non-itchy and may last for weeks, may be months.

Subcutaneous Nodules

Subcutaneous nodules are uncommon and reported in 0-10% of RF cases.

Subcutaneous nodules are round, firm painless and are 0.5-2 cm with no evidence of inflammation. They are freely mobile, appear mainly over bony prominences, e.g. elbows, wrists, knees, ankles, scalps and over spinous processes of the back. They may occur in crops and are usually associated with carditis.

Minor Manifestations

Clinical Findings

Fever and arthralgia are non-specific. Fever is present initially during acute phase and arthralgia is pain in one or more major joints without any swelling. Their diagnostic value is limited and they are used to support diagnosis of RF when one single major manifestation is present. Epistaxis and pain in abdomen may also occur-but are not included as minor manifestations.

Diagnosis

The diagnosis of acute rheumatic fever is based principally on clinical findings. In 1944, Dr. Ducket Jones formulated criteria for diagnosis of acute rheumatic fever. These criteria were modified (1955) revised (1965,1984) and updated (1992) by American Heart Association (Table 9.3) as (i) major manifestations; (ii) minor manifestations and (iii) supporting evidence of an antecedent group A streptococcal infection.

Apart from clinical manifestations, serological tests commonly used are:

Antistreptolysin O(ASO) titre and antideoxyribonuclease (DNAse) B titer which peak 3-4 weeks after GAS pharyngitis and 80-85% of acute patients will have elevated titer.

An ASO titre of 320 Todd units in children and 240 Todd units in adults and Anti DNAse B titres 240 Todd units in children and 120 Todd units in adults are considered elevated. ASO titre is well standardized and is the most sensitive and widely used test. It is elevated in 80% of cases of activity and a low ASO titre does not rule out acute rheumatic fever. A rising titre 2-4 weeks apart is evidence of a recent streptococcal infection. Anti-streptokinase and anti-hyaluronidase tests may also be obtained if available.

Differential Diagnosis

- Juvenile rheumatoid arthritis
- Other collagen disorders-systemic lupus erythematosus and serum sickness
- Pyogenic or tubercular arthritis

- Reactive arthritis
- Arthritis due to viral infection-rubella, parvovirus, hepatitis B virus
- Hematological-Hemophilia, leukemia, sickel cell anemia.

Management

Investigations

1. Complete blood count
2. Acute phase reactants-erythrocyte sedimentation rate (ESR) and C-reactive protein-both are elevated in presence of activity. They are both minor criteria and invariably seen in patients with RF arthritis and/or carditis. Thus, measurement of acute phase reactants is useful in differentiating acute carditis from indolent RHD (presenting after inflammation has resolved). The degree of inflammation at presentation is of prognostic importance since acute carditis is more likely than chronic RHD to resolve over time. It is known that ESR may be low in patients with heart failure, only to rise as cardiac status improves. In chorea, there is no elevation in acute phase reactants.
3. Throat swab culture
4. Antistreptolysin O titer
5. X-ray chest-cardiomegaly and pulmonary congestion in presence of carditis
6. Electrocardiogram - Tachycardia
    - Prolonged PR interval-1st degree heart block
    - T-wave inversion and reduced voltage in presence of pericarditis
7. Echocardiography - Two-dimensional and Doppler echocardiography is central to the diagnosis and management of valvular disease and should be performed in all patients with acute or chronic RHD.

The mitral valve prolapsed seen in RF patients differs from the redundant myxomatous mitral valve prolapse seen in Barlow syndrome. In rheumatic carditis, only the coapting portion of anterior leaflet prolapses and there is no billowing of the medial portion or body of the leaflet.[44] This results in abnormal leaflet coaptation, a regurgitant orifice and a jet of mitral regurgitation that is typically posterolaterally directed. Rarely chordal rupture results in a flail leaflet and severe mitral incompetence. Echocardiography may detect aortic regurgitation in patients with RF who have no evidence of clinical carditis on physical examination (no murmur). The World Health Organization recommends the following criteria to differentiate pathologic from physiologic mitral and aortic regurgitation.
   a. Color jet > 1 cm in length.
   b. Color jet evident in atleast two imaging planes.
   c. Color jet mosaic with peak velocity > 2.5 m/s.
   d. Doppler signal holosystolic for mitral regurgitation and holodiastolic for aortic regurgitation.[45]

Furthermore, WHO recommends silent but significant MR and AR should be considered probable RHD and be given secondary prophylaxis. Chronic established RHD should have echocardiographic follow up. In addition, echocardiography also gives evidence of cardiac dilatation, valve abnormalities, myocardial function can be evaluated and presence of pericardial effusion can be confirmed.

Treatment

General

1. The patient should be admitted for observation.
2. Bed-rest is advisable for atleast 2 weeks and should be gradually allowed to return to normal activity till the acute phase reactants return to normal.
3. Extraneous physical exercise should be avoided till carditis is present.
4. If heart failure is present then bed rest has to be enforced with salt free diet, digoxin, diuretics, oxygen inhalations, etc.
5. Diet-salt-free nutritious, high calorie, high protein, supplemented with vitamins and minerals.
6. Though throat swabs may be rarely positive, penicillin therapy has to be given to eradicate streptococci.
   - Procaine, penicillin-40,000 units/kg over a day for 10 days
   - Long acting Benzathine Penicillin once in 21 days.
   - Up to 6 years of age-60,000 units
   - Beyond 6 years-1,20,000 units (1.2 mega units) till 25-30 years.

Anti-rheumatic Therapy

Since the pathogenesis of rheumatic fever is not clear, no curative treatment is available and treatment is aimed at suppressing the anti-inflammatory response.

1. *Polyarthritis:* Salicylates (Aspirin) given at the dosage of 80-100 mg/kg in 4 divided doses for 6 weeks and a therapeutic salicylate level of 20-30 mg/dl should be maintained. If the joint pain does not respond to salicylates within 24-48 hours, then diagnosis of rheumatic fever should be re-evaluated. Aspirin toxicity may manifest in form of tinnitus, nausea, vomiting and anorexia and so dose of aspirin should be regulated.
2. *Carditis:* Corticosteroids are the drug of choice for any form of carditis in India because the cardiac involvement is severe and only corticosteroids help in preventing life threatening sequelae.

   Prednisolone (2 mg/kg) is given for a period of 12 weeks in mild carditis but in those with pericarditis and in congestive cardiac failure, prednisolone is continued for a total period of 4-6

months, and is to be given with antacids to prevent any gastric irritation. Congestive cardiac failure is treated with usual decongestive measures, e.g. digoxin, diuretics and potassium supplements with salt free diet.
3. Cardiac treatment
   - Depends on severity of involvement and symptoms.
   - Moderate to severe-salt and fluid restriction, diuretics and ACE-inhibitors.
   - Intractable heart failure-surgery.
4. Follow up–follow up of acute phase reactants (ESR, C – reactive proteins).

Treatment of Chorea

- Physical and emotional stress should be reduced.
- Drugs
  - Sodium valproate-15-20 mg daily twice a day and increased over 1 week and given for a total duration of 3 months.[12]
  - Halo peridol-0.05 mg/kg/day is now also being used.
  - Phenobarbitone, chlorpromazine and diazepam are sometimes used.
- Anti-inflammatory drugs are not necessary, but prophylaxis should be continued.

Prevention

Primary Prophylaxis (Table 9.4)

Aim of primary prevention is the prophylaxis against initial attack of rheumatic fever by early treatment of streptococcal infection.
- To differentiate group A streptococcal pharyngitis from others can only be done by throat swab culture. But since this takes time, nowadays rapid diagnostic tests are available, allowing children to be diagnosed at the first visit and throat swab cultures are only done when such tests are negative. In the developing countries, since these tests are beyond reach of some, a strategy of treating all children of pharyngitis with one dose of injectable benzathine penicillin has been adopted.
- Penicillin is the drug of choice for treatment of group A streptococcal pharyngitis. It has a narrow spectrum, is inexpensive and resistance to GAS has not been documented. It can prevent primary attacks of rheumatic fever even if started 8 days after start of throat infection.

Table 9.4: Treatment of streptococcal pharyngitis (Primary prophylaxis)[46]

Benzathine penicillin G
- 600,000 units intramuscularly once for patients < 27 kg.
- 1.2 million units intramuscularly once for patients > 27 kg.

or

Phenoxymethyl penicillin (penicillin V)
- 250 mg orally BD or TID for 10 days for children
- 500 mg orally BID or TID for 10 days for adolescents and adults

Penicillin-allergic patients

Erythromycin estolate
- 20-40 mg/kg/day (max. 1g/day) orally + BID to QID for 10 days.

Erythromycin ethyl succinate
- 40 mg/kg/day (max. 1g/day) orally + BID to QID for 10 days.

Cephalosporin (1st generation) : dosage regimen depends on agent

Approximately 15% of penicillin-allergic individuals are also allergic to cephalosporins.
Modified from Dajani A, Taubert K, Ferrieri P, et al. Treatment of acute streptococcal pharyngitis and prevention of rheumatic fever: A statement for health professional. Committee on Rheumatic Fever, Endocarditis and Kawasaki disease of the Council on Cardiovascular Disease in the young, The American Heart Association, Pediatrics 1995:96:758-764, with permission

- If sensitive to penicillin-erythromycin is to be used.

The new macrolide azithromycin has a similar susceptibility pattern to that of erythromycin against group A streptococci, and gastrointestinal side effects are less. Furthermore, it can be given once daily and gives a high tonsillar concentration after 3 days.

Secondary Prevention (Table 9.5)

Secondary prophylaxis is aimed at prevention of streptococcal infections which precipitate recurrences of rheumatic fever. Studies have shown that if recurrences are prevented, 70% of patients who develop carditis in the initial attack will eventually lose their murmurs and have normal hearts. A GAS infection need not be symptomatic to trigger a recurrence. Furthermore, a RF recurrence can occur even when symptomatically RF has been optimally treated. That is why prevention of recurrent RF requires continuous antimicrobial prophylaxis rather than recognition and treatment of acute attacks of rheumatic fever. A full therapeutic course of penicillin (Table 9.4) should first be given to patients with acute rheumatic fever to eradicate residual GAS even if a throat culture is negative at that time. Streptococcal infections occurring in family members of rheumatic patients should be treated promptly. Choice of antibiotics-Intramuscular injection of long acting benzathine penicillin once in 3 weeks-provides the most effective secondary prophylaxis (Table 9.6).

Table 9.5: Duration of secondary prophylaxis in patients with rheumatic fever[22]

Category	Duration
• Rheumatic fever with carditis and residual vascular disease	At least 10 years after last episode and at least till initial age of 40 and sometimes lifelong prophylaxis.
• Rheumatic fever with carditis but no residual valvular disease	10 years or well into adulthood, whichever is longer
• Rheumatic fever without carditis	5 years or until age 21, whichever is longer.

Table 9.6: Secondary prophylaxis after rheumatic fever

Benzathine penicillin G
- 1.2 million units intramuscularly every 3-4 weeks

or

Phenoxymethyl penicillin (penicillin V)
- 250 mg orally BID

or

Sulfadiazine or sulfisoxazole
- 0.5 g orally daily for patients < 27 kg.
- 1 g orally daily for patients > 27 kg

Penicillin and sulfa allergic patients

Erthromycin
- 250 mg orally BID

Category	Duration
RHD (clinical or Echocardiographic)	> 10 year since last episode and at least until age 40 years; possibly lifelong
RF with carditis, but no RHD	10 year or well into adulthood a*
RF without carditis	5 year or until age 21 years

*Whichever is longer.

Modified from Dajani A, Taubert K, Ferrieri P, et al. Treatment of acute streptococcal pharyngitis and prevention of rheumatic fever: A statement for health professional. Committee on Rheumatic Fever, Endocarditis and Kawasaki disease of the Council on Cardiovascular Disease in the young, The American Heart Association, Pediatrics 1995:96:758-764, with permission

Bacterial Endocarditis Prophylaxis

Patients with rheumatic fever and rheumatic heart disease require additional short term antibiotic prophylaxis before certain surgical or dental procedures to prevent possible development of bacterial endocarditis. Patients with prosthetic valves or previous endocarditis are at particularly high risk.

Antibiotic regimens used for prevention of rheumatic fever are inadequate for prevention of bacterial endocarditis and are likely to be resistant to penicillin group of antibiotics, clindamycin, clarithromycin or azithromycin are recommended.

Prognosis

Presence or absence of permanent cardiac damage determines the prognosis. The development of residual heart disease is influenced by the following factors:
- *Cardiac status at the initial period:* The more severe is the cardiac involvement initially, greater is the incidence of rheumatic heart disease.
- *Recurrence of rheumatic fever:* Severity of valvular involvement increases with each recurrence.
- *Regression of heart disease:* Evidence of cardiac involvement in the first attack may disappear in 25% of patients if anti-inflammatory therapy is given in adequate dosage for the required period and not stopped early. Valvular heart disease resolves more frequently when secondary prophylaxis is followed strictly.[15]

SUMMARY

- RF and RHD continue to be major problems in developing countries, resulting in significant morbidity and mortality.
- Factors related to streptococcal organism, the environment and host susceptibility influence the likelihood of an individual developing RF.
- The pathogenesis of RF is likely related to an abnormal immune response to a preceding GAS infection. Both humoral and cell mediated immune responses contribute to the clinical manifestations including acute carditis and chronic RHD.
- The most common clinical manifestations of RF are arthritis, carditis and chorea; carditis and subsequent RHD are responsible for long term morbidity and mortality.
- Diagnostic criteria (updated Jones criteria and World Health Organization should serve as guideline to assist in the diagnosis of both initial and recurrent attacks of RF.
- Valvular dysfunction is the important abnormality in both acute rheumatic carditis and chronic RHD.
- Echocardiography–should be performed on all patients with RF. It is useful for confirming, quantifying valvular regurgitation, differentiating RHD from innocent murmur or CHD for serial evaluation of patients with known RHD and for identifying subclinical rheumatic cardiac involvement.

REFERENCES

1. Steer AC, Carapetis JR, Nolan TM, et al. Systemic review of rheumatic heart disease prevalence in children in developing countries: The role of environmental factors. J Paediat Child Health 2002;38:229-34.
2. Ibrahim A, Rahman AR. Rheumatic heart disease. How big is the problem? Med J Malaysia 1995;50:121-24.
3. Carapetis JR, McDonald M, Wilson NJ. Acute Rheumatic Fever. Lancet 2005;366:155-68.
4. Majeed HA. Acute Rheumatic Fever: Medicine–International Cardiovascular Disorders. 1977,18:100-05.
5. Bitar FF, Hayek P, Obeid M, Gharzeddine W. Rheumatic fever in children: A 15 year experience in a developing country Ped Cardiol 200;20(2):119-22.
6. Massell BF. Factors in pathogenesis of rheumatic fever recurrences. J Maine Med Assoc 1962;53:88-93.
7. Bisno AL. Group A streptococcal infection and acute rheumatic fever. N Engl J Med 1991;325:783-93.
8. RK Kumar, Rammohan R, Narula J, et al. Epidemiology of streptococcal pharyngitis, rheumatic fever and rheumatic heart disease. In Narula J, Virmain R, Reddy KS, et al. eds. Rheumatic Fever Washington DC: American Registry of Pathology 1999;41-68.
9. Stollerman GH. Rheumatogenic Group A streptococci and the return of rheumatic fever. Adv Intern Med 1990;39:1-2.
10. Veasy LG, Tain LY, Hill HR. Persistence of acute rheumatic fever in the inter-mountain area of the United States J Pediatr 1994;124:9-16.
11. Smoot JC, Korgenski EK, Daly JA, et al. Molecular analysis of group A streptococcus type 18 isolated temporally associated with acute rheumatic fever outbreaks in salt lake city Utah J Clin Microbial 2002; 40:1805-10.
12. Veasy LG, Tani LY, Daly JA, et al. Temporal association of the mucoid strains of streptococcal pyogenes with a continuing high incidence of rheumatic fever in Utah. Pediatrics 2004;143:168-73.
13. Olivier C. Rheumatic fever–Is it still a problem? Anti microb Chemother 2000;45(Suppl.):13-21.
14. Tani LY, Veasy LG, Minich LL, et al. Rheumatic fever in children younger than 5 years: Is the presentation different? Pediatrics 2003;112:1065-68.
15. Stollerman GH. Rheumatic fever. Lancet 1997;349:935-42.
16. Wilson MG, Schweitzer Md, Rubshez R. The familial epidemiology of rheumatic fever. J Pediatr 1943;22:46-492.
17. Taranta A, Torosdag S, Metrakos JD, et al. Rheumatic fever in monozygotic and dizygotic twins. Circulation 959;20:778.
18. Kurahara D, Tokuda AM, Grandinetti A, et al. Ethnic difference in risk for pediatric rheumatic illness in a culturally diverse population. J Rheumatic 2002;29:379-83.
19. Massell BF, Chute CG, Walker AM, et al. Penicillin and marked decrease in morbidity and mortality from the rheumatic fever in limited states. New Engl J Med 1988;318:280-86.
20. Stollerman GH, Lewis AJ, Schultz I, et al. Relationship of immune response to group A streptococci to the course of acute, chronic and recurrent rheumatic fever Am J Med 1956;20:163-69.
21. Denny FW, Wannamaker LW, Briuk WR, et al. Prevention of rheumatic fever; treatment of the preceding streptococcal infection. JAMA 1950;143:151-53.
22. Massell BF. Management of rheumatic fever, therapy of acute attack and prevention of recurrences–Pediatc Clin of North Am 1958;5:1143-59.

23. Oltolini MG, Burnett MW. History of US military contributions to the study of respiratory infections. Mil. Med 2005;170:66-70.
24. Zabriskie JB, Leveoby D, Williams RC Jr, et al. Rheumatic fever associated cell alloantigens as identified by monoclonal antibodies. Arthritis Rheum 1985;28:1047-51.
25. Weisz JL, McMohan WM, Moore JC, et al. D8/17 and CD 19 expression on lymphocytes of patients with acute rheumatic fever and Tourettis disorder. Clin Diagn Lan Immune 2004;11:330-36.
26. Gross L, Ehrlich JC. Studies on myocardial Aschoff body. Life cycle, sites of predilection and relation to clinical course of rheumatic fever. Am J Path 1934;10:489-503.
27. Saphir O. The Aschoff nodule. Am J clin Pathol 1959;31:534-39.
28. Guilherme L, Cury P, Dmarelin LM, et al. Rheumatic heart disease: Proinflammatory cytokines play a role in the progression and maintenance of valvular lesion. Am J Pathol 2004;165:1582-91.
29. Zabriskie JB, Hsu KC, Seegal BC. Heart reactive antibody associated with rheumatic fever. Characterization and diagnostic significane. Clin Exp Immunol 1970;7:147-59.
30. Roberts S, Rosanke S, Terrence Duan S, et al. Pathogenic mechanisms in rheumatic carditis: Focus on valvular endothelium. J Infect Dis 2001;182:507-11.
31. Guilherme L, Kalie J, Cuaningham M. Molecular mimicry in the autoimmune pathogenesis of rheumatic heart disease. Autoimmunity 2006;39:31-39.
32. Fae KC, daSilva DD, Oshiro SE. Mimicry in recognition of cardiac myosin peptides by heart intralesional T cell clones from rheumatic heart disease. J Immunol 2006;176:5662-70.
33. Guideline for the diagnosis of rheumatic fever. Jones criteria 1992 update. Special writing group for the committee on Rheumatic fever, Endocarditis and Kawasaki disease of the council on Cardiovascular disease in the young of the American Heart Association JAMA 1992;268:2069-73.
34. Massell BF. The diagnosis and treatment of rheumatic fever and rheumatic carditis. Med Clin North Am 1958;42:1343-60.
35. Kinstein AR, Stern EK, Spagnuolo M. The prognosis of acute rheumatic fever. Am Heart J 1964;68:817-34.
36. Rosenthal A, Czoniczer G, Massel BF. Rheumatic fever under 3 years of age. A report of 10 cases. Pediatrics 1968;41:612-19.
37. Coombs CF. Rheumatic heart disease. New York. William Woods 1924.
38. Tompkins DG, Boxerbaum B, Liebman J. Long term prognosis of rheumatic fever patients receiving regular intramuscular benzathine penicillin. Circulation 1972;45:543-51.
39. Burge DJ, Dehoratins RJ. Acute rheumatic fever Cardiovasc Clin 1993;23:3-23.
40. Vasan RS, Shrivastava S, Vijayakumar M, et al. Echocardiographic evaluation of patients with acute rheumatic fever and rheumatic carditis. Circulation 1996;94:73-82.
41. Arora R, Subramamjam G, Khalilullah M, et al. Clinical profile of rheumatic fever and rheumatic heart disease: A study of 2500 cases. Indian Heart J 1981;33:264-69.
42. Bisno Al. Noncardiac manifestations of rheumatic fever. In: Narula J, Virmain R, Reddy KS, et al. Rheumatic fever Washington DC, American Registry of Pathology 1999;245-56.
43. Feinstein AR, Spagnuolo M. The clinical patterns of acute rheumatic fever. A re-appraisal. Medicine 1962; 41:279-05.
44. Barlon JB. Idiopathic and rheumatic mitral valve prolapse: Historical aspects and an overview. J Heart Valve dis 1992;1:163-74.
45. Rheumatic fever and rheumatic heart disease. World Health Organ tech Rep Ser 2004;923:1-122.

CHAPTER 10

Rheumatic Heart Disease: Valvular Defects

Almost all acquired valvular heart diseases are rheumatic in origin. Mitral valve involvement occurs in about 75% and aortic valve involvement in 25% of all cases of rheumatic heart diseases.[1] Isolated aortic stenosis (AS) of rheumatic origin does not occur before the end of 20 years and rheumatic involvement of tricuspid valve almost never occurs. Therefore, only mitral stenosis (MS), mitral regurgitation (MR) and aortic regurgitation (AR) of rheumatic origin are discussed in this chapter.

Mitral Valve Disease[2]

The mitral valve is the guardian of the lungs. During diastole when the valve is open, the mitral valve has a functional area of about 5 cm^2 and thus presents no obstruction to the flow of blood from the lungs into the left ventricle. The left atrium normally acts as a conduit rather than a chamber during this time. During systole, proper closure of the mitral valve allows systemic pressure development in the left atrium. Since the hydrostatic pressure in the pulmonary capillary bed is equivalent to the left atrial pressure, a properly functioning mitral valve which is mobile, flexible and opens completely is responsible for maintaining a normal low pressure in the left atrium.

Mitral Stenosis (MS)

Classification
- Congenital
- Acquired

Congenital mitral stenosis-very rare. It can be associated with congenital aortic stenosis, coarctation aorta, connective tissue disorders (rheumatoid arthritis) and collagen tissue disorders (SLE), mucopolysaccharidosis (Hurler's syndrome), etc. Almost all acquired valvular heart disease, especially those of mitral valve are rheumatic in origin.

Prevalence

Although MS of rheumatic origin has been documented mostly in the adolescent age group (the whole pathology develops by 5-10 years), it is quite commonly seen in adult rheumatic patients.

Pathology (Figs 10.1A and B)

Rheumatic fever is an autoimmune phenomenon caused by cross-reaction and development of antibodies to streptococcal bacterial antigens with antigens found on the heart.
1. In the acute stage-there is inflammation of all the layers of the heart (pancarditis)-thickening of the leaflets and fusion of the commissures dominate the pathologic finding. Calcification with immobility of the valve results over time.
2. The left atrium and right sided heart chambers become dilated and hypertrophied.
3. Severe pulmonary venous hypertension, congestion and edema bring about alveolar wall fibrosis, loss of lung compliance and hypertrophy of pulmonary arterioles.

Clinical Manifestation (Fig. 10.2)

Normal mitral valve is 4-6 cm² in area. Symptoms begin to develop when the valve stenosis comes down to an area of 1.5 cm² and usually becomes severe once the area becomes less than 1 cm².

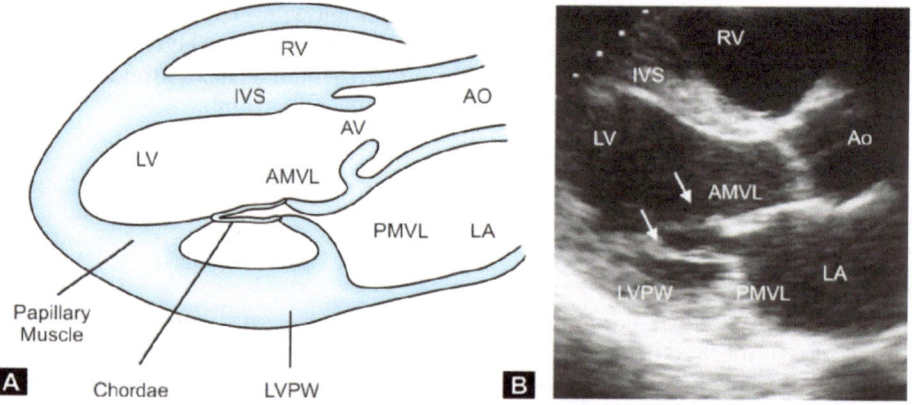

Figs 10.1A and B: 2-D picture of parasternal long axis view showing the detailed structure of mitral valve (MV), aortic valve (AV) and left ventricle (LV)

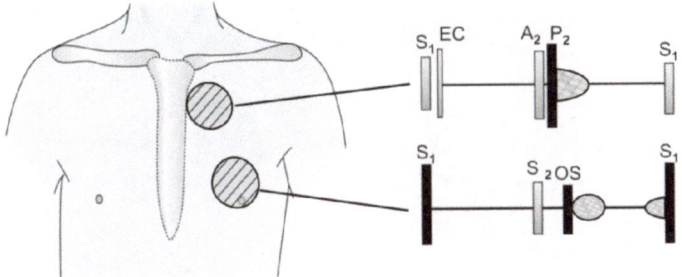

Fig. 10.2: Cardiac findings of mitral stenosis. Abnormal sounds are shown in black which include loud S_1, and ejection click (EC). A loud S_2 and an opening snap (OS). Also note the mid diastolic rumble and pre systolic murmur

1. The common manifestations in moderate to severe cases include-fatigue, palpitation, exertional dyspnea, paroxysmal nocturnal dyspnea with cough and hemoptysis occasionally.
2. When the disease is advanced-presence of RV dominance with weak peripheral pulses and elevated jugular venous pressure appear.
3. Classical auscultatory findings are:
    a. Loud opening snap in early diastole when the diseased valve snaps open forcibly by high pressure in LA. Similarly loud S_1 is heard when the A V valve closes forcibly.
    b. The opening snap is followed by a mid-diastolic murmur, which increases in length and merges with a pre-systolic murmur (atrial contraction) ending in a loud first heart sound.
    c. Pansystolic murmur is also heard because of tricuspid regurgitation which is always present in moderate to severe cases of MS. In addition there will be an early diastolic murmur due to PR (Graham Steell's murmur) in the pulmonary area which indicates long standing pulmonary hypertension.

Diagnosis

X-ray Study (Fig. 10.3)

1. Left atrial dilatation and right ventricular hypertrophy with prominent main pulmonary artery, MPA.
2. Lung fields
    - Pulmonary venous congestion.
    - Interstitial edema (kerley's B lines).
    - Redistribution of PBF to the upper lobes.

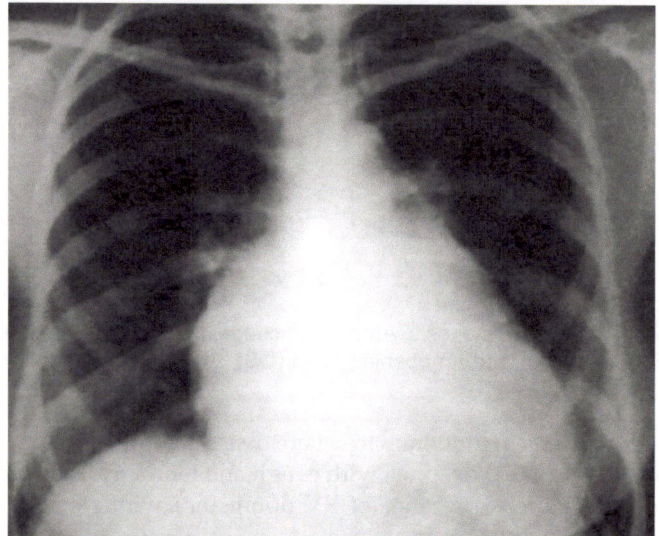

Fig. 10.3: Chest X-ray Pa view showing features of rheumatic mitral stenosis

Electrocardiogram (Fig. 10.4)

- RAD, LAH, RVH (due to pulmonary artery hypertension),
- Atrial fibrillation-uncommon in infants though common in chronic mitral valve disease.

Echocardiogram[3]

It is the most accurate non-invasive test to diagnose MS.
1. *Two dimensional (2-D) echo (Figs 10.5A and B)*
    - Doming (elbowing) of thick mitral valve leaflets.
    - A small mitral valve orifice inscribed by the thickened valve where the computer calculates the mitral valve area (MVA) planimetry.
    - Dilated LA along with dilated MPA, RV and RA.
2. *M-mode pattern*
    - Movement of leaflets restricted
    - Diminished E-F slope (reflecting slow diastolic closure of anterior mitral leaflet)

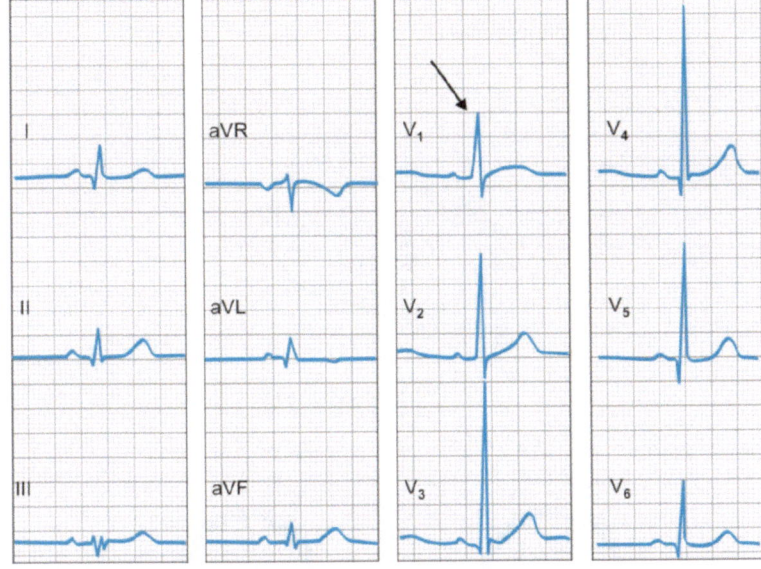

Fig. 10.4: ECG showing LAH and RVH due to mitral stenosis

- Anterior movement of posterior leaflet during diastole.
- Multiple echoes from thickened mitral leaflets-giving a fuzzy image.

3. *Doppler studies (Fig. 10.5C):* Pressure gradient across the mitral valve and the level of PA pressure (modified Bernoulli's equation).

Changes in MV area depicting severity of MS
Normal valve - 4-6 cm^2
Mild MS - 2-4 cm^2
Moderate MS - 1-2 cm^2
Severe MS - < 1 cm^2
Severe MS - Criteria for diagnosis:
   Measured valve orifice are - < 1 cm^2
   Mean pressure gradient - > 10 mm Hg
   Pressure half time - > 200 ms
   Pulmonary artery systolic pressure - > 35 mm Hg

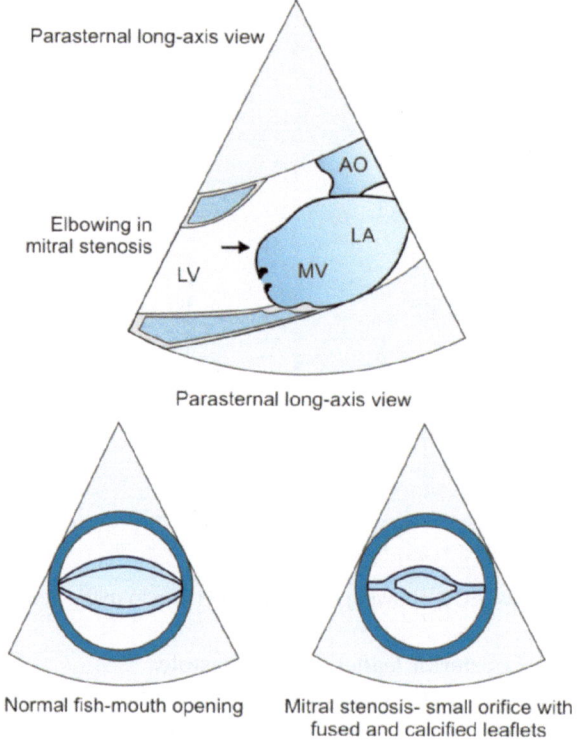

Fig. 10.5A: 2-D echo in mitral stenosis

MS Differential Diagnosis

1. LA Myxoma
2. Hypertrophic cardiomyopathy-SAM of anterior mitral leaflet.
3. MV prolapse.
4. Flail posterior leaflet.
5. Aortic regurgitation.

Natural History

1. Most children with mild to moderate MS are asymptomatic, but become symptomatic with exertion.

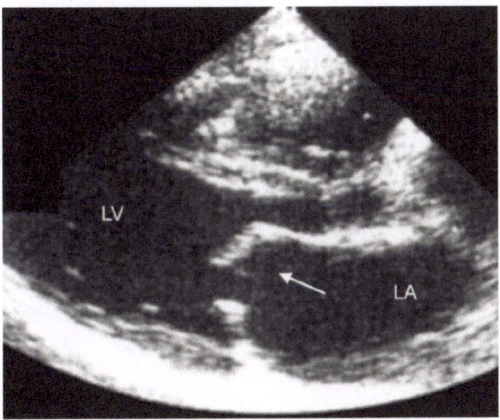

Fig. 10.5B: Parasternal long axis view – elbowing of the anterior mitral valve leaflet is shown (arrow)

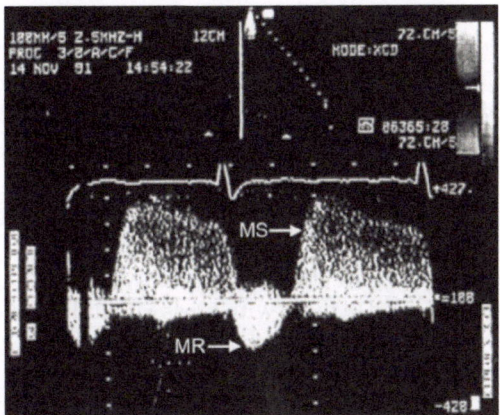

Fig. 10.5C Doppler recording of mitral flow in patients with mitral stenosis. CW Doppler in severe stenosis with the loss of EA pattern and a peak flow velocity of 4 m/s

2. Atrial flutter or fibrillations are accompaniments of chronic MS. Thromboembolism is rare.
3. Subacute bacterial endocarditis can occur as a complication.
4. Hemoptysis can occur as a result of long standing pulmonary venous hypertension.

Management

1. Good dental hygiene and antibiotic prophylaxis against SBE.
2. Prophylaxis for rheumatic fever after repeated sore-throat attacks.
3. Restriction of activity-varying degrees depending upon severity.
4. If atrial fibrillation (rare in children) develops-digoxin should be used to control ventricular response and if it persists, then cardioversion is indicated.
5. All patients with MS-should receive anticoagulation therapy.

Interventions-balloon valvuloplasty.

Indications

- Asymptomatic patients with BSA >0.5 cm^2
- Transvalvular pressure gradient> 10 mm Hg
- Symptomatic MVA< 1.5 cm^2

Surgical

Indications

- Symptomatic patient, e.g. exertional dyspnea, pulmonary edema, paroxysmal nocturnal dyspnea
- Recurrent atrial fibrillation, hemoptysis and thromboembolic phenomenon.
- Gross mitral regurgitation, calcified mitral valve.

Procedures/Mortality

1. *Closed mitral commissurotomy*-procedure of choice for mild MS, with pliable valve without calcification or MR. Mortality <1%.
2. *Open mitral commisurotomy*-in older children. Mortality <1%.
3. *Mitral valve replacement*-indicated in those with gross MR and calcified mitral valve. Homograft (Porcine valve) not indicated in children.
4. Prosthetic valves (Starr-Edward, Bjork Shiley, St. Judes) last for a longer period but require prolonged and lifelong anticoagulation therapy. Not advised in children.

Mitral Regurgitation

Prevalence

Mitral regurgitation (MR) is the most common valvular involvement in children with rheumatic heart disease.

Pathology

1. Mitral valve leaflets are shortened because of fibrosis.
2. When the degree of MR increases, LA and mitral valve ring get dilated, this leads to leakage of blood, through MV into LA during ventricular systole. It ranges between very mild to very severe, when the majority of the LV volume empties into the LA than into aorta, with each cardiac cycle.

Clinical Manifestations (Fig. 10.6)

1. Mild to moderate cases in childhood-mostly asymptomatic.
2. Rarely, fatigue (reduced cardiac output), and palpitation (intermittent atrial fibrillation) are the manifestations.
3. In severe MR-hyperdynamic pulsatile precordium-exertional dyspnea, palpitation and manifestations of CCF may be present.
4. A soft/absent first heart sound with loud second sound (pulmonary component) and also third heart sound are heard. Hollow regurgitant systolic murmur, radiating to the axilla and back. A short low frequency diastolic murmur may also be present.

Evaluation

Electrocardiography

1. Mild cases-ECG is normal.
2. Severe cases-LVH with LAH, with occasional atrial fibrillation.

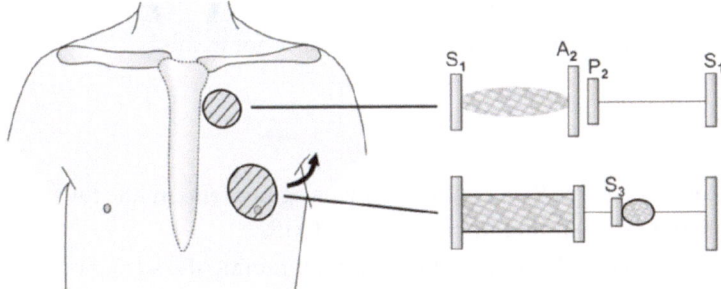

Fig. 10.6: Cardiac findings of mitral regurgitation. Arrow near the apex indicates the direction of the radiation of the murmur towards the axilla

X-ray Chest (Fig. 10.7)

1. LA and LV enlargement depending upon severity.
2. Pulmonary venous congestion-may develop if pulmonary edema or CCF supervenes.

Echocardiography (Fig. 10.8)

2D Echo	- Mitral valve morphology-flail MV leaflet with AML prolapse/vegetation.
	- Dilated LV with rapid filling.
	- Septal and posterior wall motion becomes more vigorous.
Color flow and Doppler	- LA size increased-mitral regurgitant jet is seen (Fig. 10.8).

Echo Assessment of Severity of MR

Features of Chronic MR

1. Volume overload of LV-dilatation with hyperdynamic movement.
2. Volume overload of LA-dilatation.
3. Large regurgitation volume and if it is < 4 m/s-likely to be mild.
4. Abnormal valve function, vegetation, prolapse, etc.

Natural History

1. Patients are relatively stable for a long time but MS eventually supervenes in most patients.
2. Infective endocarditis is a rare complication.
3. Pulmonary hypertension and LV failure may occur if not treated.

Management

Medical

1. Preventive measures against SBE and prophylaxis against rheumatic fever-mandatory.
2. Restriction of activity-depending upon severity of MR.
3. After load reducing agents (captopril)-helps in maintaining the stroke volume.
4. Decongestive measures-digoxin and diuretics are given if CCF develops.
5. If atrial fibrillation develops-then digoxin is given and if it fails, DC cardioversion is indicated.

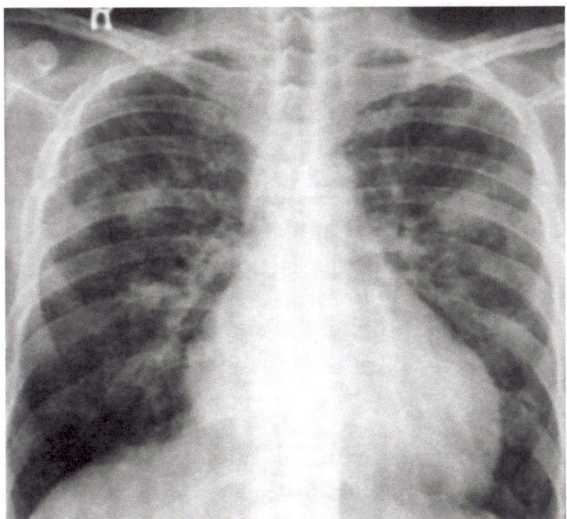

Fig. 10.7: Posteroanterior (A and Lateral) views of chest X-ray in a patient with moderately severe mitral regurgitation of rheumatic origin

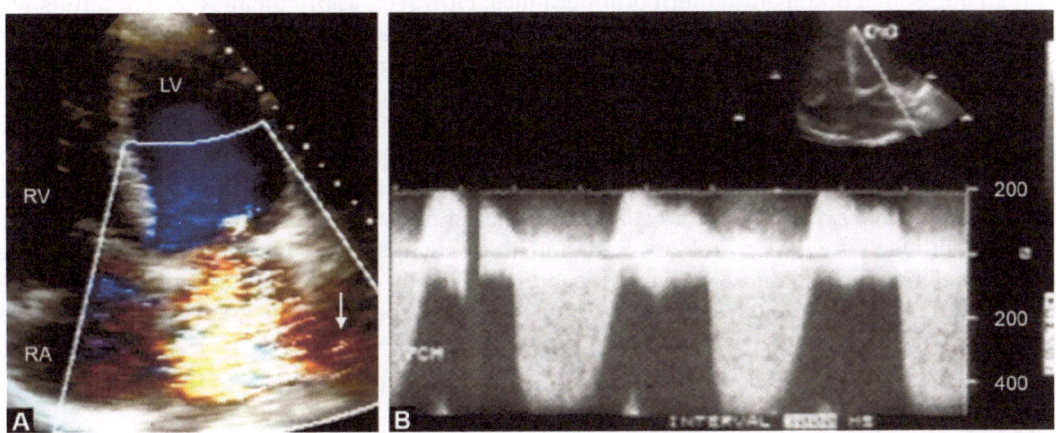

Figs 10.8A and B: Severe mitral regurgitation. (A) Color flow mapping and (B) Continuous wave Doppler recording

Surgical

Indications

1. Intractable CCF, progressive cardiomegaly with symptoms and pulmonary hypertension are some of the indications.

Procedures and Mortality

1. Mitral valve repair - in mild MR, mortality < 1%.
2. MV replacement - necessary if the valve is scarred and grossly deformed. Porcine homograft is the usual alternative.
   Prosthetic valves - Bjork-Shiley tilting disk and St. Jude Pyrolite carbon valve
   Surgical mortality - 2-7%. life long anticoagulation-essential.

Mitral Valve Prolapse[5]

Mitral valve prolapse (MVP) is the most common valvular heart disease in industrialized nations affecting approximately 3-5% of population-at large, mostly in older children and adolescents and male to female ratio is 1 : 2.

Mitral valve prolapse (MVP) is a genetically transmitted disease. Although, the genetic defect has not been definitively identified, transmission in both genders from an affected parent is consistent with an autosomal dominant-pattern of inheritance. However, approximately 2/3 of adults with mitral valve prolapse are women, which favors a gender related penetrance of the disease.

The unusual appearance of mitral valve prolapse in children and biochemical findings in myxomatous valves favor the "injury repair" hypothesis. That is the underlying abnormality present in MVP which predisposes the valve to injury and repeated episodes of injury and repair over time result in irreversible damage and valvular dysfunction. In mitral valve prolapse, collagen bundles in spongiosa layer undergo myxomatous proliferation with resultant fibrosis of the atrial and ventricular surface of the valves. Disruption of collagen bundles and myxomatous degeneration involve the chordae tendineae as well. On gross examination, these changes result in mitral leaflet and chordae tendineae elongation and thickening and depending on the magnitude of these pathologic changes, which interfere with normal competence of mitral valve apparatus. The posterior leaflet is more commonly and more severely affected than the anterior leaflet.

Etiology

1. Mitral valve prolapse (MVP) is idiopathic in more than 50% of cases.
2. Congenital heart disease (CHD) is present in 1/3 of patients with MVP. ASD secundum is the most common defect, VSD and Ebstein's anomaly are associated rarely.

3. Of all the patients with MVP, 4% have Marfan's syndrome and nearly all patients with Marfan's syndrome have MVP, which may also be seen in association with other connective tissue disorders.
4. MVP is familial in the primary form with an autosomal dominant mode of inheritance.

Clinical Manifestations

1. MVP is usually asymptomatic but a history of non-exertional chest pain, palpitation may be present.
2. Occasional family history of MVP present.
3. Asthenic built with a high incidence of thoracic skeletal anomalies (80%), including pectus excavatum (50%) straight back syndrome (20%) and scoliosis (10%).
4. Typical auscultatory findings include-mid systolic click with or without a late systolic murmur best heard at the apex-hallmark of the syndrome. The click and murmur may be made more prominent by held expiration, left decubitus or leaning forward position.

Electrocardiography

1. Inverted T. waves in LII and AVF occurs in 20-60% of patients.
2. Arrhythmias (e.g., SVT are uncommon and conduction disturbances (10° AV block, WPW syndrome, prolonged QT interval or RBBB are occasionally reported).
3. LVH or LAH is rarely present.

X-ray Study

1. X-ray films are unremarkable except for LA enlargement in severe MR.
2. Thoracoskeletal abnormalities (e.g., straight back, pectus excavatum, scoliosis) may be present.

Echocardiography

Echo-finding for adult patients with MVP have been established but for pediatric patients are not clearly defined.
1. M-mode echocardiograpy-mid to late posterior excursion (>3 mm) of posterior and/or anterior leaflet-considered diagnostic.
2. Two-dimensional echo-more reliable. Parasternal long axis view-shows prolapse of one or both mitral valve leaflets into the left atrium (Fig. 10.9).
3. MV leaflets may be thick and MR is occasionally demonstrated by color flow mapping and Doppler examination.
4. MVP is a progressive disease with a less than full manifestation in children.

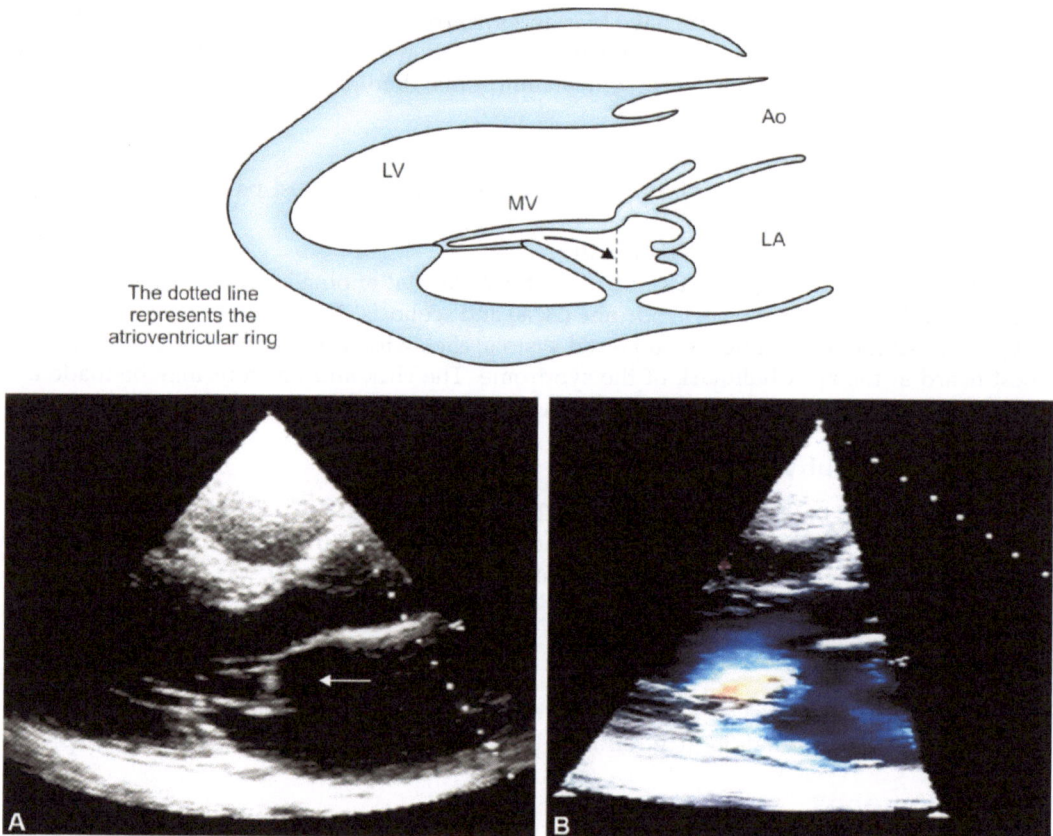

Figs 10.9A and B: Mitral valve proplapse. (A) Parasternal long axis view showing prolapse of anterior mitral valve (MV) leaflet and (B) Colour flow mapping showing mitral regurgitation

Natural History

1. MVP in children-are usually asymptomatic and no restriction of activity is necessary.
2. Complications are reported in adult patients, which includes sudden death and stroke, (probably from ventricular arrhythmias) SBE, progressive MR, rupture of chordae tendinae, arrhythmias and conduction disturbances.

In majority of patients, MVP is by and large benign. However, several studies have demonstrated significant complications over a prolonged period which includes endocarditis, severe MR requiring surgery and stroke in about 12-15% of patients.

Management

1. Asymptomatic patients require no treatment or restriction of activity.
2. Preventive measures against SBE especially when MR is present are recommended.
3. Patients who are symptomatic (palpitation, syncope, dizziness) or those who manifest with arrhythmias should undergo ambulatory ECG monitoring and/or treadmill testing.
4. Beta-blockers-Propranolol/metoprolol or/atenolol-drug of choice for ventricular arrhythmias.
5. Chest pain may be treated with propranolol and reassurance is very essential in such patients.
6. Surgical management.

Severe mitral regurgitation due to MVP requires surgery. Valve replacement especially mechanical valves with ongoing anticoagulation therapy, though give very good results but create problems for young women during pregnancy because warfarin is a proven teratogenic agent.

In patients with sinus rhythm, valve repair offers an attractive alternative to valve replacement, obviating the need for chronic anticoagulation and other co-inherent risk associated with prosthetic valve replacement.

Follow-up

Patients with mitral regurgitation should be monitored closely before and after surgery. Severe regurgitation with symptoms of congestive cardiac failure is a clear indication for operative intervention because systolic function of the myocardium has to be monitored even after surgery because MVP is a progressive disorder.

AORTIC VALVE DISEASE [1,4]

Aortic valve is located at the junction of the LV outflow tract and the ascending aorta. Since aortic regurgitation is the commonest aortic valve lesion encountered in rheumatic heart disease in children, aortic regurgitation will be discussed in some detail (Fig. 10.10).

Aortic Regurgitation

Aortic valve involvement in rheumatic heart disease results in aortic regurgitation, because by the time aortic stenosis develops, the patient is well beyond the pediatric age-group. Though pure AR is less common than MR and has been documented in 5-8%, most patients with AR have associated mitral valve disease.

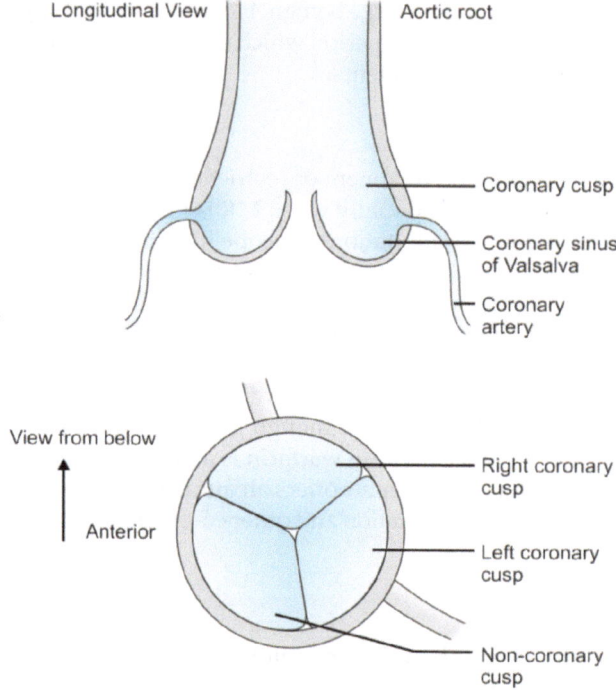

Fig. 10.10: Normal aortic valve and root

Pathology

Semilunar cusps are deformed and shortened and the valve ring is dilated so that the cusps fail to oppose tightly. The commissures are usually fused to a certain degree.

Hemodynamics

In AR, there is backward leak of blood from the aorta into the left ventricle, increasing its volume of blood and thereby dilating it. This leads on to disturbance of forward flow and it is compensated by peripheral vasodilatation and increased pulse pressure depending on the severity of the regurgitation.

Clinical Picture (Fig. 10.11)

1. Patients with mild AR are usually asymptomatic.

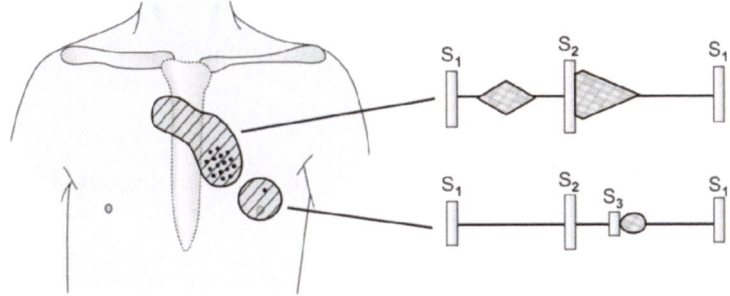

Fig. 10.11: Cardiac findings of aortic regurgitation. The S_1 is abnormally soft (black bar). The predominant murmur is a high pitched, diastolic decrescendo murmur at the third left intercostals space

2. Moderate to severe AR-Palpitation with exercise intolerance with occasional chest pain, leading on to CCF.
3. On examination
   a. Manifestations of hyperdynamic circulation-pulsatile apex with intercostal pulsations and a wide pulse pressure-water hammer pulse.
   b. On auscultation-high pitched diastolic decrescendo murmur, heard best at the third and fourth left intercostal space-is the auscultatory hallmark. And it is more easily audible when the patient bends forward. A mid diastolic rumble may be audible at the mitral area (Austin Flint murmur) when the AR is severe.
   c. Peripheral manifestations of wide pulse pressure in severe AR include
      - Prominent carotid pulsations-(Corrigan's sign).
      - Pistol shot sounds-heard over femoral arteries.
      - Wide pulse pressure in the radial artery-Water hammer pulse.

Natural History

1. Patients remain asymptomatic for a long time, once symptoms begin to develop, then deterioration sets in very rapidly.
2. Anginal pain with CCF and associated arrhythmias are unfavorable signs.
3. Infective endocarditis is a rare complication.

Management

Investigations

ECG-in mild cases, ECG is normal.
In severe and prolonged AR,-L VH and LAH are both present.

X-ray Chest (Fig. 11.12)

Cardiomegaly, because of LV dilatation in severe AR. Pulmonary venous congestion when LV dysfunction sets in.

Echocardiography (Figs 10.13A and B)

LV diastolic dimension is proportional to the severity of AR. Color flow and Doppler give a correct estimation of the severity of AR.

Treatment

Medical

1. Good oral hygiene and antibiotic prophylaxis against SBE.
2. Secondary prophylaxis with long acting penicillin against recurrence of rheumatic fever.
3. In mild to moderate AR-angiotensin-converting enzyme-inhibitor (Enalapril/Captopril) has been shown to reduce the dilatation and hypertrophy of LV in AR without LV dysfunction.
4. When CCF sets in digoxin, diuretics and afterload reducing agents are given but with little benefit.

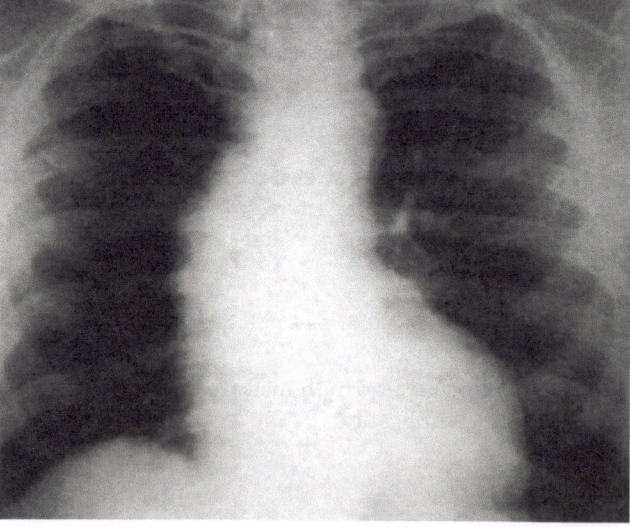

Fig. 10.12: Chest X-ray showing the features of aortic regurgitation

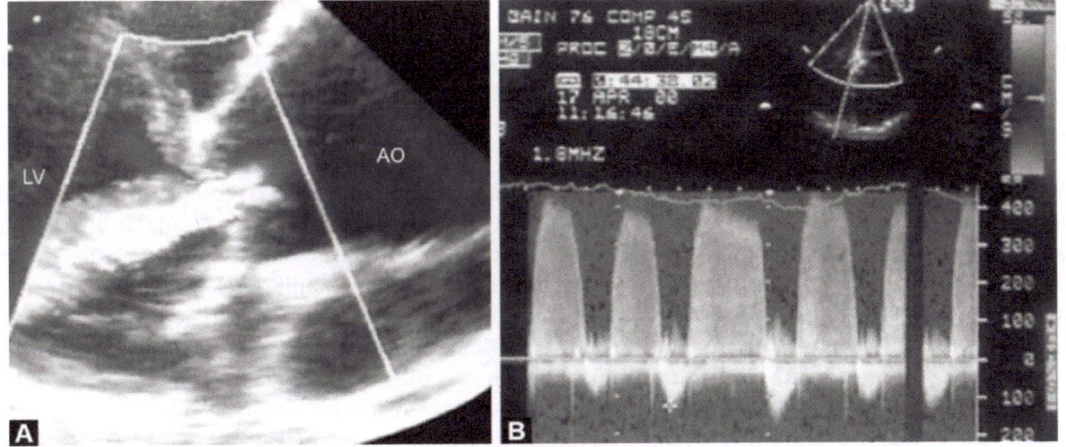

Figs 10.13A and B: Severe aortic regurgitation (A) Color flow mapping and (B) Continuous wave Doppler recording of aortic regurgitation

Surgical

Ideally aortic valve replacement should be performed before irreversible dilatation of LV develops.

Indications

1. Anginal pain associated with exertional dyspnea.
2. Significant cardiomegaly (>55%) with ejection fraction < 40% or stress test induced symptoms.

Procedure and Mortality

Aortic valve replacement is performed under cardiopulmonary bypass mortality rate-2-5%.
1. Antibiotic sterilized aortic homograph is the device of choice.
2. Prosthetic valves-require anticoagulants and so are not indicated in children.
3. Pulmonary root autograft (Ross procedure)-an attractive alternative in adolescents and young adults. The patient's own pulmonary valve and artery replace the diseased aortic valve and artery with the coronaries detached and attached to the pulmonary artery.

Complications

1. Postoperative acute cardiac failure-is the most common cause of death.
2. Thromboembolism, chronic hemolysis and anticoagulant induced hemorrhage may occur with a prosthetic valve.

Tricuspid Regurgitation

It is seen in 20-50% of patients of rheumatic heart disease in pediatric age group in India. It is difficult to differentiate between organic or functional regurgitation.

Hemodynamics

Tricuspid regurgitation results in systolic back flow from right ventricle to right atrium which leads to systolic murmur and volume load in right ventricle and right atrium. This results in increase in size of both these chambers pushing the right ventricle downwards and outwards. Patients with tricuspid regurgitation have pulmonary arterial hypertension. The systolic back flow under pressure leads to prominent systolic 'v' wave in the jugular venous pulse and liver. In patients with rheumatic heart disease, the tricuspid regurgitation lies in association with mitral stenosis or with mitral regurgitation. If associated with-mitral regurgitation it is most likely to be organic because mitral regurgitation is severe enough to cause pulmonary hypertension which brings about a functional TR. When associated with mitral stenosis, TR may be functional or organic.

Clinical Picture

There are no specific symptoms:
1. Pain in the right hypochondrium due to congested liver.
2. Fatigue due to decrease in systolic output.
3. V waves in jugular venous pulsations.
4. Systolic pulsation at the liver.
5. Systolic murmur in the lower right sternal border increasing in intensity during inspiration.
6. In severe TR, grade III-IV pansystolic murmur not varying in intensity during inspiration and association with thrill can be heard.
7. Right ventricular third sound or a short tricuspid delayed diastolic murmur may be audible in severe TR.
8. In association with mitral stenosis, severe TR results in right ventricular dilatation.

Investigations

ECG-shows severe right ventricular hypertrophy.
Echocardiography and Doppler can document and quantitate the severity of TR (Fig. 10.14).

Management

1. Anticongestive measure-help in reducing the severity. Further management depends upon associated mitral valve involvement.

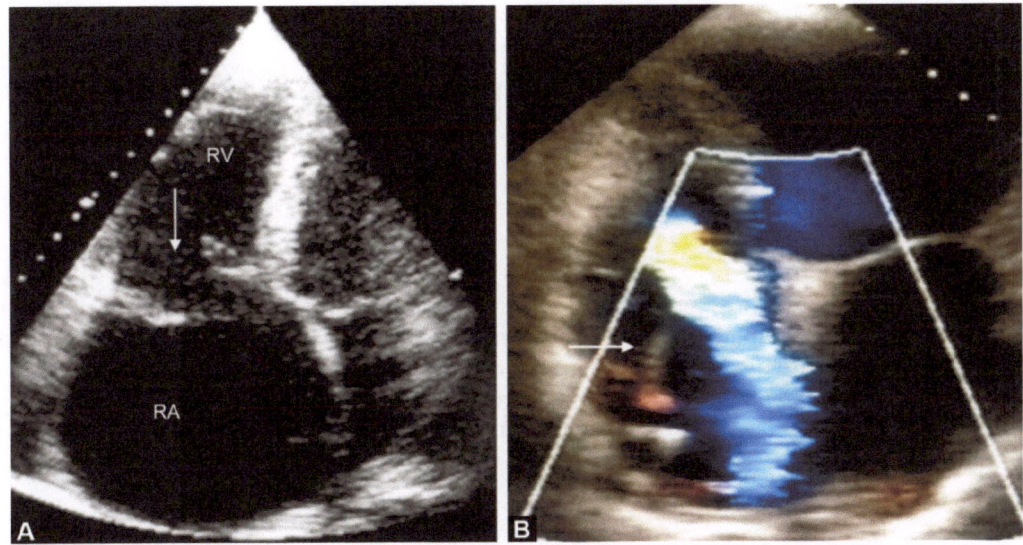

Figs 10.14A and B: Tricuspid regurgitation. (A) Apical chamber view showing prolapsed leaflet of tricuspid valve and (B) eccentric jet of tricuspid regurgitation

2. Patients with mitral stenosis-with all features of TR, mitral valvotomy is indicated.
3. Patients with severe MR and TR should be treated conservatively initially and subsequently the affected valve has to be surgically replaced.

REFERENCES

1. Park MK. Pathophysiology of obstructive and valvular regurgitant lesions: Pediatric Cardiology for practitioners (3rd edn). Mosby, St Lewis, Baltimore, Boston 1995;107-13.
2. Roger Hall, Mitral Valve Disease. Medicine International-Cardiovascular disorder: Chapter Editor-Roger JC Hall, Aduian Banming 1997;18:96-99.
3. Valves. Mitral valve in Echo made easy ed. Sam Kaddonra Churchill Livingstone. Harcount Publishers Ltd 2002;23-37.
4. MK Park Valvular Heart Disease: Pediatric Cardiology for Practitioners (3rd edn). Mosby 1995;310-19.
5. Faren R Angella, Lewis Jannet F. Mitral Valve Prolapse-Gender difference in evaluation and management. Cardiology in Review 1999;7(3):161-67.

CHAPTER 11

Myocardial Disorders

Myocardial disorders are those which are primarily disorders of the myocardium itself, and not associated with any congenital, valvular or ischemic heart disease or any other systemic disorder. Myocardial disorders are broadly divided into two main groups:
1. Myocarditis-active inflammation of the myocardium.
2. Cardiomyopathies-disease of the heart muscle itself, not associated with inflammation.

PART I

MYOCARDITIS

The term myocarditis refers to inflammation of the muscular walls of the heart. In 1984 pathologists at a meeting in Dallas defined myocarditis as "process characterized by inflammatory infiltrate of the myocardium with necrosis/degeneration of adjacent myocytes not typical of ischemic damage of coronary artery disease. This definition does not take into account the underlying cause.[1] In general, the disease may go unrecognized in many patients whose illness resolves spontaneously, or it may lead to a fulminant form with a rapid downhill course or to a chronic state possibly resulting in dilated congestive cardiomyopathy.

Epidemiology

Myocarditis is generally a sporadic disease, although epidemics have been reported.[2] Epidemics are usually seen in newborns most commonly associated with Coxsackie Virus B (CVB).

Intrauterine myocarditis occurs during epidemics as well as sporadically.[3] The World Health Organization (WHO) reports that this ubiquitous family of viruses results in cardiovascular sequelae in < 1% of infections, although it becomes 4% when CVB is considered.[1] Other important viruses, e.g. adeno viruses[3] and influenza A are transmitted through air. Males seem to be slightly more predisposed to develop myocarditis although the true incidence or prevalence in the general population is unknown. It is estimated that 5% of a virus infected population may experience some form of cardiac involvement associated with acute form of illness. These symptoms may be minor or as non-specific as transient electrocardiographic changes particularly in adult patients. In neonates and children, a fulminant presentation is more likely. Not unexpectedly as many as 20% of young subjects with sudden cardiac deaths have been found to have histologic evidence of myocarditis. Concerning the general category of cardiotropic viruses, CVB is ubiquitous: approximately 50% of general population is reported to be antibody positive, less commonly with Coxsackie A virus (1%) and ECHO virus (0.7%). Those associations are based on either serologic studies or the isolation of virus from extracardiac sources. It should be noted that it is extremely rare to isolate the virus from the myocardium during active infection, given the brief period of actual viral replication (< 2 weeks).

The Coxsackie virus B organisms use receptors that are not shared with other enteroviruses to attach to their target cells. These receptors are believed to be an element essential for viral replication and may help determine tissue tropism. After birth, spread occurs by the fecal/oral or air-borne route. CVB antigens have been demonstrated with the use of an immuno-fluorescent technique in 41 % of 29 infants and children who at routine autopsy were found to have had interstitial myocarditis.

Etiology

Acute myocarditis has both infectious and non-infectious causes (Table 11.1). It is considered that most recognized cases of acute myocarditis are secondary to infections with the so-called cardiotropic viruses.[4] These are a group of viruses (i.e., enteroviruses, adenoviruses) with a predilection for infecting the myocardium. In the developed countries, enteroviruses are considered to be the most common infectious agents that cause acute myocarditis: and within this group, the Coxsackie B viruses (CVB) have been implicated most frequently.[5] Most recently Parvovirus B19 has become

Table 11.1: Viral cause of myocarditis

Enterovirus	Varicella
Coxsackie A	Mumps
Coxsackie B	Measles
Echovirus	Rabies
Poliovirus	Hepatitis B,C
Adenovirus	Rubella
Parvovirus B19	Rubeola
Cytomegalovirus	Respiratory syncytical virus
Herpesvirus	Human immunodeficiency virus
Influenza A	Epstein-Barr virus

commonly identified in subjects with suspected myocarditis.[6] However many other viral causes of myocarditis have been described in children which include influenza, cytomegalovirus (CMV), hepatitis, rubella, herpes simplex virus (HSV), varicella, mumps, HIV and respiratory syncytial virus.

Bacterial, fungal, spirochetal organisms rarely cause acute cardiac inflammation, usually however such causes are just one component of a major systemic illness (Table 11.2). One important exception is Chagas disease, which is caused by the protozoa *Trypanosoma cruzi*. The immunologic response to infection and subsequent myocardial injury is similar to that observed in viral myocarditis. This infection remains the most common cause of myocardial inflammation and cardiomyopathy worldwide. Chagas disease is endemic in rural and central South America and it usually manifests with heart failure secondary to dilated cardiomyopathy.

Table 11.2: Non viral causes of myocarditis

Rickettsial	Protozoal	Fungi and Yeasts
Rickettsia rickettsii	*Trypanosoma cruzi*	Actinomycosis
Rickettsia tsutsugamushi	Toxoplasmosis	Coccidioidomycosis
	Amebiasis	Histoplasmosis
		Candida
Bacterial	**Other Parasites**	
Meningococcus	*Toxocara canis*	
Klebsiella	Schistosomiasis	
Leptospira	Heterophyiasis	
Mycoplasma	Cysticercosis	
Salmonella	*Echinococcus*	
Clostridia	Visceral larva migrans	
Tuberculosis	Trichinosis	
Brucella		
Legionella pneumophila		
Streptococcus		
Smallpox		

During the human immunodeficiency virus (HIV) epidemic, various cardiac manifestations have been recognized including myocarditis. Acute myocarditis in the HIV patient may be secondary to the HIV-I. virus alone or to other associated infection such as cytomegalovirus or *Toxoplasma gondii*.

Table 11.3: Causes of myocarditis: non-infectious etiologic agents

Toxic	Hypersensitivity/Autoimmune
Scorpion	Rheumatoid arthritis
Diphtheria	Rheumatic fever
	Ulcerative colitis
	Systemic lupus erythematosus
	Mixed connective tissue disease
	Scleroderma
	Whipple disease
Drugs	Others
Sulfonamide	Sarcoidosis
Phenylbutazone	Kawasaki disease
Cyclophosphamide	Cornstarch
Neomercazole	
Acetazolamide	
Amphotericin B	
Indomethacin	
Tetracycline	
Isoniazid	
Methyldopa	
Phenytoin	
Penicillin	

Various drugs including antimicrobial medications, hypersensitivity, autoimmune or collagen vascular diseases such as systemic lupus erythematosus, rheumatoid arthritis, rheumatic fever, scleroderma, toxic reactions to infectious agents e.g. mumps or diphtheria or Kawasaki disease (Table 11.3).[8]

Mason classified myocarditis into six distinct categories (Table 11.4). These are active viral infection, postviral/lymphocytic myocarditis, hypersensitivity to drugs and other exogenous agents, autoimmune (systemic lupus erythematosus and possibly peripartum myocarditis), other infectious causes and giant cell myocarditis.

Lymphocytic myocarditis is believed to result from a pathologic immune response to a recent enteroviral infection (often CVB) and is the most common form detected by endomyocardial biopsy. This form of myocarditis is also referred to as idiopathic or viral myocarditis and is the commonest form of myocarditis which is referred to generally.

Table 11.4: Myocarditis

Classification (Mason)	
Active viral	
Post viral (lymphocytic)	– Common form of acute myocarditis
Hypersensitivity	– Drugs
Autoimmune	– SLE, peripartum myocarditis
Infectious	
Giant cell myocarditis	

Pathophysiology

Infectious agents cause myocardial damage by three basic mechanisms:
1. Invasion of myocardium.
2. Production of myocardial toxin, e.g. diphtheria.
3. Immunologically mediated myocardial damage.

The present knowledge of immunopathology of acute myocarditis is derived from animal models e.g., murine (rat) enteroviral model (using CVB) has been used most commonly and provides a reasonable description of the complicated immunologic process that follows virus induced myocardial injury.

Viral infection triggers interstitial inflammation or myocardial injury, resulting in cardiac enlargement and an increase in ventricular end-diastolic volume.[9] Flow chart 11.1 identifies the following domino effects of various changes that occur which lead on to the pathophysio response in patients with carditis.

1. Interaction with sympathetic nervous system, leads on to vasoconstriction and thereby elevated afterload which results in tachycardia and diaphoresis.
2. Congestive heart failure ensues with disease progression. The progressive increase in endiastolic volume and pressure results in increased left atrial pressure, which if left untreated, results in acute pulmonary oedema.
3. Concomitantly, all cardiac chambers dilate especially the left ventricle. The dilation leads on to worsening of ventricular function and results in pulmonary edema. The ventricular dilation results in stretching of mitral annulus resulting in mitral regurgitation thereby increasing left atrial pressure further.
4. During the healing stage of myocarditis, fibroblast replace normal myofibers which result in scar formation. Reduced elasticity and ventricular performance can result in persistent heart failure. In addition, ventricular arrhythmias commonly accompany fibrosis.[10]

The ultimate result of dilated cardiomyopathy may depend on the virulence of viral strain, host genetic factors as well as other known risk factors that alter the severity of myocarditis including host age, nutritional age and prior chest radiation.

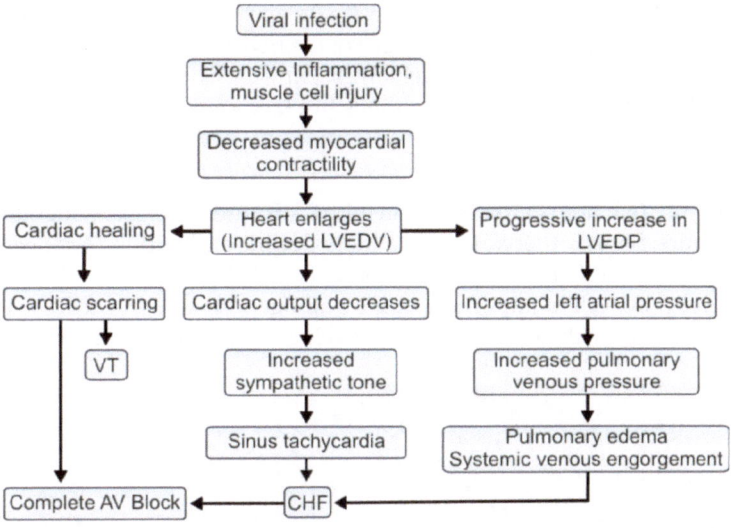

Flow chart 11.1: Pathophysiology of myocarditis

AV, atrioventricular; CHF, congestive heart failure; LVEDP, left ventricular end-diastolic; LVEDV, left ventricular end-diastolic velocity; VT, ventricular tachycardia

Pathology

Pathologic findings are non specific. See the four chambers are affected; the muscle is flabby and pale, with petechial hemorrhage often seen on the epicardial surfaces, especially in cases of coxsackie virus B (CVB) infection. A bloody pericardial effusion also may be seen relating to the often combined finding of pericarditis. The endocardium and valves are not involved.

In cases of chronic myocarditis the valves may be glistening white suggesting that endocardial fibroelastosis (EFE) may be the result of an *in utero* viral myocarditis. The children with myocarditis are usually symptomatic for < 2 weeks; whereas those with EFE had symptoms for > 4 months. Mumps and CVB 3 have been identified in the myocardium of infants with EFE.[11]

An interstitial collection of mononuclear cells, including lymphocytes, plasma cells and eosinophils (Fig. 11.1) is typical of early myocarditis,[5] though polymorphonuclear cells are rare. Exclusive necrosis, striation in the muscle fibers and edema is seen in severe infections, especially with coxsackie virus.

Diphtheria myocarditis is frequently complicated by arrhythmias and complete A-V block.[12] The diphtheria exotoxin attaches to conduction tissue and interferes with protein synthesis and triglycerides accumulate producing fatty changes of the myofibers. Bacterial myocarditis produces micro-abscess and patchy focal suppurative changes. Parasitic myocarditis caused by *Trichinella* has a focal infiltrate with lymphocytes and eosinophils but larvae are not identified.[13]

Immunology

Twenty four to seventy two hours after infection with CVB, viremia exists with maximum growth in tissues for 72-96 hours. Shortly thereafter virus titers decline and antibody concentrations increase and macrophages appear 5-10 days after infection with CVB.[5]

The natural killer (NK) cell is important in the pathogenesis of myocarditis. Those depleted of NK cells prior to infection with coxsackie virus develop a more severe myocarditis.[14] NK cells are

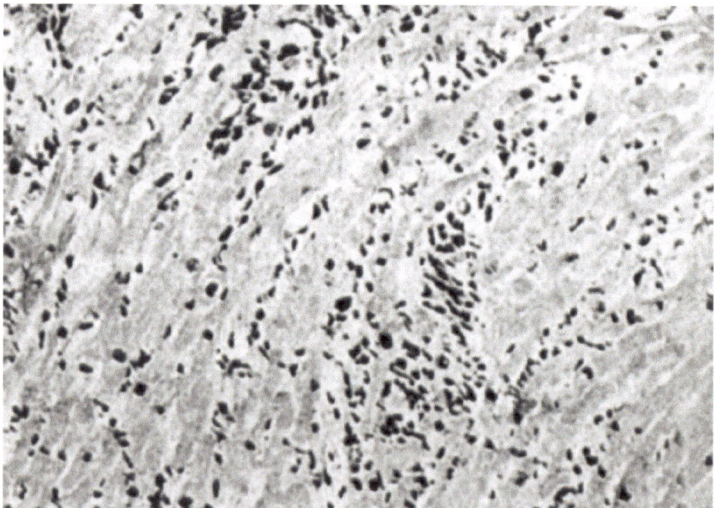

Fig. 11.1: Endomyocardial biopsy histology demonstrates lymphocytic infiltrates, myocardial edema and necrosis

activated by interferon, which is an indirect modulator of myocardial injury. The NK cells specifically limit the now enveloped virus infection by killing the virally infected cells.

T cells can affect injury by accumulation of activated macrophages, production of antibody and antibody-dependent cell-mediated cytotoxicity, direct lysis by antibody and complement and direct action by cytotoxic T cell.[15] Defective cell mediated immunity occurs in patients with myocarditis and DCM when compared with healthy controls. Adenoviral myocarditis differs from CVB because inflammatory exudate is substantially less.[16] Several adenovirus encoded proteins can interact with host immune components (E3), which can protect cells from tumor necrosis factor (TNF) mediated lysis and EIA proteins are capable of promoting the induction of apoptosis[17] and inhibiting interleukin 6 (IL-6) expression. These functions of EIA may be pertinent to the development of myocardial pathology seen in DCM.

Role of Cytokines in Myocarditis and Dilated Cardiomyopathy

Recent animal studies suggest that a relationship may exist between subclinical viral infection and subsequent development of DCM. This process is presumed to occur by an autoimmune like mechanism triggered by the initial viral insult. Cytokines contribute to regulation of antibody production. Susceptible murine strains when infected with CVB3 develop myocytic necrosis and an acute inflammatory response. After the initial viral infection, resolution of inflammation eventually occurs.

In other strains however, a second autoimmune phase of myocarditis appears later, with findings of diffuse mononuclear cell infiltrates within the heart. These mononuclear cells are a significant source of cytokine IL-1 and TNG and they release large amount of TNG α and IL-1B by human monocytes when exposed to CVB3.[18] Both of these cytokines are known to participate in leukocyte activation, which may be beneficial in promoting a specific lymphocyte response to viral infection. These cytokines may also promote cardiac fibroblast activity. Therefore, it has been speculated that local secretion of cytokines in the myocardium perpetuates the inflammatory process, which secondarily leads to fibrosis associated with DCM and results in deterioration of cardiac function.

Clinical Presentation

The clinical picture of myocarditis varies greatly. The presentation may be non-specific and a high index of suspicion is required to make a diagnosis of acute myocarditis. Acute myocarditis may manifest in following manner:
1. Asymptomatic–transient and non specific electrocardiographic changes.
2. History of viral fever 10-15 days prior to the presentation. Initial manifestations include lethargy, low grade fever and pallor with decreased appetite and also abdominal pain. Diaphoresis

palpitation, rashes and exercise intolerance are common manifestations.[19] Later in course of illness, respiratory distress, syncope and sudden cardiac arrest may occur.
3. It may mimic acute myocardial infarction (Flow chart 11.2) acute chest pain with the presence of Q wave in ECG and segmental wall motion abnormalities-seen in echocardiogram. Endomyocardial biopsy does not show any abnormality.
4. Myocarditis is usually associated with systolic heart failure and dilated cardiomyopathy giving rise to diastolic and systolic dysfunction.
5. Less common manifestations include arrhythmias in the form of tachyarrhythmias and bradyarrhythmias and also conduction abnormalities manifesting as Stokes Adam's attacks (Figs 11.3A to C).
6. In newborns-abrupt onset in the first 8-9 days of life with episodes of diarrhea and lack of appetite with lethargy, presence of greyish pallor and mild icterus. Tachycardia, dyspnea and cyanosis with cardiomegaly and hepatomegaly are manifestation of cardiac failure. Sudden death may occur in this group of infants 20% have histologic evidence of myocarditis.[19]
7. It is important to note that younger the child, it is more likely that intrauterine myocarditis is now expressed as a chronic disease.[20]

Diagnosis and Noninvasive Testing

Since there is no sensitive clinical or laboratory clue to the diagnosis of acute myocarditis when there is history of recent viral illness with unexplained congestive cardiac failure, acute myocarditis should be suspected and investigated to prove it.
1. *Chest radiography:* Cardiomegaly with prominent vascular markings of pulmonary edema (Fig. 11.2).

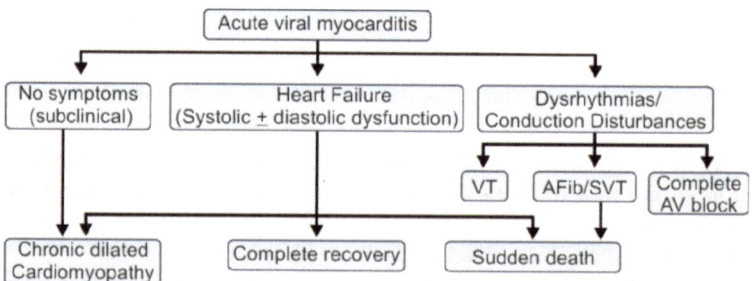

Flow chart 11.2: Clinical presentation of myocarditis

aFib, atrial fibrillation; AV, atrioventricular; SVT, supraventricular tachycardia; VT, ventricular tachycardia

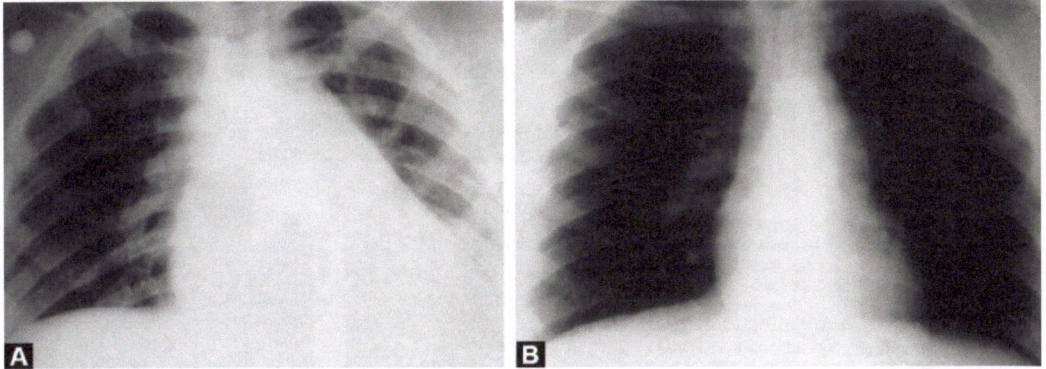

Figs 11.2A and B: Chest radiograph in a child with acute myocarditis. Left: Initial radiograph demonstrating cardiomegaly and increased pulmonary vascular markings consistent with pulmonary edema. Right: Radiograph obtained 6 months after initial presentation demonstrates normalization of heart size and lung markings

2. *Electrocardiography*
    a. Sinus tachycardia with low voltage QRS complexes with inverted T waves are classically described (Fig. 11.3).
    b. A pattern of myocardial infarction with wide Q waves and ST segment changes may also be seen[21] (Fig. 11.3B).
    c. Ventricular tachycardia, supraventricular tachycardia, atrial fibrillation or atrio–ventricular block are seen in some children (Fig. 11.3C).
3. *Echocardiography (Figs 11.4A to C):* A dilated and dysfunctional left ventricle consistent with DCM is seen in two dimensional and M Mode views. Global hypokinesia is predominant with pericardial effusion. Doppler commonly demonstrates mitral regurgitation used at one time or the other to diagnose myocarditis. Although magnetic resonance imaging, echocardiography and indium-III-monoclonal antimyosin antibody imaging continue to be researched actively, they lack the specificity that endomyocardial biopsy does in diagnosing myocarditis.
4. *Endomyocardial biopsy:* Endomyocardial biopsy from right ventricle despite its' limitations (complications of sampling, low negative predictive value) remains the standard for diagnosing myocarditis. The inflammatory infiltrate is usually patchy and scattered in ventricular myocardium. A mononuclear cell infiltrate is diagnostic of myocarditis, although the cause is not evident. Myocardial biopsy is diagnostically sensitive in 3-63% of cases.[22] Because of insensitive biopsy reporting to identify 80% of cases, 17 or more specimens must be obtained.[23] Because of risk involved with biopsy especially in children, the procedure has been abandoned in many centers.

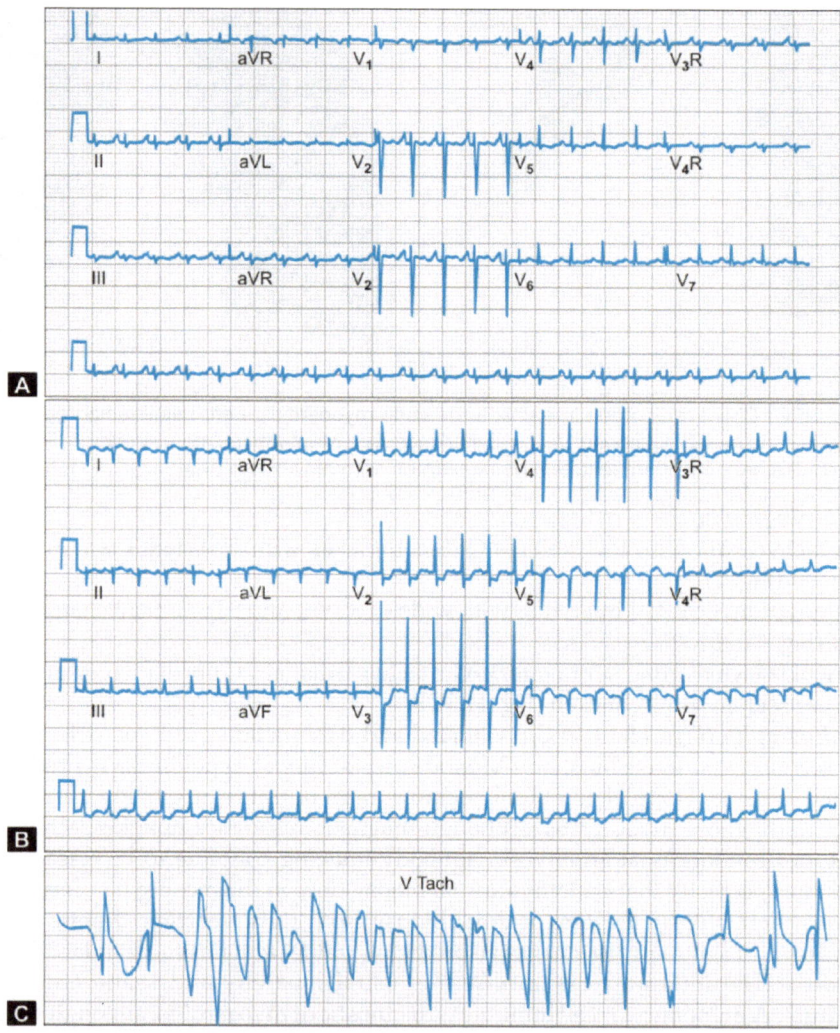

Figs 11.3A to C: Electrocardiogram in a case of myocarditis. (A) Sinus tachycardia and low voltage QRS complexes with inverted T waves. (B) Pattern of myocardial infarction with wide Q waves in leads I and aVL, and ST segment changes consistent with ischemia noted throughout. (C) Ventricular tachycardia

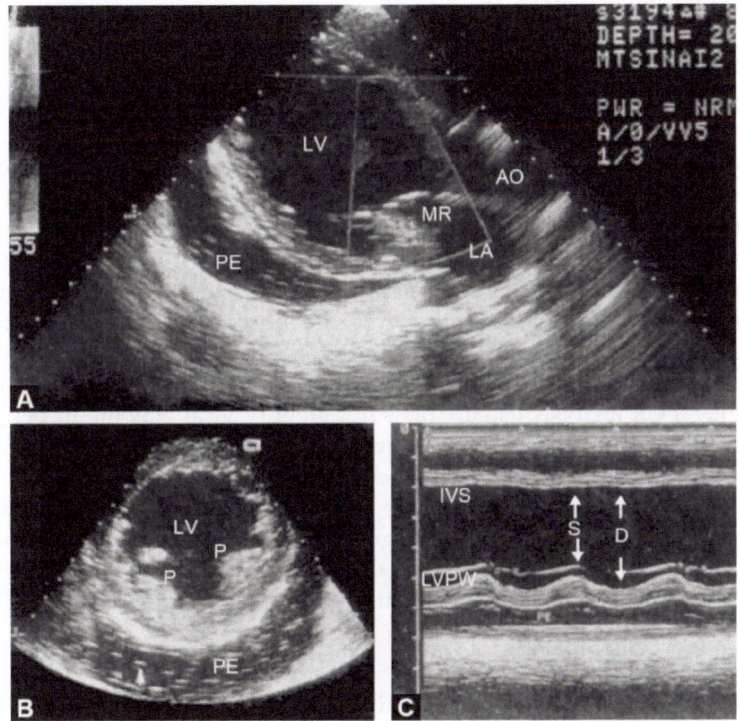

Figs 11.4A to C: Echocardiographic features of myocarditis: (A) Two-dimensional parasternal long-axis view demonstrating left ventricular (LV) dilation and a pericardial effusion (PE). Color Doppler interrogation provides evidence of mitral regurgitation. (B) Parasternal short-axis view demonstrating LV dilation and normal papillary muscles (P). (C) M mode demonstrating systolic dysfunction with flattened interventricular septal motion (IVS), fair LV posterior wall excursion (LVPW), LV dilation with increased LV end-diastolic dimension (D), and reduced systolic function (S) and PE. Ao, aorta; LA, left atrium; MR mitral regurgitation

The Dallas criteria: An expert panel of pathologists in Dallas established the standard criteria for diagnosing myocarditis by endomyocardial biopsy–Dallas criteria–"a process characterized by an inflammatory infiltrate of the myocardium with necrosis/and or degeneration of adjacent myocytes not typical of ischemic damage, owing to coronary artery or other disease.[24] At the time of initial biopsy, a specimen may be classified as active, borderline or no myocarditis depending on the degree of inflammatory infiltrate with myocyte necrosis or degeneration. Repeat endomyocardial biopsy may be indicated in cases where there is strong suspicion of myocarditis. Diagnosis may be depending on report as ongoing, resolving or resolved myocarditis.

5. *Viral studies:* A positive viral culture from myocardium has been considered the diagnostic standard in the past. A four fold increase in antibody titre correlate with infection.[25] Polymerae chain reactions (PCR) amplifies viral sequence from cardiac tissue samples is extremely sensitive and typically specific.[26] PCR amplification process which identifies specific portion of a viral genome is quite specific and 20 to 50% of cases were reported to identify enterovirus PCR positive results and adenovirus has also been identified as enterovirus from heart tissue specimens of myocarditis or DCM. Additional viral genomes identified using PCR include cytomegalovirus, parvovirus, respiratory syncytical virus, Epstein–Barr virus, herpes simplex virus and influenza A virus.[4] Mumps virus is responsible for endocardial fibroelastosis, an important cause of heart failure 20 years ago. Over the past 2-3 years parvovirus B19 has become the predominant viral genome identified in the heart[6] and in Japan, hepatitis C virus has been shown to be a common etiologic agent.[28] PCR analysis usually does not identify viral genome in peripheral blood of patients with myocarditis, but it has been shown to be identified in tracheal aspirate of incubated children with myocarditis thus reducing need for endomyocardial biopsy.[29]

6. *Molecular biology techniques:* To evaluate biopsy specimens is of significant research interest and may provide future insight into both the diagnosis and the pathogenesis of myocarditis. Insulin hybridization was performed on myocardial tissue using probes for Coxsackie virus.[27] But since it is difficult to use in a hospital setting, this investigation lost favor.

Differential Diagnosis

Any cause of acute circulatory failure may mimic myocarditis. Table 11.5 lists the differential diagnosis of congestive heart failure based on age of child.

Treatment

Care of patient presenting with a clinical picture strongly suggesting of myocarditis depends on severity of myocardial involvement.[30]

The general principles of management include:

1. *Exercise restriction:* Data from the animal models have shown that exercise increases myocardial inflammation and necrosis with myocarditis and so it is recommended that patients with myocarditis abstain from vigorous exercise for several months. Bed rest prevents an increase in viral replication and is strongly advocated.
2. *Decongestive measures:* Inotropic drugs-Digoxin and diuretics, etc. are the prime drugs to bring about dramatic improvement in decongestion. When oral therapy is possible, an after

Table 11.5: Differential diagnosis of myocarditis by age

Newborn and Infant	Child
Sepsis	Idiopathic dilated cardiomyopathy
Hypoxia	X-linked dilated cardiomyopathy
Hypoglycemia	Autosomal dominant dilated cardiomyopathy
Hypocalcemia	Anomalous left coronary artery from the pulmonary artery
Structural heart disease	
Idiopathic dilated cardiomyopathy	Endocardial fibroelastosis
Barth syndrome	Chronic tachyarrhythmia
Endocardial fibroelastosis	
Anomalous left coronary artery from the pulmonary artery	Pericarditis
Cerebral arteriovenous malformation	

Table 11.6: Clinical characteristics of patients with acute myocarditis [From Myocarditis Treatment Trial (1995) (n=111)][33]

Age	5-4 years
Sex	62% males
Ejection fraction	0.24+0.10
Flu-like symptoms	59%
Increased ESR	61%
Fever	18%
Leukocytes	24%
Chest pain	35%

load reducing drug such as captopril (1-3 mg/kg/day every 8 hours) or enalapril (0.2 mg/kg/day divided every 12 hours) should be given.[31] Sodium nitroprusside has been used to regulate systemic resistance and more recently phosphor-diesterase inhibitors such as intravenous milrinone has been used for inotropy.

3. *Anticoagulation:* Systemic anticoagulation may be required because inflamed endomyocardium may be predisposed to thrombosis. Greater frequency of thrombosis has been observed in human echocardiographic studies.
4. *Arrhythmias:* In presence of life threatening ventricular arrhythmias—long term solutions (e.g., ICD, permanent pacemaker implantation) should be considered only if temporary measures fail. Chronic arrhythmias may persist after acute disease has passed, so the patients have to be followed.[32]

5. *Mechanical assistance:* When myocarditis is refractory to standard medical therapy, intensive medical support and mechanical assistance should be used before heart transplantation is considered.
6. *Immunosuppressive therapy:* The Myocarditis Treatment Trial–largest randomized trial to date-designed specifically to address the efficacy of immunosuppression in myocarditis. A total of 111 patients with myocarditis who were diagnosed by endomyocardial biopsy under Dallas criteria-had an LV ejection fraction (LVEF) of < 45% were randomized to conventional therapy alone and also to conventional therapy combined with immunosuppression (prednisolone in all patients combined with either azathioprine or cyclosporin) for 6 months. The primary outcome measure was change in LVEF at 28 week follow up.

    The results of the trial showed no difference in the change in mean LVEF between the two treatment groups and also no difference in survival between the two groups was observed. These results did not identify any clinical benefit of immunosuppressive therapy for myocarditis and so routine immunosuppressive therapy cannot be recommended.

    The results of the myocarditis trial also have significantly influenced current approaches to the evaluation of myocarditis, and in most centers frequency of endomyocardial biopsy has also decreased.

    As far as the use of immunosuppressive therapy in myocarditis is concerned, the issue remains controversial, given the immunological mechanism of the disease, particularly when the clinical course is one of fulminant myocarditis. Currently, although no guidelines are in place, many physicians still initiate immunosuppression in patients with biopsy proved myocarditis in whom clinical deterioration continues despite standard heart failure treatment. The recognized approach by most physicians is that immunosuppression should be reserved for extraordinary circumstances and should not be considered a routine treatment.
7. *Investigational therapies:* Immune modulatory therapy with intravenous immunoglobulin was shown to be associated with improved cardiac function in a small cohort of adult patients with myocarditis and acute cardiomyopathy. The role of virus in initiating and maintaining the immunologic response is of interest, as is the significance of the persistence of viral ribonucleic acid fragments and their relationship to disease-progression to dilated cardiomyopathy.

    Interferon: Recently use of interferon has been reported. Kuhl et al[35] reported efficacy of interferon treatment in myocarditis with viral clearance and prevention of progressive deterioration of left ventricular function. Similarly, Daliento et al[36] reported similar success with interferon in patients with enterovirus induced myocarditis.

    Cardiac assist devices: Finally left ventricular assist device and aortic balloon pumps have been used in some cases, whereas extracorporeal membrane oxygenator has been used in others.

8. *Heart transplantation:* When no treatment helps and the clinical deterioration is progressive, the search should be on for a compatible donor for heart transplantation, more so in dilated cardiomyopathy, than in myocarditis.

Prognosis

Prognosis of acute myocarditis in newborn is poor.[37] 75% mortality was reported in 25 infants with suspected CVB myocarditis and mostly death occurred in the first week of illness. Older infants and children have a better prognosis with mortality rate between 10-25% of recognizable cases.

Vaccination

Vaccination has been used successfully to prevent diseases. A broadly specific enteroviral vaccine or atleast a CVB specific vaccine could be beneficial for reducing the incidence of myocarditis or DCM.[38] Endocardial fibroelastosis (EFE) was the commonest form of DCM seen in late 60s and EFE used to result from in utero mumps infection of myocardium. The mumps vaccine has all but eliminated this form of DCM.

Specific Causes of Myocarditis

Chagas Disease

American trypansomiasis or Chagas disease is one of the common causes in the western countries of congestive cardiac failure in childhood. This condition results from infection with *Trypanosoma cruzi* and is endemic in rural central and South America and some states of United States of America. In the chronic phase, the autonomic ganglia of the gastrointestinal tract are affected, leading to megacolon and megaesophagus. The characteristics of the cardiac disease include congestive heart failure, heart block and arrhythmias.

Diagnosis

1. Cellular and humoral immune response of myocardial injury.
2. Various anti-heart antibodies detected in high frequency.
3. Endomyocardial biopsy may show active myocarditis-shows organisms as well as polymorphic, lymphocytes, macrophages and eosinophils.
4. Echocardiography—segmental wall motion abnormalities, specifically apical aneurysms.
5. Electrocardiography—may show complete heart block, AV block or right bundle branch block.
6. Antibiody titers to *T. cruzi*—suggests the diagnosis.

Treatment

1. Nifurtimox-should be administered if not already treated and also for preventing recurrence.
2. Pacemaker implantation for complete heart block.
3. Amiodarone-for ventricular arrhythmias.
4. Decongestive therapy-for CCF-Digoxin, diuretics, ACE inhibitors.
5. Immunosuppressive therapy-controversial.

Toxoplasmosis

Acute infection by *Toxoplasma gondii* leads onto acute myocarditis. Diagnosis established by endomyocardial biopsy-identification of toxoplasma cysts in areas of focal myocyte necrosis, edema and a mixed inflammatory infiltrate including plasma cells, macrophages, lymphocytes and eosinophils. The organisms are seen within the myocytes (Figs 11.5A and B). Rise in antibody titer to *T. gondii* is commonly detected.

Treatment

This form of myocarditis is treatable if detected early. Usually treated with pyrimethamine and sulphadiazine.

Cytomegalovirus

Cytomegalovirus may lead to myocarditis in the general population, but it is usually asymptomatic and self limited.

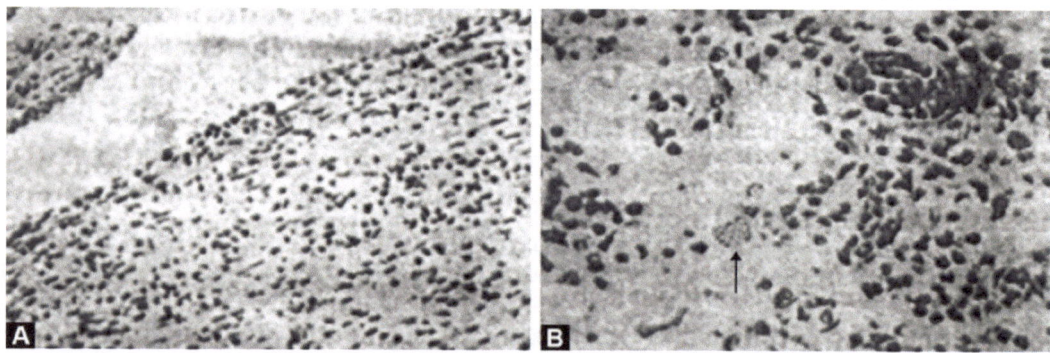

Figs 11.5A and B: (A) Low power microscope view of section of the heart in a patient with myocarditis showing diffuse cellular infiltration in the myocardium. (B) Higher power microscopic view of section of myocardium showing cellular infiltration and toxoplasma (arrow)

But in immunosuppressed patients, the myocarditis may take a serious form resulting in cardiac dysfunction.

It is proposed that infection of either sub-intimal fibroblasts or endothelial cells results in immunologic injury that predisposes to this potentially fatal condition.

Treatment

Intravenous gauciclavir, which effectively eradicates the virus.

Lyme Disease

Infection with spirochete *Borrelia burgdorferi* introduced by a tick bite results in Lyme disease.

Clinical features include-erythema chronica migrans, myalgias, and arthralgias, headache, fever, lymph-adenopathies and fatigue.

Occasionally it may progress to lyme carditis which presents with complete heart block. Left ventricular dysfunction is unusual.

Endomyocardial biopsy may reveal acute myocarditis and in one report spirochetes were identified in the myocardium.

Treatment

Tetracycline has been found to be of use in the early phase, followed by corticosteroids when carditis stage has set in.

Giant Cell Myocarditis (Fig. 11.6)

Giant cells in endomyocardial biopsies is particularly an aggressive form of myocarditis. It has the histological appearance of multinucleated giant cells of unknown etiology. It has an erratic clinical course with a worse prognosis, not consistently responding to immunosuppression. It is often associated with ventricular arrhythmias and refractory heart failure. The clinical implications of biopsy proven diagnosis are that cardiac transplantation should be considered as an essential measure even though giant cell myocarditis may recur in the allograft also.

This condition may be associated with autoimmune diseases such myasthenia gravis, autoimmune hemolytic anemia or polymyositis.

HIV Infection and Myocarditis

Involvement of the myocardium and pericardium with both common and unusual opportunistic infections and neoplasms such as Kaposi's sarcoma and lymphoma have been recognized. At times

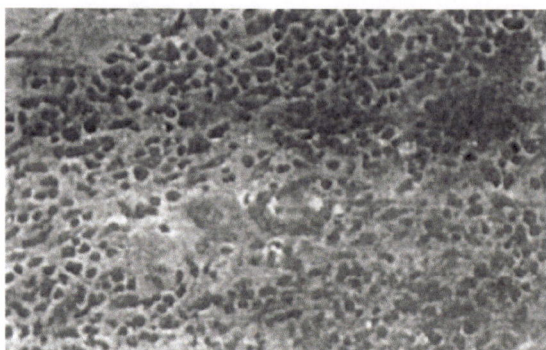

Fig. 11.6: Photomicrograph showing mixed cellular infiltrate and giant cells characteristic of giant cell myocarditis (H and E × 50)

this involvement appears to be incidental and associated with presence of organisms in many tissues including the heart and at times as intense myocarditis. Opportunistic infection has included viruses (*R. simplex,* Cytomegalovirus and Coxsackie virus) bacteria, protozoa (*Toxoplasma gondii*) and fungi (*Candida albicans*). Identification of organism is important because of potential for treatment, for instance amphotericin B and flucytosine for cryptocercosis.

There is a wide variation of association of lymphomas, Hodgkin's and non-Hodgkin's lymphomas in AIDS patients. Unfortunately, they tend to be histologically aggressive turnouts, involving many organs and responding poorly to treatment.

Echocardiography-revealing infiltration into myocardium and/or myocardial or pericardial masses. It is most helpful in establishing a diagnosis.

Non-infectious Inflammatory Myocarditis

Collagen Diseases

Systemic lupus erythematosus: Cardiovascular manifestations are not uncommon and approximately 40% demonstrate signs and symptoms of cardiac disease. Pericarditis and pericardial effusion are most commonly encountered, whereas myocarditis, conduction disturbances and heart failure occur less frequently.

Polyarteritis nodosa: Uncommon in children. Hypertension, tachycardia, heart failure and dysrrhythmias, more fulminant than adults.

Mucocutaneous Lymph Node Syndrome

Kawasaki disease: Kawasaki disease (KD) first described in Japan in 1967, but is now encountered worldwide.[39] Despite intensive research, its cause remains unknown. By mid 1970s, 2% of the affected children died suddenly in the convalescent stage of illness, mostly owing to myocardial infarction caused by acute thrombosis of aneurysmal coronary arteries.

Kawasaki disease-epidemiology
1. It occurs mostly in young children. Eighty percent of patients are younger than 5 years and 50% are younger than 2 years of age.
2. Males are more susceptible than girls with an approximate ratio of 1.5:1.
3. Children of all racial and ethnic groups are affected although. Most commonly affected are Asians, Pacific islanders (32.5/100,000 children under 5 years of age) moderate in black Americans, Hispanic and least commonly seen in white American (91/100,000 under 5 years of age).[40]
4. The recurrence rate of Kawasaki disease is approximately 3% and the proportion of positive history is 1%. Siblings have a relative risk that is tenfold and half of them develop Kawasaki within 10 days of first case.[41] The risk of developing Kawasaki is 100 times higher in twins.[41] These data support the role of genetic factors in susceptibility to Kawasaki disease. In USA, the familial incidence of Kawasaki disease is much lower than in Japan.

Etiology and Pathogenesis

1. The etiologic agent has not been identified. The disease is pobably driven by abnormalities of immune system initiated by infectious insult.
2. Genetic predisposition of the host appears to be as important as an external etiologic trigger, most probably combination for pathogenesis of Kawasaki disease.
3. Immunoregulatory abnormalities during acute phase include:
   a. Activation of monocytes and macrophages CD4+, T helper cells and β lymphocytes.
   b. Increased spontaneous production of immunoglobulins.
   c. Upregulations of cytokines–interleukin IL-1, IL-2, IL-6 and tumor necrosis factor (TNF), Proinflammatory cytokines appear to render vascular endothelium suceptible to lysis by antibodies.[42]
   d. Immunoglobulin Ig A secreting plasma cells have been identified from the cardiovascular system of a number of patients who died of Kawasaki disease. The same investigators have demonstrated immunohistochemical evidence of antigens within respiratory epithelium and macrophages which react with IgA antibodies genetically engineered from plasma cells.[43]

Pathology[44]

1. Generalized microvasculitis–first 10 days.
2. Myocarditis in first 3-4 weeks–mononuclear cell infiltration and edema in the myocardium.
3. Inflammation persists in walls of medium and large arteries especially coronary arteries, characterized by edema, mononuclear cell infiltration and progressive fibrosis with disruption in the internal elastic lamina which forms aneurysms. These are prominent in left anterior descending and branching points of coronary arteries. They may be fusiform, saccular, cylindrical or beaded.
4. More than 50% of the aneurysms regress within 1-2 years. Factors favoring aneurysm regression include, (i) onset age less than 1 year, (ii) female sex, (iii) fusiform shape and (iv) aneurysm diameter < 8 mm.

Aneurysms with internal diameter > 8 mm (giant aneurysms) present disproportionately higher risk of myocardial infarction as compared to smaller ones. Rarely anuerysms may rupture and cause sudden death. Postmortem examination in a few cases where death owing to unrelated causes occurs many years after acute Kawasaki disease showed extensive fibrosis and intimal proliferation in coronary arteries. Vasculitis with aneurysm formation which may lead to scar formation and calcification. Occasionally myocardial infarction may result in death.

5. In addition there are pericarditis (100%) and myocarditis (69%) also.
6. Elevated platelet count-contributes to coronary thrombosis.

Clinical Picture

Clinical course divided into three phases: Acute, subacute and convalescent.

Acute Phase (First 10 days)-Diagnostic Criteria

1. Fever (up to 40°C) for 5 days.
2. Bilateral non-exudative conjunctival injection.
3. Diffuse reddening of oral cavity, erythema and cracking of lips, strawberry tongue.
4. Induration and erythema of hands and feet–fusiform swelling of proximal interphalangeal joints–painful.
5. Polymorphous exanthema–rash begins in the diapered area and spreads to torso and extremities.
6. Cervical lymphadenopathy (>1.5 cm), usually unilateral.
7. Non–suppurative–gangrene of fingers and toes–rare. Seen in non Asians.
8. Aseptic meningitis–rare.

Sub Acute Phase (11-25 days after Onset)

1. Desquamation of tips of fingers and toes in sub-ungual region-characteristic.
2. Fever, rash and lymphadenopathy disappear.

3. Cardiovascular manifestations, e.g. pericardial effusion, myocarditis giving rise to CCF, myocardial ischemia manifest at this stage. Approximately 20% of the patients reveal coronary artery aneurysm on echocardiogram.
4. Hepato biliary–hepatomegaly, transient jaundice and abnormal liver function tests.
5. Arthralgia and arthritis in some which may last for months.
6. Transient diarrhea, abdominal discomfort.
7. Signs of urethritis accompanied by dysuria proteinuria and sterile pyuria.
8. Transient and isolated peripheral nerve involvement, e.g. facial palsy, phrenic nerve paralysis or sensorineural hearing loss may occur.
9. Thrombocytosis occurs beyond 2 weeks.

Convalescent Phase

This phase lasts till ESR and platelet count return to normal.

Echocardiography

To detect coronary artery aneurysm and other reported cardiac dysfunction:
1. Normal caliber of the coronary arteries is 2 mm in infants and 5 mm in teenagers in proximal 10 mm of the arteries, normal coronary arteries are uniform in caliber. Large aneurysm can be documented (Figs 11.7 and 11.8).
2. Depressed LV function (systolic/diastolic dysfunction) with decreased fractional shortening and ejection fraction.
3. Regurgitation of tricuspid/mitral and aortic valves present in 50% of patients.
4. Pericardial effusion may be present.

Laboratory Studies

1. Blood–marked leukocytosis with a shift to left. Neutrophilia with vacuoles and toxic granules–common in first week.
2. Thrombocytosis-in subacute phase.
3. Acute phase reactants-elevated ESR and C-reactive protein.
4. Elevated myocardial enzyme levels.

Natural History

Kawasaki's disease is a self limiting disease for most patients. Cardiovascular involvement is the most serious complication of the disease.

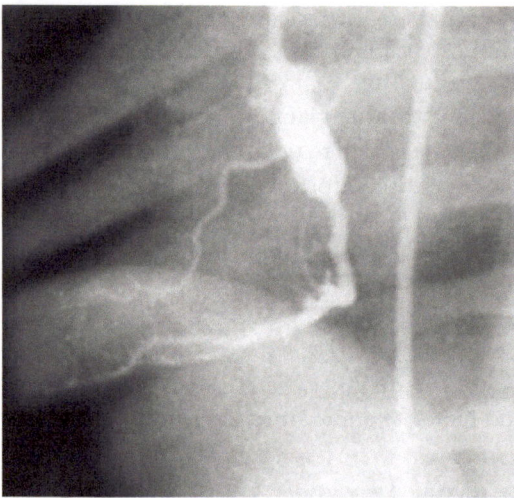

Fig. 11.7: Angiogram of right coronary artery, showing giant aneurysm[44]

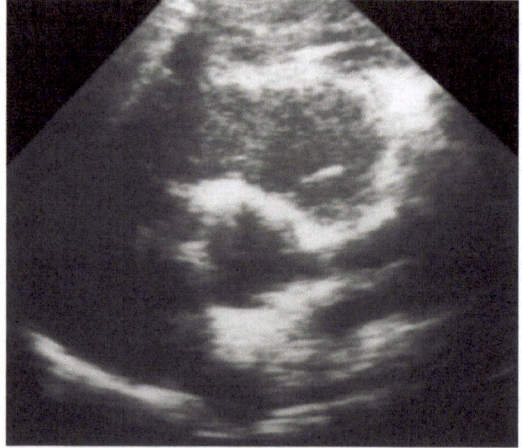

Fig. 11.8: Parasternal short-axis view from a patient with Kawasaki's disease. There is a large circular aneurysm (Arrow) of the left coronary artery

1. Coronary aneurysm occurs in 15-25% of patients and is responsible for myocardial infarction (5%) and mortality (1-5%). Giant aneurysm (>8 mm) is associated with greater morbidity and mortality (because of thrombotic occlusion or stenotic obstruction and subsequent myocardial infarction).
2. Coronary aneurysm tends to regress by 1 year in 50% but in some coronary stenosis may take place.
3. If the coronary arteries remain normal throughout the first month, then subsequent development of new aneurysm is unlikely.

Treatment

No specific therapy is available. Two goals of therapy are reduction of inflammation within the coronary artery and myocardium and prevention of thrombosis by inhibition of platelet aggregation.

1. Single dose I/V immune globulin (IVIG) (2 gm/kg/day) as a single infusion[45] with Aspirin (80-100 mg kg/day) for 10 days-treatment of choice. Because of presence of myocardial dysfunction IVIG is administered slowly over 8-12 hours to minimize side effects in four divided doses.
2. Reduction of Aspirin to 3-5 mg/kg/day (antiplatelet dose) in single dose on 14th day of illness. Aspirin should be discontinued by 6-8 weeks after onset of disease.
3. Blood salicylate levels and liver function tests should be monitored to avoid salicylate intoxication.
4. Serial Echo monitoring is important for evaluation of cardiac status.
5. Occasionally coronary angiography is indicated in presence of large aneurysm.
6. On rare occasions, coronary artery bypass surgery-may be indicated.
7. Influenza vaccine is recommended for all children on chronic aspirin therapy.[46]

REFERENCES

1. Wynn J, Brannwald E. The cardiomyopathies and myocarditis. In Brannwald E ed. Heart disease: A text book of cardiovascular medicine. Philadelphia: WB Saunders 1997:1404-63.
2. Berkovich S, Rodrignez–Jerres R, Din JS. Virologic studies in children with acute myocarditis. Am J Dis child 1968;11:207-11.
3. Van de Veyver IB, NiJ, Bowles, et al. Detection of intrauterine viral infection using polymerase chain reaction (PCR). Mol Genet Metab 1998;63:85-95.
4. Bowles NE, Bowles KR, Towbin JA. Viral genome detection and outcome in myocarditis. Heart Failure clinics 2005;1:407-17.
5. Woodruff JF. Viral Myocarditis. A review Am J Palthol 1980;101:427-84.
6. Pankuweit S, Lamparter S, Schoppet M, et al. Parvovirus B19 genome in endomyocardial biopsy specimen. Circulation 2004;109:e179.
7. Prolikov GF, Minkovich BM. A case of respiratory syncytial virus infection in a child by interstitial myocarditis with lethal outcome. Arkh Pathol 1972;34:70-73.

8. Lash AD, Wittman AL, Quismorio FP Jr. Myocarditis in mixed connective tissue disease: clinical and pathological study of 3 cases and review of literature. Semin Arth. Rheumatic 1986;15:288-96.
9. Friedman RA, Schoengerdt KO, Towbin JA. Myocarditis in Bricher Jt, Garson A Jr, Fisher DJ, et al (Eds). The science and practice of Pediatric cardiology: 2nd ed. Baltimore: William and Wilkins 1998:1777-94.
10. Towbin JA. Myocarditis. In Allen HD, Driscott DJ, Shaddy RE, Fettes TF, eds. Moss and Adams Heart Disease in infants, children and adolescents including the fetus and young adult. Seventh Edition Philadelphia: Wotters Kluwer, Lippincott. Williams and Wilkins 2008:1207-24.
11. Sasaki K, Sakata K, Kachi E, et al. Sequential changes in cardiac structure and function in patients with Duchenne type muscular dystrophy: A two dimensional echocardiographic study. Am Heart J 1998; 135:937-44.
12. Milasin J, Muntoin F, Severini GM, et al. A point mutation in the 5; splice site of the dystrophin gene first intron responsible for X-linked dilated cardiomyopathy. Hum Mol. Genet 1996;5:73-79.
13. Bessendo R, Marrie TJ, Smith ER. Cardiac involvement in trichionosis. Chest 1981;79:698-99.
14. Godemy EK, Gauntt CJ. Murine natural killer cells limit coxsackie virus B3 replication. J Immuno, 1987; 139:913-18.
15. Wong CY, Woodruff JJ, Woodruff JF. Generation of cytotoxic T lymphocytes during Coxsackie B-3 infection. II: Characterization of effective cells and demonstration of cytotoxicity against viral infected fibers J Immunol 1997;118:165-169.
16. Panshinger M, Bowles NE, Fuontes–Garcia FJ, et al. Detection of adenoviral genome in the myocardium of adult patients with idiopathic left ventricular dysfunction. Circulation 1999;99:1348-54.
17. Narula J, Haider N, Virmain R, et al. Apoptosis in myocytes in end stage heart disease. N Engl J Med 1996;335:1182-89.
18. Kubota T, Mc Tiernan CF, Frye CS, et al. Cardiac specific over expression of tumor necrosis factor-alpha causes lethal myocarditis. J Card Fail 1997;3:117-24.
19. Shimiz C, Ramband C, Cheron G, et al. Molecular identification in sudden infant death associated with myocarditis and pericarditis. Pediatr. Infest Dis J 1995;14:584-88.
20. Ni J, Bowles NE, Kim YH, et al. Viral infection of myocardium in endocardial fibroelastosis: Molecular evidence for the role of mumps virus as an etiologic agent. Circulation 1997;9:133-39.
21. Towbin JA, Bricker Jt, Garson A Jr. Electrocardiographic criteria for diagnosis of acute myocardial infarction in childhood. Am J Cardiol 1992;69:1545-48.
22. Mason JW. Distinct forms of myocarditis. Circulation 1491;83:1110-11.
23. Chow LH, Radio SJ, Sears TD, et al. Insensitivity of right ventricular biopsy in the diagnosis of myocarditis. J Am Coll Cardiol 1989;14:915-20.
24. Aretz HT, Myocarditis: The Dallas Criteria Hum Pathol 1987;18:619-24.
25. Shingu M. Laboratory diagnosis of viral myocarditis. A review. Jp Circ J 1989;53:87-93.
26. Martin AB, Webber S, Fricker FJ, et al. Acute myocarditis: Rapid diagnosis by PCR in children. Circulation 1994;90:330-33.
27. Bowles NE, Richardson PJ, Olsen EGJ, et al. Detection of Coxsackie B virus specific RNA sequence in myocardial biopsy samples from patients with myocarditis and dilated cardiomyopathy. Lancet 1986; 1:1120-23.

28. Matsumori A. Hepatitis C virus infection and cardiomyopathies. Circ Res 2005;96:144-47.
29. Akhtar N, Ni J, Stromberg D, et al. Tracheal aspirate as a substitute for polymerase chain reaction detection of viral genome in childhood pneumonia and myocarditis. Circulation 1999;99:2011-13.
30. Parril JE. Myocarditis: How should we treat in 1998? J heart lung transplant 1998;17:941-44.
31. Rezkalda S, Kloner RA, Khatil G, et al. Beneficial effects of Captopril in acute coxsackie virus B3 murine myocarditis. Circulation 1990;81:1039-46.
32. Friedman RA, Kearney DL, Moak JP, et al. Persistence of ventricular arrhythmia after resolution of occult myocarditis in children and young adults. J Am Coll Cardiol 1994;24:780-83.
33. Mason JW, O'Connell JB, Herokowitz A, et al. The myocarditis treatment trial investigators. A clinical trial of immunosuppressive therapy for myocarditis. N Engl J Med 1995;333:269-75.
34. Drucker NA, Colan SD, Lewis AB. Gamma globulin treatment of acute myocarditis on the pediatric population. Circulation 1994;89q:252-57.
35. Kuhl V, Panschinger M, Schwimmbeck PL, et al. Interferon B treatment eliminates cardiotropic viruses and improves left ventricular function in patients with myocardial persistence of viral genomes and left ventricular dysfunction. Circulation 2003;107:2793-98.
36. Daliento L, Calabrese F, Tona F, et al. Successful treatment of enterovirus induced myocarditis with interferon alpha. J Heart Lung transplant 2003;22:214-17.
37. Bengtssen E, Lamberger B. Five year follow-up study of cases suggestive of acute myocarditis. Am Heart J 1966;72:751-63.
38. Zhang HY, Morgan-Capner P, Latif N, et al. Coxsackie virus B3 induced myocarditis characterization of stable attenuated variants that protect against infection with the cardiovirulent wild type strain. Am J Pathol 1997;150:2197-207.
39. Kawasaki T, Kosaki F, Okawa S, et al. A new infantile acute febrile mucocutaneous lymph node syndrome (MLNS) prevailing in Japan. Pediatrics 1974;54:271-76.
40. Holman RC, Curns AT, Belay ED, et al. Kawasaki syndrome hospitalizations in United states, 1997 and 2000. Pediatrics 2003;112:495-501.
41. Fujita Y, Nakamura S, Sakaqta K, et al. Kawasaki disease in families. Pediatrics 1989;84:666-69.
42. Leung DYM, Geha RS, Newburger JW, et al. Two monokines, interleukin and tumor necrosis factor, render cultured vascular endothelial cells susceptible to lysis by antibodies circulating during Kawasaki syndrome. J Exp Med 1986;164:1958-72.
43. Rowley AH, Baker SC, Shulman ST, et al. Detection of antigen in bronchial epithelium and macrophages in acute Kawasaki disease by use of synthetic antibody. J Infect Dis 2004;190:856-65.
44. Fujiwara H, Hamashima Y. Pathology of the heart in Kawasaki disease. Pediatrics 1978;61:100-07.
45. Terai M, Shulman ST. Prevalence of coronary artery abnormalities in Kawasaki disease highly dependent on gamma globulin dose but independent of salicylate dose. J Pediatr 1997;131:888-93.
46. Takahashi M, Mason W, Thomas D, et al. Reye Syndrome following Kawasaki syndrome confirmed by histopathology. In Kato H, ed. Kawasaki Disease. Proceedings of 5th International Kawasaki Disease symposium Amsterdam: Elsevier Science 1995;436-44.

PART II

CARDIOMYOPATHY

The term cardiomyopathy refers to any structural or functional abnormality of the ventricular myocardium not associated with coronary artery disease, high blood pressure, valvular, congenital heart disease or pulmonary vascular disease. With increasing awareness of this condition, cardiomyopathy is being recognized as a significant cause of morbidity and mortality.

It can be broadly divided into 2 main categories, primary and secondary. The latter is that where it is associated with a systemic disorder and is termed "specific heart muscle diseases" (Table 11.7). Primary(idiopathic), cardiomyopathies are classified into 3 main groups. Dilated (Congestive), Hypertrophic and Restrictive, which can further be classified based on the underlying pathology (Table 11.7). The summary of clinical characteristics of cardiomyopathies are elaborated in Table 11.8.

Dilated Congestive Cardiomyopathy (DCM)

Cardiac dilation and decreased systolic function are the uniform diagnostic features of dilated cardiomyopathy. DCM with a prevalence of (36.5 per 100,000 population[1]) is a final common

Table 11.7: Cardiomyopathy in children–classification (WHO)

Primary		
Dilated	-	Idiomyopathic dilated cardiomyopathy
	-	Endocardial fibroelastosis
Hypertrophic	-	Obstructive
		Non-obstructive
Restrictive	-	Endomyocardial fibrosis
	-	Loffler's eosinophilic endomyocardial disease
	-	Hemochromatosis, sarcoidosis
Arryhthmogenic	-	Right ventricular dysplasia
Secondary		
Infection	-	Myocarditis – all varieties
Metabolic	-	Diabetes mellitus, thyrotoxicosis
Systemic diseases	-	Aorto-arteritis, coarctation of aorta
Heredofamilial	-	Duchenne's muscular dystrophy
Hypersensitivity and Toxic reactions	-	Sulfonamides penicillins, steroids, chloramphenicol

Table 11.8: Summary of clinical characteristics of cardiomyopathies (Fig. 11.9)[23]

	Hypertrophic	*Dilated*	*Restrictive*
Etiology	Inherited (AD in 60%) Sporadic (new mutation) +	Pleuricausal (e.g., toxic metabolic, infectious, Alcohol, doxorubicin)	Myocardial fibrosis Hypertrophy, or infiltration (amyloid)
Hemodynamic Dysfunction	Diastolic dysfunction (with normal systolic function) (abnormally Stiff LV with impaired Ventricular filling)	Systolic contractile dysfunction (↓ cardiac output ↓ stroke volume- ↑ - LVEDP)	Diastolic dysfunction (rigid ventricular walls impede ventricular filling)
Echo (morphology)	Thickened LV wall Small or normal LV chamber dimension Supernormal LV contractility HOCM and/or ASH	Biventricular dilatation (LVDD, LVSD) Atrial enlargement in proportion to ventricular enlargement, Decreased LV contractility, Apical thrombus (+)	Biatrial enlargement Normal LV and RV volume Normal LV systolic function until advanced stage atrial thrombus (+)
Doppler	Reduced relaxation pattern (Fig. 11.12)	Reduced relaxation pattern (Fig. 11.12)	"Restrictive" pattern (Fig. 11.12)
Treatment	β – Adrenoreceptor blockers Calcium antagonists digitalis/ nitrates contraindicated diuretics may worsen symptoms	Vasodilator therapy (ACE-inhibitors Digitalis plus, diuretics β – Adrenoceptor blockers (+) - Anticoagulants Antiarrhythmics (+) Cardiac transplant (+)	Diuretics Anticoagulants (+) Corticosteroids (+) Permanent pacemaker for advanced heart block (+) Cardiac transplant (+)

AD, autosomal dominant; LVEDP, LV end diastolic pressure; ASH, asymmetric septal hypertrophy, LVDD, LV diastolic dimension; LVSD, LV Systolic dimension

pathway for diverse disease processes that lead to heart failure. Most patients with idiopathic DCM have clinically silent disease in childhood, becoming symptomatic only in years beyond childhood.[2] Primary cause of sporadic and hereditary DCM in childhood is unknown and in over 70%[3] of DCM cases has shown a high incidence of myocardial inflammation but not so in children. Reports have shown an increase in structural abnormalities of mitochondrial DNA in a high percentage of patients with DCM. Experimental reports suggest that an immunologic abnormality may be implicated in the pathogenesis of the disease. Usually the pathologic process involves the myocardium in both ventricles in a uniform fashion resulting in generalized cardiac dilatation. The myocardium is pale

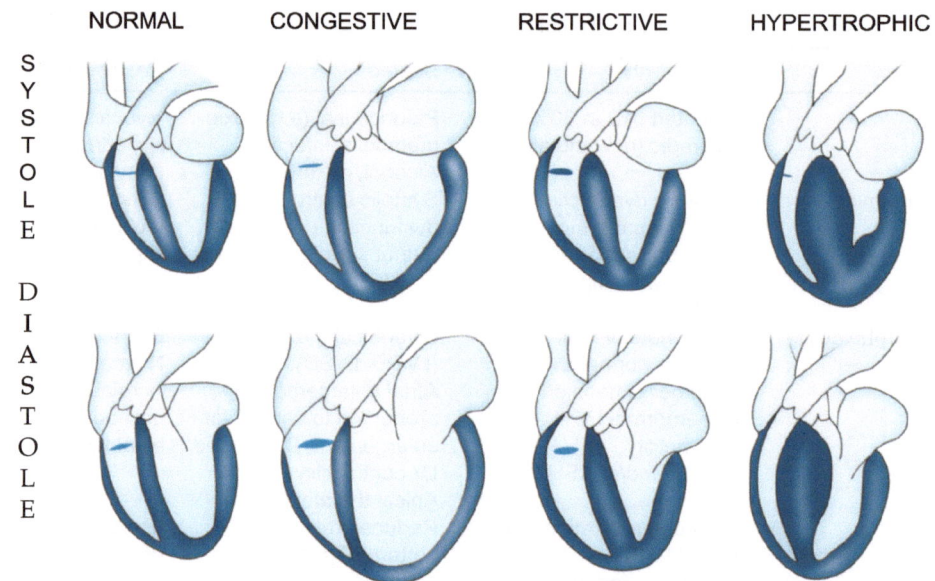

Fig.11.9:[10] Diagram of the 50 degree left anterior oblique view of the heart in different types of cardiomyopathy at end-diastole. "Congestive" corresponds to "dilated" cardiomyopathy as used in the text

and thinned out and the endocardium is translucent. Microscopic examination shows interstitial fibrosis, myofiberhypertrophy, degeneration and necrosis. Sensitive preclinical markers of DCM unfortunately are lacking. Despite an insidious onset, advanced myocardial disease with substantial re-modeling is often present and late diagnosis of end-stage disease is often confounded by lack of guideline for treatment of heart failure due to DCM in children.[4] Prognosis in individual patient is often unpredictable ranging from intractable heart failure to occasional spontaneous recovery.[5] Improved treatment and prevention of DCM will require identification of pre-clinical markers, new insights into disease mechanisms, risk classification and optimal therapies that alter pathologic molecular and cellular processes prior to the development of end-stage myocardial disease.

Etiopathogenesis (Fig. 11.10)

It is likely that DCM represents a common expression of myocardial damage that has been produced by a variety of as yet unestablished myocardial insults (Table 11.9):

Table 11.9: Causes of dilated cardiomyopathy

- Acute and chronic myocarditis – coxsackievirus, adenovirus, HIV
- Collagen vascular disease
- Drugs – alcohol, sympathomimetics, anthracyclines
- End-stage hypertrophic cardiomyopathy
- Endocrine – growth hormone deficiency, hyperthyroidism, hypothyroidism, hypocalcemia, diabetes mellitus pheochromocytoma
- Hereditary – autosomal dominant, automsomal recessive, X-linked, mitochondrial
- Inborn errors of metabolism
- Ischemic – atherosclerosis, Kawasaki disease, anomalous origin of left coronary artery
- Muscular dystrophies
- Nutritional deficiency – selenium, carnitine, thiamine
- Peripartum
- Structural heart disease – AR, MR, TR
- Systemic hypertension
- Toxins – cobal, lead

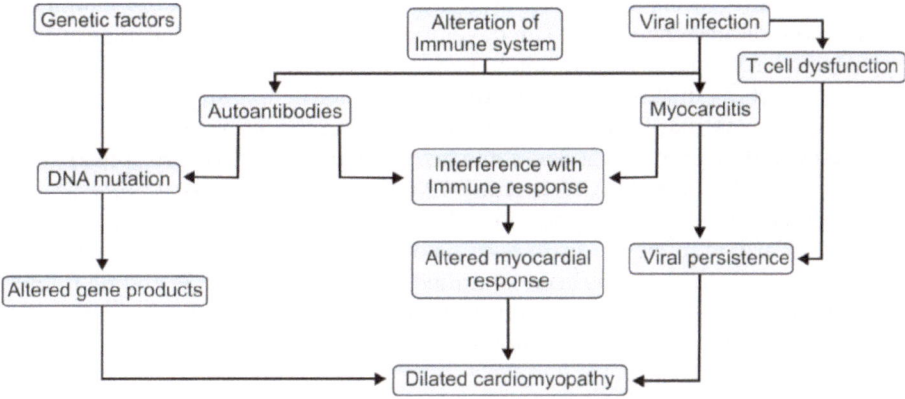

Fig. 11.10:[1] Etiopathogenesis of dilated cardiomyopathy

Although the cause is still unclear, interest has centered on 3 basic mechanisms (Fig. 11.10).
– Familial and genetic factors
– Viral myocarditis
– Immunological abnormalities

Familial linkage of DCM occurs more commonly and in 20% of patients, a first degree relative also shows presence of DCM, suggesting that familial transmission is relatively frequent.[6] Most familial cases demonstrate autosomal dominant transmission, but the disease is quite genetically heterogenous and autosomal recessive and X-linked inheritance has also been documented. This has fuelled speculation that a resulting deficiency of cardiac dystrophin is the cause of dilated cardiomyopathy. One intriguing familial metabolic deficiency is that of carnitine with improvement occurring in the myopathy with carnitine repletion. In idiopathic DCM, cardiac dilation initially or eventually becomes maladaptive and cardiothoracic ratio on chest radiography is predictive of mortality.[1] It is unknown whether dilation initially is an adaptive response to myocardial dysfunction or a primary pathologic process of ventricular remodeling. In either case unless wall thickness increases dilation leads to increased wall stress (Laplace's law) and mismatch of myocardial oxygen supply and demand. In fact, decreased posterior wall thickness in DCM is associated with a worse prognosis.[1]

Pathology

On postmortem examination, there is enlargement and dilatation of all 4 chambers, though ventricles are more dilated than atria. The development of left ventricular hypertrophy appears to have a protective role in dilated cardiomyopathy, presumably because it reduces systolic wall stress and this protects against further cavity dilatation. Microscopic study reveals extensive areas of interstitial and perivascular fibrosis particularly involving the left ventricular subendocardium. There is marked variation in myocyte size, some myocardial cells are hypertrophied and others are atrophied (apoptosis). Myocyte loss in chronic DCM occurs by two general processes – apoptosis, programmed cellular self destruction[7] and subclinical necrosis detected by release of cardiac enzymes in bloodstream.[8] Cardiac myocyte death is a major pathologic process in DCM and correlates with worse prognosis.[9] No virus has been identified in tissues from DCM and no immunological, histochemical, morphological, ultrastructural or biological markers have been identified to establish the diagnosis of idiopathic dilated cardiomyopathy.

Clinical Picture

Patients with DCM usually develop symptoms correlating with the degree of myocardial dysfunction.
1. Initial presentation is gradual, preceded by upper respiratory infection or gastroenteritis/gastritis in 33-50% of cases.
2. Manifestations of congestive cardiac failure in older childen—feeding difficulties, tachypnea, excessive perspiration leading on to failure to thrive – manifestations of low output state and pulmonary venous congestion. In severe cases, fulminant pulmonary edema may occur.

3. Some present with ventricular or supraventricular tachycardia.
4. In infants, the symptoms are vague. They present with tachypnea, dyspnea, irritability and poor feeding. History of dry skin and peripheral edema indicate/hypothyroidisms

Physical Examination

1. Ill looking child in moderate to severe respiratory distress, anxious, grunting, diaphoretic and with tachycardia.
2. Moderate to severe pallor.
3. Manifestations of low output state—weak peripheral pulses with low blood pressure and narrowed pulse pressure.
   "Pulsus alternans"—a common finding—where volume of each pulse alternates"
4. Thoracic overdistension and rarely prominence of left hemithorax.
5. On auscultation—muffled heart sounds with presence of gallop rhythm. Initially murmurs are absent but soft apical pansystolic murmur of mitral regurgitation often appears after a few days, once the cardiac function improves.
6. Other signs of congestive cardiac failure—enlarged tender liver, facial edema in an infant. Neck vein distension and pedal edema are rarely found in infants but are frequently present in older children and adolescents.

Laboratory Investigations

1. *Chest radiography:* Cardiomegaly secondary to dilatation of left atrium and left ventricle and evidence of pulmonary venous congestion. Left atrial enlargement may cause elevation of left main stem bronchus. The pattern of increases pulmonary vascular markings is reticular (Figs 11.11A and B).
2. Electrocardiogram, sinus tachycardia with LV hypertrophy and T wave changes are seen in most patients.
   - Atrial or ventricular tachycardias and A V conduction disturbances may also be seen.
3. *Echocardiography:* It is the most important tool in the diagnosis of this condition and is important in the longitudinal follow up of patients.
1. The LV and RV are both dilated. The end-diastolic and end-systolic dimensions of the LV are both increased with a reduced fractional shortening and ejection fraction (Figs 11.11A and B).
2. Pericardial effusion and intracavitary thrombus may be seen.
3. Mitral inflow Doppler tracing demonstrates a reduced E velocity and a decreased. E/A ratio compared with normal subjects (Fig. 11.12).
4. Mitral regurgitation is well demonstrated by color flow Doppler imaging.

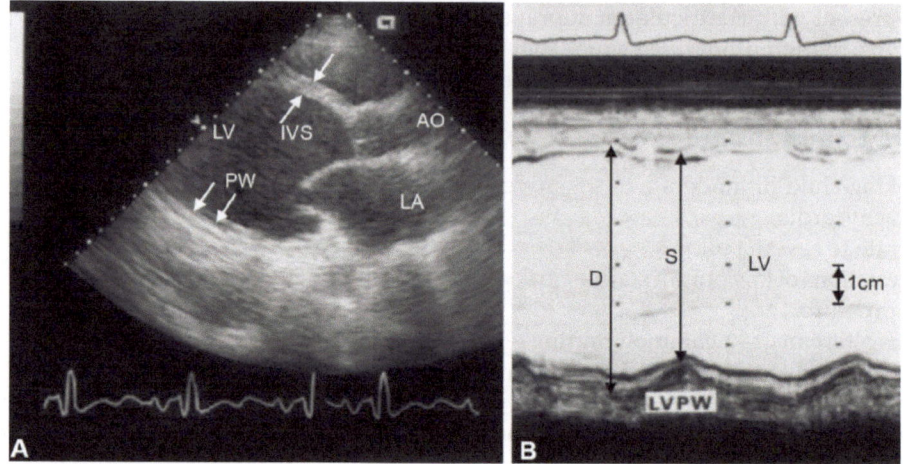

Figs 11.11A and B: Dilated left ventricle with impaired systolic function due to dilated cardiomyopathy

Natural History

1. Progressive deterioration in the clinical condition and about 60% die of intractable heart failure in about 3-4 years after the onset of symptoms of heart failure.
2. Atrial and ventricular arrhythmias develop in the course of the disease process diagnosed by 24-hour ambulatory monitoring.
3. Systemic and pulmonary embolism resulting from dislodgement of intracavitary thrombus occurs in the late stages of the disease.
4. Causes of death include congestive cardiac failure. Sudden death may also result from arrhythmias and massive embolization.

Treatment

Treatment is aimed at increasing cardiac output, enhancing tissue oxygen delivery and sustaining vital organ function. An optimal inotropic agent would be one that improves systolic and diastolic dysfunction, decreases systemic and pulmonary vasoconstriction, has little or no side effects and improves quality of life.[10]

1. Control congestive cardiac failure.
    a. Bed rest, restricted fluid intake. Careful monitoring of daily weight gain
       Infants-Parenteral nutrition-75-80% of their fluid requirement

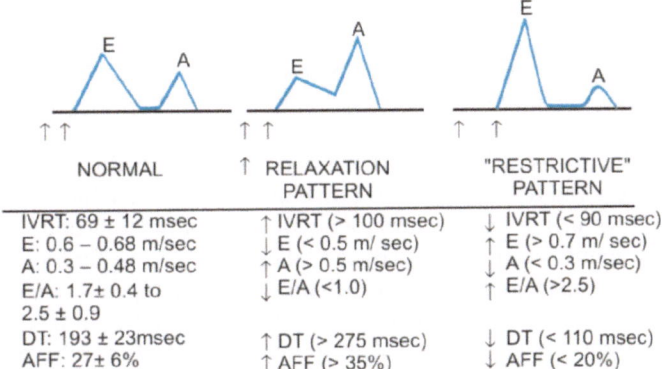

Fig. 11.12: Examples of diastolic dysfunction seen in various forms of cardiomyopathy. A, A wave (the velocity of a second wave that coincides with atrial contraction); AFF, atrial filling fraction; DT, deceleration time; E, E wave (the velocity of an early peak); E/A, ratio of E wave to A wave velocity; IVRT, isovolumic relaxation time

    b. Diuretics-Controls the cardiac load. Frusemide -1-2 mg/kg, then oral feeding -can be given with potassium chloride supplementation. Spironolactone can be added to reduce potassium loss. Other potent diuretics include ethacrynic acid and bumetanide and they also act at loop of Henle.
    c. Inotropic agents
       i. Digoxin -0.06 mg -0.04 mg/kg/24 hours followed by maintenance -1/5 -1/4 of maintenance dose
      ii. Sympathomimetic amines -dopamine and dobutamine –faster mode of action.
     iii. Type III phosphodiesterase inhibitor: Amrinone/Milrinone -improves contractility and reduces after load in both ventricles. Because of some side effects, amrinone is no longer used. Milrinone, a bipyridine compound and derivative of amrinone is the primary agent of choice. This drug is said to promote increase in intracellular calcium concentration by inhibition of phosphodiesterase III. Milrinone in combination with dobutamine may increase cardiac output and also may help in pulmonary vascular resistance. The half life varies between 1-4 hours and the dose should be adjusted if there is renal impairment.
        Levosimendan is a calcium sensitizing agent and has been evaluated in children in congenital heart disease and has been found to be useful in treating chronic congestive heart failure.[11] It binds to troponin-C in cardiac myocytes and improves cardiac contractility.
    d. Afterload reducing agents.
       Hydralazine (0.25 -1.00 mg/kg 4 times a day)

Prazosin (50 -100 µg/kg 4 times a day)

These drugs dilate peripheral vessels and decrease afterload, increase cardiac output and decrease filling pressures. Other effective orally administered afterload reducing agents include angiotensin converting enzyme inhibitors. Captopril and Enalapril are used most commonly in children.

The action of ACE-inhibitors include decreased synthesis of angiotensin II, a potent vasoconstriction and decreased breakdown of bradykinine which are potent vasodilators. They also reduce urinary potassium loss by inhibiting aldosterone secretion.

e. Beta blocking agents – Carvedilol, a drug that has both β receptor blocking and vasodilating actions, improve left ventricular performance. Both metaprolol and carvedilol have been used in children. Nesiritide is a recombinant β type natriuretic peptide that causes a balanced dilation of arteries and veins, enhances glomerular filtration rate, produces diuresis and natriuresis and causes neurohormonal of suppression sympathetic and rennin – angiotensin – aldosterone systems.[12]
f. Arrhythmias
   – Anti-arrhythmic agents -amiodarone, adenosine
   – Radiofrequency ablation – useful in chronic atrial fibrillation.
g. Anticoagulation in presence of atrial fibrillation -heparin, warfarin, etc. – Anti-platelet drugs have a role to play in treatment of DCM.
h. Immunosuppressive agents: Role of steroids and azathioprine or cyclosporine -controversial
   They are indicated in only those children who have myocardial inflammation on endomyocardial biopsy.
i. Cardiac transplantation.
   Those children who fail to respond to medical therapy
   NYHA class IV symptomatology—life expectancy of 6 months
   The greatest risk for death or transplantation was age, younger than 1 year or older than 12 years and female gender. With transplantation, 1 year and 5 years survival for children with dilated cardiomyopathy was 90% and 83% respectively.[13]

Prognosis

– For infants and small children with idiopathic DCM -prognosis is poor
– Mortality -35% - 60% -mostly in the first year
– Those who manifest before 2 years of age—better chance of survival
– Mode of death - intractable heart failure, arrhythmias
– About 50% recover completely and others continue with LV dysfunction

Endocardial Fibroelastosis

Epidemiology

Endocardial fibroelastosis (EFE) is detected in less than 1 % of infants with CHD. Girls are affected 1.5 times more than boys. The prevalence has declined in the past 2 decades for unknown reasons. It used to account for 4% of all cardiac autopsy cases in children.

Etiopathogenesis

1. The etiology of primary fibroelastosis is not known. It has been associated with intrauterine mumps infection, and because of immunization, incidence of mumps has also gone down significantly. It may be a reaction to many different mechanisms producing endocardial and myocardial stress during fetal life. The disease is 700 times more common in siblings of affected children, underlying the importance of genetic factors.
2. Endocardial fibroelastosis is a form of dilated cardiomyopathy in children. It is characterized by diffuse changes in endocardium with a white opaque glistening appearance. Left atrium and ventricle are dilated and hypertrophied. Right sided chambers are rarely involved. Papillary muscles and chordae tendineae are deformed and shortened (producing MR) and similar pathology appears secondary to obstructive lesions of the left heart, such as AS, coarctation of aorta and HLHS (secondary fibroelastosis). Patients with aortic atresia and a patent mitral valve, may also have associated endocardial firboelastosis which is probably due to subendocardial ischemia. Presence of tricuspid insufficiency may be an additional feature. Arrhythmias associated with endocardial fibroelastosis may both contribute to an increased mortality risk.

Clinical Manifestations

Manifestations of congestive cardiac failure (feeding difficulties, easy fatigability, sweating, tachypnea, failure to thrive) appear in infancy and on examination also the findings of CCF, e.g., tachycardia, tachypnea, hepatomegaly and sometimes systolic murmur of MR would be heard.

Electrocardiography

LVH with "Strain" is typical of the condition. Occasionally myocardial infarction pattern, arrhythmias and varying degrees of AV blocks may be present.

X-ray Study

Marked generalized cardiomegaly with normal or congested pulmonary vascularity is usually present.

Echocardiography

LA and LV are markedly dilated with poor contractility with no structural heart defects. Bright endocardial echoes are characteristic of this condition.

Treatment

1. Early diagnosis and long term decongestive therapy with digoxin, diuretics and after load reducing agents, e.g. hydralazing are mandatory.
2. Prophylaxis against SBE should be observed, especially when MR is present.

Prognosis

When proper treatment is instituted, about one third of the patients deteriorate and another 1/3 remain with persistent symptoms. The remaining one third exhibit complete recovery.

Hypertrophic Cardiomyopathy

Hypertrophic cardiomyopathy (HCM) is a congenital disease that may manifest in infancy, childhood, adolescence or young adulthood. Recent studies have confirmed the genetic predisposition of HCM and with appropriate therapy; most patients can enjoy a reasonable lifestyle with little fear of sudden cardiac death. If undiagnosed, HCM may cause disability and death at virtually any age and is the most common cause of sudden cardiac death in young including competitive athletes.

Clinical Screening – Strategies in Families

In clinical practice, prospective screening of HCM family members (Table 11.10) to ascertain affected or unaffected genetic status usually takes place without doing DNA analysis by doing ECG, history taking and echocardiography.

Prevalence

HCM occurs in at least 0.2% in general population (1:500)[14], though it is rather uncommon in general pediatric population.[15]

Genetics

Hypertrophic cardiomyopathy is quite heterogeneous. Even members of the same family with a common genetic substrate can exhibit markedly diverse evolution and natural history of the disease. This disease can progress in siblings at different rates, one presenting with congestive cardiac failure in infancy and the other becoming symptomatic during adolescence.

Table 11.10: Clinical screening strategies with echocardiography (and 12 lead ECG) for detection of HCM in family members

- < 12 years old
  Optional unless:
    Malignant family history of premature HCM, death or other adverse complication.
    Competitive athlete in an intense training program
    Onset of symptoms
    Other clinical suspicion of early LV hypertrophy
- 12 to 18 years old[a]
  Every 12-18 months
- > 18-21 years old[b]
  Probably about every 5 years, or at more frequent intervals with family history of late-onset hypertrophy and/or malignant clinical course

[a] In the absence of laboratory based genetic testing
[b] Age range takes into consideration the acknowledged individual variability in achieving physical maturity.

Several genotypes result in HCM, and the pattern of inheritance has been demonstrated to be both autosomal dominant and autosomal recessive. The underlying factors determining the etiopathogenesis of the progression and degree of hypertrophy are unclear, but it is clearly multifactorial. There is evidence to suggest that the progression of the disease is regulated by genetic mechanism. The angiotensin-converting enzyme genotypes and endothelin-1 appear to have some influence on the phenotypic expression of hypertrophy because both angiotensin-converting enzyme and endothelin-1 are emitted during periods of rapid somatic growth, when there tends to be largest increase in hypertrophy.

The co-existence of other genetic diseases with HCM is evidence also for its genotypic heterogeneity. There have been at least 4 foci identified in families with HCM resulting in defects in cardiac troponin T, the myosin binding protein C and the alpha and beta myosin heavy chain. The genetic footprints and extrapolating this to phenotypic expression can be done in a mouse model of HCM that mimics the human form of the disease.

Pathology and Pathophysiology

1. The most characteristic abnormality is hypertrophied LV, with ventricular cavity, usually small or normal in size. Although asymmetric septal hypertrophy (ASM) a condition formerly known as idiopathic hypertrophic subaortic stenosis (IHSS) is very common, the hypertrophy may be concentric or localized to a small segment of septum. Although a truly symmetric (concentric)

pattern of LV hypertrophy may occur occasionally, the distribution of hypertrophy in HCM is characteristically asymmetric in which some portions of LV wall shows greater thickening than other areas.[16] Microscopically, an extensive disarray of hypertrophied myocardial cells, myocardial scarring and abnormalities of small intramural coronary arteries are also present (Fig. 11.13).

2. In some patients, an intracavitary pressure gradient develops during systole partly because of systolic anterior motion (SAM) of the mitral valve against the hypertrophied septum, which is called hypertrophic obstructive cardiomyopathy (HOCM). The SAM probably is created by the high outflow velocities and venturi forces (Fig. 11.15).

3. The myocardium itself has an enhanced contractile state but diastolic ventricular filling is impaired by abnormal stiffness of the LV which may lead to LA enlargement and pulmonary venous congestion producing congestive symptoms (exertional dyspnea, orthopnea, paroxysmal nocturnal dyspnea).

4. In about 60% of cases, HCM appears to be genetically transmitted as an autosomal dominant trait and it occurs sporadically in the rest.

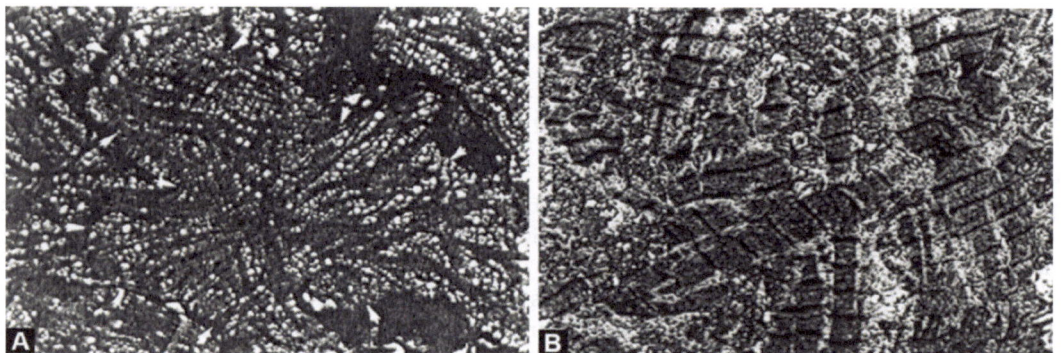

Figs 11.13A and B: Left ventricular (LV) architecture in hypertrophic cardiomyopathy. A: Light micrograph of a section of ventricular septum. A hypertrophied and stellate-shaped muscle cell containing obliquely and transversly oriented myofibrils is shown in the center (cell outline is indicated by arrow beads). This cardiac muscle cell maintains intercellular connections with several adjacent cells. (Alkaline toluidine blue stain; 675 X magnification.) B; Electron micrograph of an area of a cell similar to that shown in A. Myofibrils also show marked disarray and are oriented at perpendicular and oblique angles to each other. (5,900 X magnification). (From Ferrans VJ, Morrow AG, Robert WC. Myocardial ultrastructure in idiopathic hypertrophic subaortic stenosis: A study of operatively excised left ventricular outflow tract muscle in 14 patients. Circulation 1972:45:769, with permission)

5. A unique aspect of HOCM is the variability of the degree of obstruction from moment to moment. Because the obstruction of LV outflow tract results from SAM of mitral valve against hypertrophied ventricular septum, the LV systolic volume might be decreased (reduced blood volume or lowering of SVR) increases the obstruction and the measures that increase systolic volume (blood transfusion) lessens the obstruction.
6. About 80% of the stroke volume is ejected during the early part of systole, producing a sharp upstroke in the arterial pulse, a characteristic finding of HOCM. The obstruction occurs late producing a late murmur.
7. Cardiac myocytes in ventricular septum and LV free wall are chaotic and bizarre in structure, and completely disorganized in oblique and perpendicular angles to each other (Fig. 11.13). Areas of disorganized cardiac muscle cells occur in 95% of patients dying of HCM.[17] The presence of marked cellular disorganization in a few symptomatic infants with HCM, shows that this histological abnormality can be present since birth.[18] Therefore, this disorganized architecture probably serves as an electrically unstable arrhythmogenic substrate and the nidus for potentially lethal ventricular tachyarrhythmias and sudden death in HCM.[19] In addition, this distorted cellular architecture could contribute to impaired diastolic function. Abnormalities of intramural coronary arteries are present in about 80% of patient's studies at necropsy most commonly in ventricular septum.

Clinical Manifestations

Infancy

The presentation of HCM in an infant can be very different from that of an older child or a teenager.
1. These infants are usually appropriate for gestational age (AGA), products of term pregnancy with no neonatal problems.
2. Easy fatigability, dyspnea, palpitation and other signs of CCF may be present manifesting in failure to thrive.
3. Family history of sudden cardiac arrest, characteristic of HOCM, -positive in 30-60% of patients.
4. Bradycardia and central cyanosis—produced on crying.
5. A sharp upstroke of arterial pulse is characteristic. A left ventricular heave and a systolic thrill at the apex may be present.
6. An ejection systolic murmur of varying severity may be heard at the apex or along the left parasternal border.

Childhood and Adolescence

Hypertrophic cardiomyopathy is seen more frequently in adolescents and young adults with equal gender distribution. If the disease remains undiagnosed in childhood, then it manifests in adolescence in a less severe form. HCM in adolescence manifests in an obstructive or non-obstructive manner. Many adolescents with HCM become symptomatic with complaints of syncope/pre-syncope. Angina, palpitation or exercise intolerance may develop symptoms of congestive cardiac failure, probably due to functional decrease in oxygen demand and supply to the myocardium and diminished myocardial perfusion.

Natural History

1. The obstruction due to hypertrophy may be absent, stable or slowly progressive. Genetically predisposed children often show striking increases in wall thickness during childhood and adolescence.

    To monitor the progression of left ventricular hypertrophy, it can be done by a two dimensional echocardiography that divides the left ventricle into five segments: anterior and posterior ventricular septum and the anterior, posterior and lateral free wall. The wall thickness measurement of each segment is done at the level of mitral valve and papillary muscle. The progression of hypertrophy in children may be considerable increasing as much as 250% (average 100 + 61 %) during periods of rapid somatic growth as compared with the changes in left ventricular hypertrophy seen during normal growth (10%). Children who appear to be normal may quickly develop pathologic hypertrophy over a few years during periods of rapid somatic growth. Progression of left ventricular hypertrophy with HCM has been seen in patients as old as 19-21 years of age. Therefore, serial echocardiographic examinations should be done every 2-3 years in the genetically predisposed children into adulthood.

2. Sudden cardiac death may occur commonly in patients between 10-35 years of age, particularly during exercise, even in those with mild obstruction. The incidence of sudden death is 4-6% a year in children and adolescents and 2-4% in adults. Even brief periods of ventricular tachycardia on ambulatory ECG monitoring is a significant risk factor. The age at which HCM manifests is also a significant risk factor the younger the age at presentation, more severe the disease. Sudden deaths are commoner in young children where there is no control on exercises or activity.

3. Some adolescents/young adults manifest with symptoms of severe congestive heart failure following a viral illness. Echocardiographic examination reveals septal hypertrophy with left ventricular dilatation and markedly depressed ventricular function. The pathophysiology of this "burned out" HCM is progressive myocardial ischemia resulting in fibrosis and severe ventricular systolic and diastolic dysfunction.

Evaluation

1. Electrocardiography (Fig. 11.14)
    Common ECG abnormalities include:
    Left ventricular hypertrophy with strain pattern (ST-T wave changes).
    Abnormally deep Q waves/septal hypertrophy.
    Right ventricular hypertrophy is usually present in infancy.
2. *X-ray study:* Mild left ventricular enlargement with a globular shaped heart may be present. The pulmonary vascularity is normal.
3. *Echocardiography*
    a. *Echo is diagnostic (Figs 11.15A and B):* Presence of right ventricular and left ventricular hypertrophy in infancy as compared to presence of LV hypertrophy only in older childhood or adolescence.

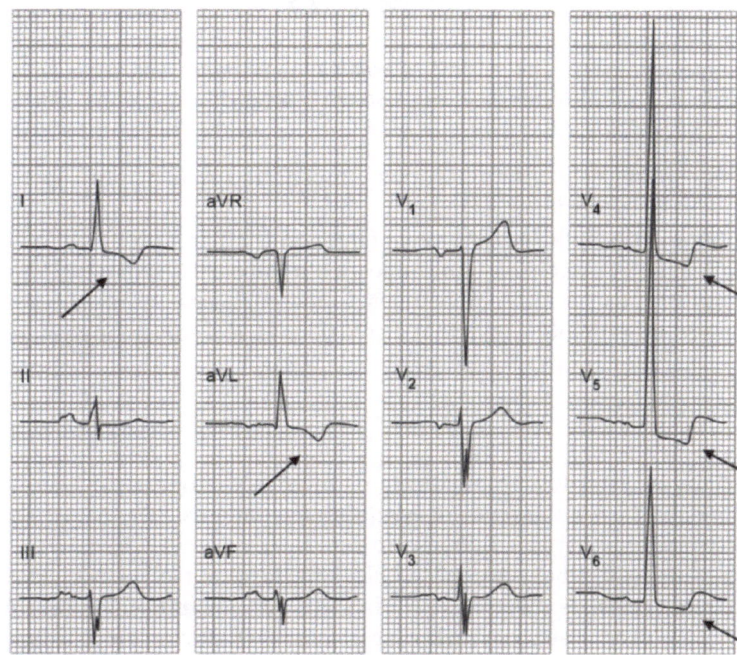

Fig. 11.14: Electrocardiogram which demonstrated severe left ventricular hypertrophy with ischemia/strain

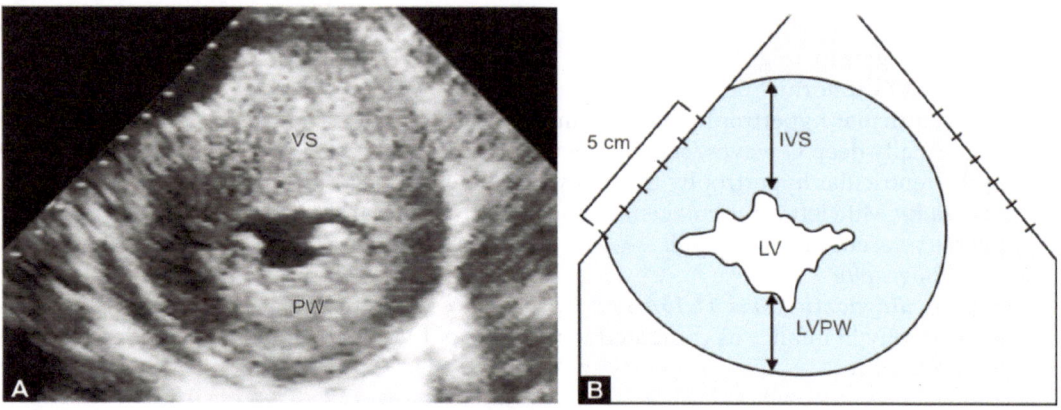

Figs 11.15A and B: Parasternal short axis-view of a 14-year old boy with hypertrophic cardiomyopathy. Marked hypertrophy of the interventricular septum (IVS) as well as the posterior wall of the left ventricle (LVPW) is present. The LV cavity is small. The interventricular septum is approximately 39 mm and the LV posterior wall is 26 mm in thickness. The thickness of both structures does not exceed 10 mm in normal persons

   Two-dimensional echo demonstrates concentric hypertrophy, localized segmental hypertrophy or asymmetric septal hypertrophy.
   b. *M Mode:* Asymmetric septal hypertrophy of interventricular septum and occasionally systolic anterior motion. (SAM) of anterior mitral leaflet in the obstructive type (Figs 11.16A and B).
   c. *Mitral inflow:* Doppler tracing demonstrates decreased E wave velocity, increased deceleration time and decreased ratio of E wave to A wave (Fig. 11.17)—diastolic dysfunction.

Management

Medical

Response of heart failure symptoms to medical treatment is highly variable, hence therapy may be individually tailored to the requirements of symptomatic patients.
1. Moderate restriction of physical activity is indicated.
2. Prophylactic therapy with either—adrenergic blockers (Propranolol) or calcium channel blocker—Verapamil is controversial. Some prefer prophylactic administration to prevent sudden cardiac death or to delay the progression of the disease process by reducing myocardial oxygen demand. Others limit prophylactic drug therapy to young patients with a family history of premature sudden death, especially those with marked LVH.

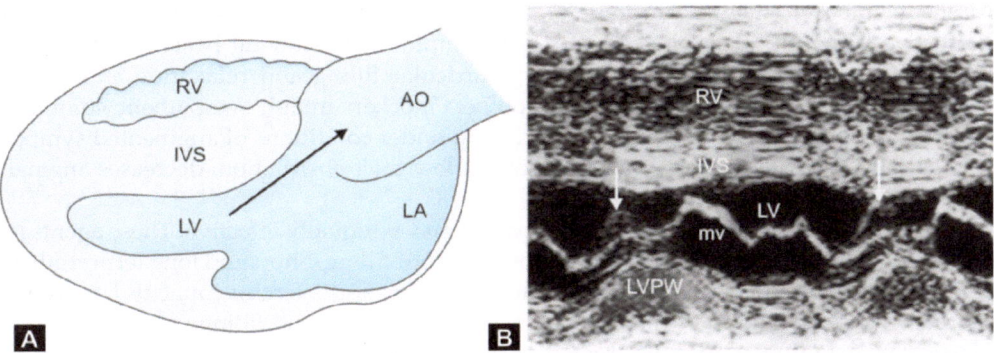

Figs 11.16A and B: Systolic anterior motion of the mitral valve. A. diagnostic illustration of systolic anterior in the presence of an asymmetric septal hypertrophy. The Venturi effect may be important in the production of systolic anterior motion. B, M-mode echo of mitral valve in a patient with hypertrophic cardiomyopathy. Systolic anterior motion of the anterior leaflet of the mitral valve is indicated by arrows

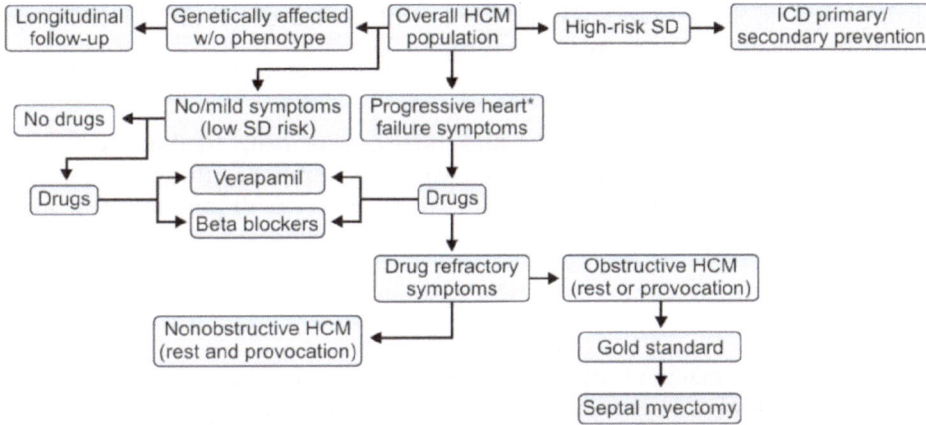

Fig. 11.17: Clinical presentations and treatment strategies for patent subgroups within hypertrophic cardiomyopathy (HCM) disease spectrum, adapted to the pediatric population. *No specific treatment or intervention indicated, except under exceptional circumstances. AF, atrial fibrillation; ICD, implantable cardioverter-defibrillator; SD, sudden death. (From Maron BJ Hypertrophic cardiomyopathy in childhood. Pediatr Clin N Am 2004;51:1305, with permission)

3. **Adrenergic blocker** (such as propranolol, atenolol or metoprolol) is the drug of choice in the obstructive subgroup. Beta blockers improve symptoms by slowing heart rate and reducing force of LV contraction, thus augmenting ventricular filling and relaxation and decreasing myocardial oxygen consumption. In addition beta blockers inhibit sympathetic stimulation of heart therapy often reducing the outflow gradient under conditions of augmented sympathetic stimulation. This drug reduces the degree of outflow tract obstruction, decreases anginal pain and has antiarrhythmic effects.
4. **Calcium channel blockers** (principally verapamil) may be equally effective. These agents reduce hypercontractile systolic function and improve diastolic filling. Short and long term studies have reported oral verapamil to improve cardiac symptoms and exercise capacity largely in non-obstructive patients due to a beneficial effect on LV relaxation and filling.
5. Ventricular arrhythmias may be treated with propranolol, amiodarone and other standard antiarrhythmic agents guided by serial ambulatory ECG monitoring.
6. Digitalis or other inotropic drugs and vasodilators should be avoided because it increases the degree of obstruction and thereby increasing the pressure gradient.
7. Diuretics are usually ineffectual. However, judicious use can help reduce congestive symptoms (e.g. exertional dyspnea, orthopnea) by reducing LV filling pressure.
8. Prophylaxis against SBE is indicated in patients with obstructive form of HCM. Vegetations commonly involve the AML or septal endocardium.

Prevention of Sudden Cardiac Death

In selected patients with evidence of high risk for sudden cardiac death, treatment with implantable cardioverter-defibrillator (ICD) is indicated. The ICD is proven to be effective in high risk HCM patients by reliably sensing ventricular tachycardiac/fibrillation (VT/VF) and restoring sinus rhythm by delivering appropriate defibrillation shocks or anti-tachycardia pacing.[20]

Surgical

Indications

Operative management remains an important therapeutic alternative for symptomatic patients who do not respond to medical management and also those who have severe obstruction with a resting pressure gradient of 50 mm Hg or more.

Procedures

1. *Morrow's myotomy-myectomy:* Transaortic LV septal myectomy (Morrow's operation) is the procedure of choice. It is performed through aorta under direct visualization, a rectangular portion

of 2-10 gm of hypertrophied ventricular septum is usually excised usually. The postoperative mortality has steadily decreased and now it is < 1% in most of experienced centers. Serious complications of surgery include complete heart block (3-5%) and surgically induced VSD (3%). More than 90% of patients who undergo myectomy experience abolition or substantial reduction in the outflow gradient under basal conditions (owing to reduction of SAM) but without important compromise in LV function.

2. *Mitral valve replacement:* Mitral valve replacement with a low-profile prosthetic valve may be indicated in those patients where the basal anterior septum is thin (less than 18 mm). The operative mortality is about 6%.
3. *Cardiac transplantation:* Patients with "burned out" cardiomyopathy are treated with afterload reduction and inotropic agents and then referred for cardiac transplantation.
4. *Pacemaker therapy:* There has been much controversy recently regarding the role of pacemaker therapy in children with HCM. Pacing of either the right ventricle or left ventricle improves left ventricular outflow tract obstruction in these patients probably as a result of alterations in regional myocardial stress, which in turn result in chronic segmented remodelling of the ventricle. Because of limited experience in children, the details of pacemaker therapy have yet to be worked out. Reduction in subaortic gradient with pacing while demonstrating in some patients is modest when compared with that achieved with myectomy.
5. *Alcohol septal ablation:* This technique has been introduced to reduce outflow tract obstruction in adults – not applicable in children.

Doxorubicin Cardiomyopathy

Doxorubicin cardiomyopathy is becoming the cause of chronic CCF in children, especially those who are being treated for oncologic disorders. It's prevalence is dose related, occurring in 2-5% of patients who have received a cumulative dose of 400-500 mg/m^2 and up to 50% of patients who have received more of 1000 mg/m^2 of doxorubicin (adriamycin).

Etiopathogenesis

1. Doxorubicin is an important cause of cardiomyopathy, it is a C-13 anthracycline metabolite and is responsible for the cardiotoxicity.
2. Children less than 4 years of age are vulnerable to cumulative effect of the drug exceeding 400-600 mg/cm^2.
3. Dilated LV, decreased contractility, elevated filing pressures and decreased cardiac output characterize the pathophysiologic features. Microscopically, interstitial edema, loss of myofibrils within the myocyte, vacuolar degeneration, necrosis and fibrosis are present.

Clinical Manifestations

1. Patients are asymptomatic till signs of CCF appear. History of doxorubicin administration with onset of symptoms within 2-4 months.
2. Tachypnea, exertional dyspnea, palpitation, substernal discomfort, cough are the usual complaints. Signs of CCF, i.e. hepatomegaly, engorged neck veins, gallop rhythm may be present.

Evaluation

- X-ray chest—Cardiomegaly with pulmonary venous congestion.
- ECG—Sinus tachycardia with non-specific ST -T wave changes.
- Echo studies—reveal the following:
    1. LV is dilated with thinned out walls, decreased fractional shortening and ejection fraction
    2. Dobutamine stress Echo is more sensitive to evaluate the cardiac status.

Management

1. Decongestive therapy—Digoxin, diuretics and afterload reducing agents.
2. Risk factors of doxorubicin cardiotoxicity should be avoided or closely monitored by serial echo, radionuclide angiocardiography, cardiac catheterization and even endomyocardial biopsy may be carried out.
3. Modifying the dose of anthracycline therapy is controversial, if the dose is reduced, then malignancy cannot be treated.
4. Cardiac transplantation is an option for selected patients.

Prognosis

Symptomatic cardiomyopathy carries a high mortality rate. The 2-year survival rate is 20% and almost all die by about 8-9 years after onset.

Restrictive Cardiomyopathy (RCM)

Restrictive cardiomyopathy (RCM) is an extremely rare cardiomyopathy in children accounting for 2.5 – 5% of all diagnosed cardiomyopathies.[21] Restrictive cardiomypathy (RCM) is characterized by restrictive filling and reduced diastolic volume of either or both ventricles with normal or near normal systolic function and wall thicknesses. Increased interstitial fibrosis may be the additional feature and it may be idiopathic or an associated feature of another disease.[22] Overall, the incidence of cardiomyopathies is higher in children younger than 1 year of age when all of cardiomyopathies are considered,[23] although RCM may be an exception. Beyond infancy, boys have a higher incidence of cardiomyopathy than girls.[23]

Table 11.11: Causes of restrictive cardiomyopathies in children and or adults

Myocardial	Endomyocardial
Idiopathic	Endomyocardial fibrosis
Familial	Hypereosinophilia syndrome (Löffler)
Scleroderma	
Myocarditis	Endocardial fibroelastosis
Cardiac transplant	Carcinoid
Pseudoxanthoma elasticum	Metastatic cancers
Diabetic cardiomyopathy	Radiation
Amyloidosis	Drugs – anthracyclines
Sarcoidosis	Serotonin
Gaucher disease	Ergotamine
Hurler disease	Mercurials
Fatty infiltration	Busulfan
Hemochromatosis	
Fabry disease	
Glycogen storage disease	
Cystinosis (possibly)	
Emery-Dreifuss syndrome	
Coffin-Lowry syndrome	

Etiology

RCM has multiple causes including myocardial disease which may be of infiltrative and non-infiltrative processes, storage diseases, endomyocardial diseases and following cardiac transplantation. Endomyocardial fibrosis may be the most common cause of RCM in tropics and idiopathic RCM is the commonest cause outside tropics.

Pathology

1. This condition is characterized by abnormal diastolic ventricular filling resulting from excessively stiff ventricular walls. The ventricles are neither dilated nor hypertrophied and contractility is normal. The atria are dilated and they resemble constrictive pericarditis in clinical presentation and hemodynamic abnormalities. Diastolic function is primarily affected by ventricular compliance stiffness and impaired relaxation. Restrictive physiology results from increased myocardial; stiffness with decreased compliance with marked ventricular pressure rise with small change in volume.

2. There may be areas of myocardial fibrosis or the myocardium may be infiltrated by various materials such as amyloidosis, sarcoidosis, hemochromatosis, glycogen deposits, etc.

Clinical Manifestations (Table 11.12)

Table 11.12: Clinical features of children with restrictive cardiomyopathy

Family history: positive	30%
Presenting complaints	
Respiratory: DOE, "asthma", cough/pneumonia	46%
Abnormal PR: ascites, hepatomegaly, edema, gallop, loud P2, murmur	19%
Congestive heart failure (not otherwise defined)	11%
Syncope	9%
Other (includes sudden death palpitations, fatigue embolic events, incidental cardiomegaly on chest X-ray, positive family history, Musculoskeletal abnormalities)	< 10%

DOE, dyspnea on exertion; PE, physical exam

1. Family history – positive
2. History of exercise intolerance, weakness, exertional dyspnea or chest pain.
3. Hepatomegaly, elevated jugular venous pressure, loud P_2, gallop rhythm, systolic murmur of MR or TR may be present or there may be no murmur at all (Table 11.13).
4. Congestive heart failure – not otherwise defined and syncope. Each account for approximately 10% of presenting complaints. Sudden cardiac death may be the presentation, presumable secondary to familial RCM, as there were 13 family members in 5 generations.
5. Chest X-ray-cardiomegaly with pulmonary venous congestion.

Table 11.13: Cardiomegaly without heart murmur–Differential diagnosis[23]

1. Myocardial diseases: Endocardial fibroelastosis: Myocarditis (viral or idiopathic), Glycogen storage disease
2. Coronary artery diseases resulting in myocardial insufficiency: Anomalous origin of left coronary artery from PA, Collagen disease (periarteritis nodosa), Kawasaki's disease (mucocutaneous lymph node syndrome)
3. CHD with severe heart failure: Coarctation of aorta in infants, Ebstein's anomaly
4. Miscellaneous conditions: CHF secondary to respiratory disorders, SVT, pericardial effusion, severe anemia, neonatal thyrotoxicosis, tumors of the heart, malnutrition

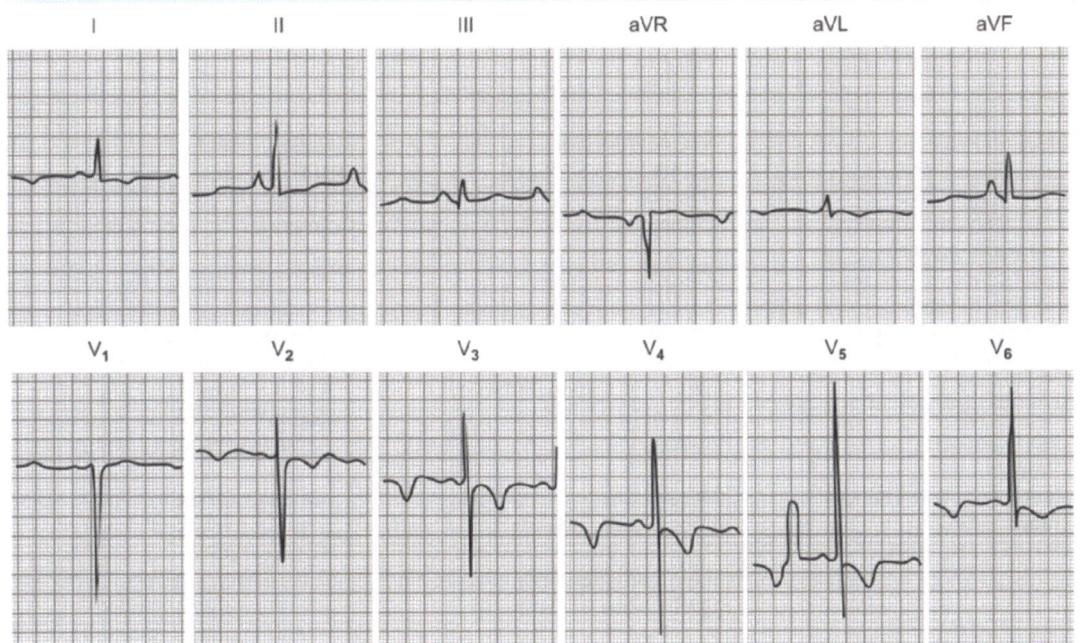

Fig. 11.18: ECG from a 2 year old with restrictive cardiomyopathy demonstrating sinus rhythm with biatrial enlargement, qr pattern in the right chest leads and ST-segment depression and T-wave inversion in the inferolateral lateral leads

6. ECG -may show paroxysms of SVT and atrial fibrillation.
   Biatrial or left atrial enlargement with ST – T waves abnormality
7. Echocardiography-characteristic biatrial enlargement with normal sized LV. Contractility remains normal till last stages (Fig. 11.18).
   - Atrial thrombus may be present.
8. Mitral inflow Doppler tracing shows an increased E velocity with decreased deceleration time and increased E/A ratio (Fig. 11.12).

Differential Diagnosis

Constrictive pericarditis (CP) is the disease process that is most commonly confused with RCM. The clinical presentation of patients with RCM and CP can be similar as can be results of tests used to differentiate between the two (Table 11.14).

Table 11.14: Restrictive cardiomyopathy versus constrictive pericarditis

	RCM	CP
ECG finding		
Atrial enlargement	Nearly universal	May be present
LVH and/or RVH	Common	Usually Absent
Low-voltage QRS	Unusual	Common
ST-T wave abnormality	Common	Common
Chest radiograph		
Calcification	Absent	< 21 %
Echocardiogram		
Pericardial thickening	Absent	May be thickened
Atrial dilatation	Marked	May be enlarged
Wall thickness	Normal to mild hypertrophy	Usually normal
Systolic function	Normal to depressed	Normal
Septal bounce	Absent	Usually present
Doppler		
Respiratory flow changes	Occasional	Usually marked
Gated MRI/CT	Normal pericardium	Usually thickened
Cardiac catheterization	PWP and LVEDP may exceed RAP and RVEDP by > 4 mm Hg RVSP often > 50 mm Hg	RAP = PWP RVEDP = LVEDP usually within 4 mm Hg RVSP usually < 50 mm Hg
RV endomyocardial biopsy	Usually abnormal (frequently non specific)	Usually normal
Thoracotomy	Normal pericardium	Usually abnormal pericardium

CP, constrictive pericarditis; LVH, left ventricular hypertrophy; RVH, right ventricular hypertrophy; PWP, pulmonary wedge pressure; LVEDP, left ventricular end-diastolic pressure; RAP, right atrial pressure; RVEDP, right ventricular end-diastolic pressure; RVSP, right ventricular systolic pressure.

Treatment

1. Diuretics are beneficial but inotropic drugs (digoxin) are contraindicated.
2. Because of 21% incidence of thromboembolics episodes, anticoagulants (Warfarin) and anti-platelet drugs (Aspirin) should be administered.
3. Risks and benefits of ACE—inhibitors and beta blocker therapy need to be evaluated in children.
4. Pacemaker implantation—for complete heart block.

5. Cardiac transplantation—only definitive therapy.
6. Strenous physical activity—avoided

REFERENCES

1. Manolio TA, Baughman KL, Rodeheffer R, et al. Prevalence and etiology of idiopathic dilated cardiomyopathy. Am J Cardiol 1992;69:1458-66.
2. Michels VV, Moll PP, Miller FA, et al. The frequency of familial dilated cardiomyopathy in a series of patients with idiopathic dilated cardiomyopathy. N Engl J Med 1992;326:77-82.
3. Nugent AQW, Daubeney PEF, Chondros P, et al. The epidemiology of childhood cardiomyopathy in Australia. N Engl J Med 2003;348:1639-42.
4. Shaddy RE. Medical management of chronic systolic left ventricular dysfunction in children. In Shaddy RE, Wernovsky G. eds. Pediatric Heart Failure Boca Raton FL: Taylor and Francis 2005;589-619.
5. Arola A, Tuominen J, RuusKanene O, et al. Idiopathic dilated cardiomyopathy in children: Prognostic indicators and outcome. Pediatrics 1998;101:369-76.
6. Taylor MR, Fain PR, Sinagra G, et al. Natural history of dilated cardiomyopathy due to lamin a/c gene mutations. J Am Coll Cardiol 2003;41:771-80.
7. Davies MJ. Apoptosis in cardiovascular disease. Heart 1997;77:498-501.
8. Missov E, Calzolari C, Pan B. Circulatory cardiac troponin I in severe congestive heart failure. Circulation 1997;96:2953-58.
9. Dec GN, Fuster V. Idiopathic dilated cardiomyopathy N Engl J Med 1994;331:1564-75.
10. Rosenthal D, Chrisant MRK, Edeus E, et al. International society for heart and lung transplantation: Practice guideline for management of heart failure in children. J Heart Lung Transplant 2004;23:1313-33.
11. Earl GL, Fitzpatrick JT, Levosimendan. A novel inotropic agent for treatment of acute decompensated heart failure. Ann Pharmacother 2005;39:1888-96.
12. Mahle NT, Cuadrado AR, Kirshbom PM, et al. Nesiritide in infants and children with congestive heart failure. Pediatr Critc Care Med 2005;6:543-46.
13. Tsirka AE, Trinkans K, Chen SC, et al. Improved outcomes of pediatric dilated cardiomyopathy with utilization of heart transplantation. J Am Coll Cardiol 2004;44:391-97.
14. Maron BJ, McKenna WJ, Danielson GK, et al. American College of Cardiology/European Society of Cardiology Clinical Expert consensus Document on Hypertrophic cardiomyopathy. J Am Coll Cardiol 2003;42:1687-1713.
15. Maron BJ, Paterson EE, Maron MS, et al. Prevalence of hypertrophic cardiomyopathy in an outpatient population referred for echocardiographic study. Am J Cardiol 1994; 73: 577-80.
16. Maron BJ. Hypertrophic cardiomyopathy: A systematic review. JAMA. 2002; 287: 1308-20.
17. Maron BJ, Roberts WC. Quantitative analysis of cardiac muscle cell disorganization in the ventricular septum of patients with hypertrophic cardiomyopathy. Circulation 1979; 59: 689-706.
18. Maron BJ, Tajik AJ Ruttenberg HD et al. Hypertrophic Cardiomyopathy in infants, clinical features and natural history. Circulation 1982; 65: 7-17.

19. Maron B, Fananpazir L. Sudden Cardiac death in hypertrophic cardiomyopathy. Circulation 1992; 85 (Suppl.) 1: 57-63.
20. Maron BJ, Shen WK, Link MS et al. Efficacy of implantable cardioverter defibrillators for the prevention of sudden death in infants with hypertrophic cardiomyopathy. N Engl J Med 2000;342:365-73.
21. Denfield SW, Rosenthal G, Gajarski RJ et al. Restrictive cardiomyopathies in childhood, etiologies and natural history. Tex heart Inst J 1997;24:38-44.
22. Celta F, O'Seary PW, Seward JB et al: Idiopathic restrictive cardiomyopathy in childhood: diagnostic features and clinical; course. Mayo Clin Proc 1995;70:634-40.
23. Lipshultz SE, Sleeper CA, Towbin JA et al. The incidence of pediatric cardiomyopathy in two regions of United States. N Engl/J Med 2003;348:1647-55.

CHAPTER 12

Cardiac Infections

Cardiac infections include infections of the 3 layers of the heart:
1. Myocarditis has been dealt with in a Chapter on Myocardial Disorders.
2. Infective endocarditis.
3. Pericarditis included in pericardial diseases.

INFECTIVE ENDOCARDITIS

Infective endocarditis (IE) is one of the most dreaded complications of structural heart disease. Over the years, since the advent of echocardiography-and further development and refinement of echocardiographic techniques have contributed to a better diagnosis and management of endocarditis. More precise criteria for the diagnosis of IE have been established that assist physicians in making a more objective assessment of the varied clinical manifestations of this process.

Definition

Infective endocarditis (IE) is defined as an "endovascular microbial infection of cardiovascular structures".[1] Despite advances in diagnosis and management since its first description by Wilhaim Oster, IE is associated with considerable morbidity and mortality. Native or prosthetic heart valves are the most frequently involved sites but can also involve septal defects, mural endocardium or intravascular devices such as intracardiac patches, surgically constructed shunts and intravenous catheters.

The epidemiology of IE has changed over the past few decades. The proportion of patients with congenital heart disease remained stable throughout the four decades, whereas the proportion of patients with rheumatic heart disease has decreased because of the declining incidence of rheumatic fever in the industrialized countries in the past few decades. On the contrary, endocarditis remains an important complicating factor in at least 10% of patients with rheumatic valvular heart disease.

At least 70% of IE cases occur in children complicating congenital heart disease. But in the last 2 decades, a number of cases of neonatal IE have been reported[2] in structurally normal hearts with the vegetations being right sided. This reflects on the use of prosthetic indwelling intravascular catheters used for resuscitation. Children with underlying cardiovascular disease may develop endocarditis at any age, in childhood, adolescence or adulthood. The mortality due to IE ranges from 16 to 25%[3,4] and almost 20% of patients require emergency surgery[5]. In a review of several published studies between 1986 to 1995, estimated incidence in children was 0.3/1,00,000 children per year with mortality of 11.66%.[6]

Careful review of available reports suggests that the incidence of endocarditis in children may be increasing in recent years because of improved survival of children of CHD following surgery and increased use of indwelling catheters, valves and prosthetic tubes during surgery. In general cardiac lesions associated with steep pressure gradients pose a particularly high risk for IE, e.g. VSD, PDA, MR or aortic regurgitation. Tetralogy of Fallot and bicuspid aortic valve are the other lesions who may be predisposed to IE (Table 12.1).[7]

Table 12.1: Relative risk of endocarditis for various underlying conditions

High risk
Prosthetic valves
Previous episodes of endocarditis
Complex cyanotic CHD's (TGA, TOF, single ventricle)
Surgically constructed systemic to PA shunts
Intravenous drug abuse
Indwelling central venous catheters
Moderate Risk
Uncorrected PDA, VSDs
Bicuspid aortic valve
Atrial septal defect (Primum)
Mitral valve prolapse with regurgitation
Rheumatic mitral and aortic valve disease hypertrophic cardiomyopathy

Pathogenesis

A complex interaction between host vascular endothelium, hemostatic response and circulating bacteria has to occur for development of IE
1. Two factors are important in the pathogenesis of infective endocarditis: the presence of structural abnormality of the heart and great vessels with a significant pressure gradient or turbulence (resulting endothelial damage and platelet-fibrin thrombus formation) and bacteremia, even if it is transient.

2. Almost all patients with IE have underlying heart disease, e.g. even bicuspid aortic valve whose presence one is not aware of, might be a predisposing factor. Drug addicts or those with intravenous catheters may develop IE in the absence of cardiac anomalies.
3. All CHDs with exception of ASD secundum predispose to endocarditis. More frequently encountered defects are TOF, VSD and aortic valve disease. Rheumatic mitral insufficiency is responsible in a small number of patients of IE. Patients with MVP (with MR) and HOCM (IHSS) are also vulnerable to IE Those with prosthetic valve or prosthetic material in the heart are particularly at high risk to develop endocarditis (Table 12.1).
4. Any localized infection, abscesses, osteomyelitis, pyelonephritis predispose to bacteremia, which also frequently results after dental procedures of carious infected teeth. Good dental hygiene is more important in prevention of IE than antibiotic coverage before dental procedures. Bacteremias associated with various tissue manipulations, e.g. interventions (gastrointestinal or cardiac/genitourinary) are more vulnerable.

Pathology

The greater the turbulence of flow around a cardiac lesion, e.g. VSD, higher is the risk of infective endocarditis. This is because endothelial damage results in platelet and fibrin deposition, which can subsequently become infected to form vegetations (Fig. 12.1). A vegetation is usually found in the low pressure side of the defect, either around the defect or on the opposite surface where the jet effect of the flow damages the endothelium. Vegetations are found in pulmonary artery in patent ductus arteriosus or systemic PA shunts. They can be seen on the atrial surface of mitral valve in

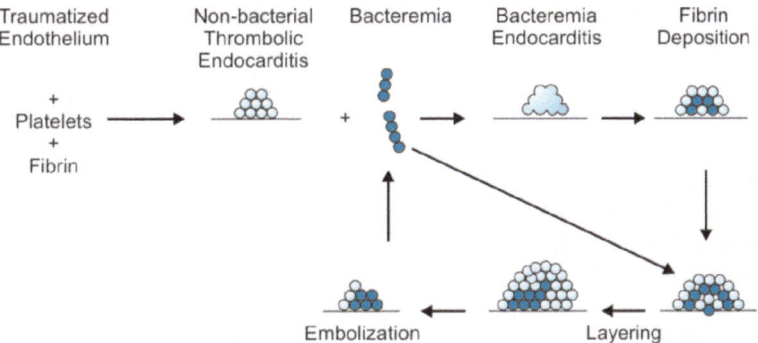

Fig. 12.1: Evolution of infected vegetation on a traumatized valve

mitral regurgitation and ventricular surface of aortic valve. In valvular aortic stenosis, intact cardiac endothelium is a poor stimulation of block coagulation and is weakly receptive to bacterial attachment whereas damaged endothelium is a potent inducer of thrombogenesis resulting in a vegetation.

Microbiology (Table 12.2)

The majority of cases of endocarditis are caused by a relatively small number of micro-organisms, and some bacteria are more commonly associated than others, because the intriguing explanation relates to bacterial adherence. The bacteria most frequently responsible for endocarditis (e.g., streptococcus viridans) displayed a propensity for adherence to canine or human valves.[7] For endocarditis, gram positive cocci have a predilection for sub-endocardial connective tissue especially, fibronectin that gets exposed when endocardium is damaged. In contrast, gram-negative organisms that are seldom responsible adhere rather poorly. Systemic gram positive cocci account for about 90% of recoverable bacteria, haemolytic streptococcus being the commonest causative organism in all age groups. Staphylococci (*S. aureus* and coagulase negative staphylococci) are the second largest group.[8] In review of pediatric literature, prevalence of definite IE due to S.aureus was approximately 12% and possible IE was 20% probably due to infected intraventricular device.[9]

Table 12.2: Etiologic agents of infective endocarditis in infants and children[11]

Agent	Frequency
Streptococci	
α-Haemolytic (Viridian's)	Most common
β-Haemolytic enterococci	Uncommon
Pneumococci	Rare
Staphylococci	
S.aureus	Second most common
Coagulase -negative	Uncommon but increasing
Gram negative agents	
Enterics	Rare
Pseudomonas species	Rare
Haemophilus species	Rare
Neisseria species	Rare
Fungi	
Candida species	Uncommon
Others	Rare

Gram-negative organisms cause less than 10% of endocarditis in children, but they predispose to endocarditis in neonates, immunocompromised patients and drug addicts. *Haemophilus* species are more common of the gram-negative organisms, which affect the damaged valves, bring about a subacute course of endocarditis which frequently results in embolization. In narcotic addicts, organisms commonly isolated include *S. aureus* and gram-negative organisms (particularly *Pseudomonas* species) and occasionally *Candida* or other fungal species. Fungal endocarditis (candida, histoplasma, *Cryptococcus*) are resistant to treatment and may occur in neonates, where it may be a complication following intensive care measures. Mortality rate from fungal endocardiac is high even with intensive medical or surgical therapy.[10]

Approximately 5% of patients with endocarditis have negative blood cultures. The clinician should carefully evaluate such cases and consult the microbiologist for fastidious organisms.

Clinical Features

Most clinical manifestations and complications of endocarditis are directly related to hemodynamic changes caused by local infection, embolization from vegetations or immunologic reactions from the host. It should be a part of differential diagnosis of any prolonged pyrexia of unknown origin in patients with underlying heart disease, and if not diagnosed early, it may leave behind irreparable damage.

In majority, and also in adults, endocarditis are valvular in origin but in children, congenital heart lesions may often involve the right side of heart and other structures such as mural endocardium patent ductus arteriosus or other vascular mycotic sites such as surgical shunts. Endocarditis involving the left side, commonly results in peripheral embolization, leading to ischemia, infarction or myotic aneurysms. Specific clinical findings depend on the localization of the emboli. In children, embolization from right heart may be no less frequent, but such embolization is not appreciated clinically because of filtration by the lungs.

Neonates represent a unique group in that many may have relatively few specific symptoms (e.g. systemic hypotension, clinical signs compatible with generalized sepsis or focal neurological findings from central nervous system. Embolization may be due to the development of endocarditis. Neonates appear particularly prone to peripheral septic embolization and development of satellite infections including meningitis and osteomyelitis[11] (Table 12.3).

Fever is the most common finding in all patients with endocarditis with exception of neonates. When the causative organism is α-*haemolytic Streptococcus*, the fever is often low grade (subacute), but when *Staphylococcus aureus* is the causative organism, then the fever is high grade (acute) with toxic outcome.

Table 12.3: Clinical picture

History
1. History of underlying cardiac defect-in 80%
2. History of toothache or dental procedure
3. Fever (90%) low grade or high with headache, malaise, lack of appetite, myalgia
4. History suggestive of complications
   • Hematuria
   • Convulsions

Physical examination
1. Presence of heart murmur, depending upon defect, sometimes changing in character
2. Splenomegaly – 70%
3. Manifestations of heart failure
4. Skin manifestations – petechiae in 50%
5. Embolic phenomenon
   • Pulmonary emboli in patients with VSD, PDA etc.
   • Hemiparesis, renal failure, Roth's Spots (retinal hemorrhages), splinter hemorrhages
   • Osler nodes, Janeway's lesions – rare in children

Laboratory Investigations

1. *Positive blood culture:* In 90%, blood culture is the most valuable aid in making the diagnosis of endocarditis. Collection of three separate sets of blood cultures, each from a separate venepuncture over a 24 hour period is adequate in most cases : In an infant 1-3 ml of blood and 5-7 ml in an older child is optimum and inoculated into bottles for acrobolic incubation because anaerobic bacteria do not usually cause IE. If there is no growth after 24 hours, then 2 more blood cultures may be drawn if antibiotics have not been started.
2. Acute phase reactants elevated.
   • Anemia with leukocytosis with a shift to the left in acute IE.
   • Erythrocyte sedimentation rate elevated.
3. *Hematuria* Microscopic -in 30%-represents renal embolization or nephritis.
4. *Echocardiography*: Two dimensional echocardiography has become the principal diagnostic method in cases of suspected infective endocarditis with sensitivities in children reported to be >80%[12] but a negative echocardiography does not rule out IE. Echocardiography not only demonstrates the vegetation, but it also provides important information on presence of severity of valvular destruction, degree of valvular regurgitation and presence of myocardial abscess etc. Because of its immense usefulness in arriving at a diagnosis, it has been included as a major criteria for IE diagnosis.[13]

Transthoracic echocardiography (TTE) is a good enough mode for better acoustic windows in children than in adults and TTE is more likely to identify vegetation in simple CHD than complex CHD. Transoesophageal echocardiography (TEE) is of limited use in children and the indications are (Figs 12.2A and B):
1. Obese or muscular patients with chest wall deformities with poor acoustic window.
2. Patients with prosthetic valves, grafts or conduits.
3. Patients with pulmonary hyperinflation, a negative TTE with a high index of suspicion.
4. Patients with aortic valve endocarditis and suspicion of aortic root abscess on TTE.
5. Patients suspected of paravalvular damage and valve dehiscence due to prosthetic valve infection.

Echocardiography is particularly important as part of serial evaluation of a patient with IE and echocardiac assessment is essential for progressive complications including surgical intervention.

The echocardiographic findings include (Figs 12.3A to D):
1. Vegetation – mobile echodense masses implanted on a valve or mural endocardium in the trajectory of a regurgitant jet or implanted in prosthetic material.

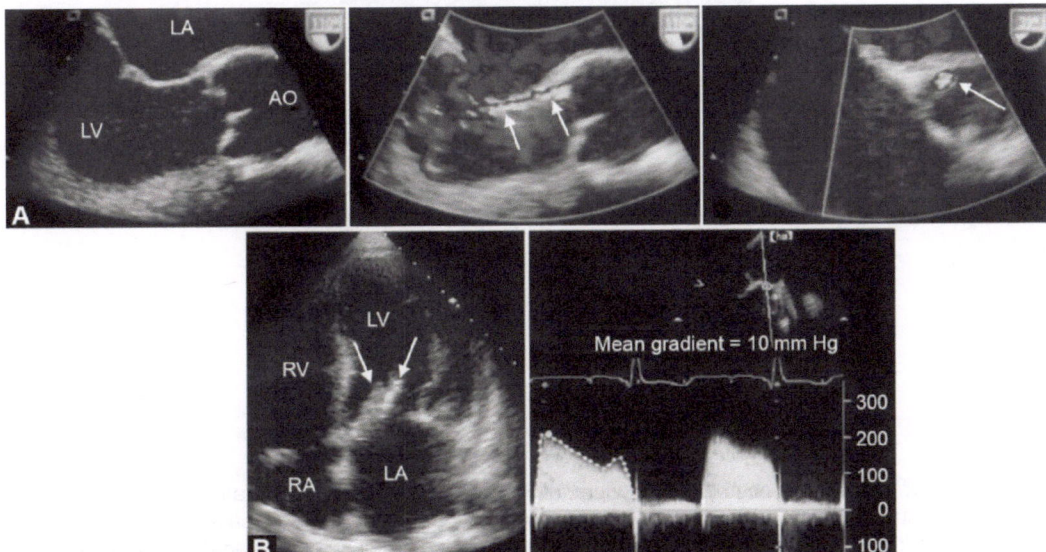

Figs 12.2A and B:[13] (A) TEE image demonstrating a vegetation attached to the noncoronary cusp of the aortic valve in systole. (B) Apical four-chamber view demonstrating a large vegetation attached to the anterior mitral leaflet in a patient with mitral stenosis

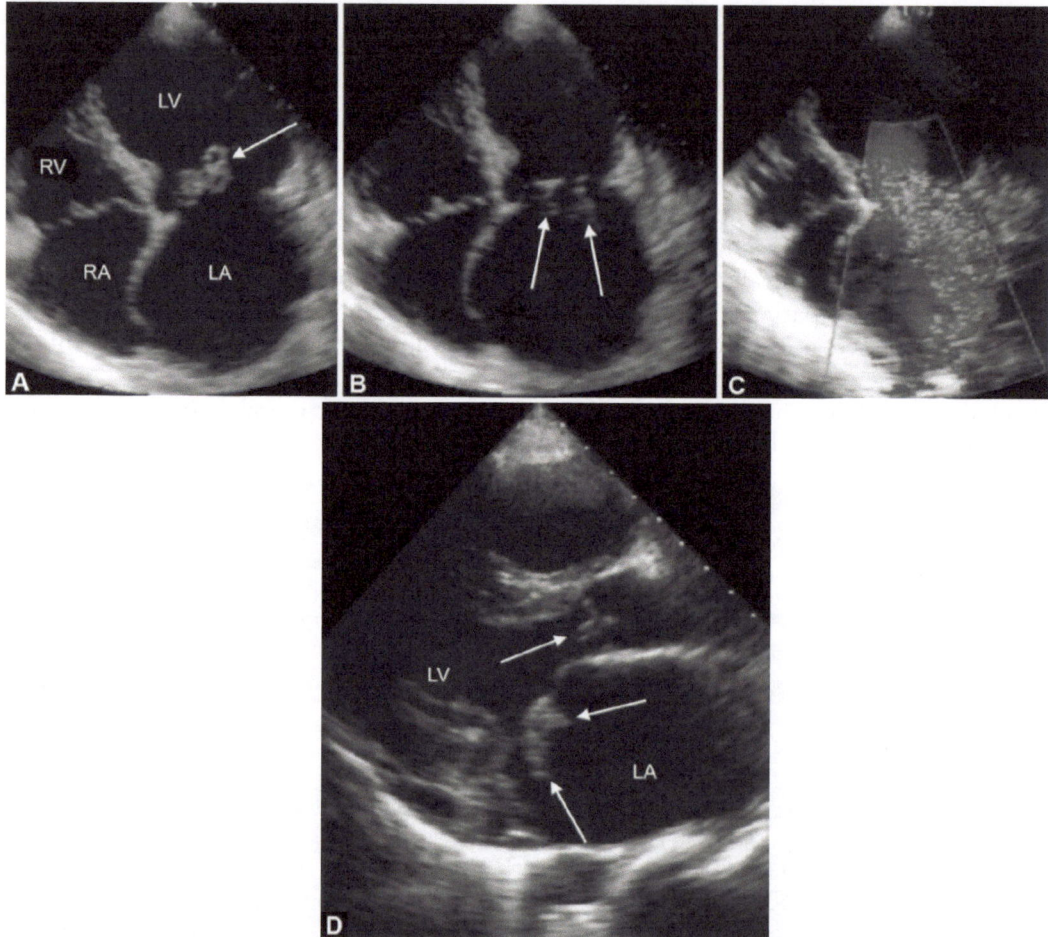

Figs 12.3A to D:[12] Apical four-chamber views demonstrating (A) multiple vegetation attached to the mitral valve leaflets and annulus in diastole; (B) prolapsing of the vegetation into the left atrial cavity (arrows); (C) Severe mitral regurgitation; (D) Parasternal long axis view demonstrating prolapse of the vegetation into the left atrial cavity (arrows)

2. Presence of myocardial abscess or
3. Presence of new dehiscence of a valvar prosthetics.

Diagnosis

The diagnosis of IE can be straightforward in patients with classical manifestation: bacteremia (fungimia), active valvulitis, peripheral emboli and immunologic vascular phenomenon.

Variability in the clinical presentation of IE requires diagnostic criteria that are both sensitive and specific. A diagnostic strategy has been developed (Duke criteria), that uses a combination of clinical, microbiologic pathologic and echocardiographic findings (Tables 12.4 and 12.5). A rapid diagnosis is of critical importance for the survival of the affected child.

Table 12.4: Modified Duke criteria for diagnosis of infective endocarditis — Definitions of terms

Major criteria
1. Positive blood culture
    a. Micro-organism consistent with IE from 2 separate blood cultures.
        - *Streptococcus viridians/bovis, haemophilus* sp.
        - *Staphylococcus aureus* in absence of primary focus.
    b. Micro-organisms consistent with IE from persistently positive blood cultures defined as follows:
        (i) Atleast 2 positive cultures of blood drawn > 12 hours apart or
        (ii) All of 3 or a majority > 4 separate culture of blood (with first and last sample drawn 1 hour apart)
    c. Single positive blood culture for *Coxiella burnetii* or anti phase -1 IgG antibody titer > 1:800.
2. Evidence of endocardial involvement
    Echocardiogram -positive for IE (TEE recommended for prosthetic valves)
    Oscillating intracardiac of mass/vegetation on valve on supporting structure, in path of regurgitant jet or an implanted material in absence of alternative anatomic explanation.
    - Abscess
    - New partial dehiscence of prosthetic valve
    - New valvular regurgitation (worsening or changing of murmur not sufficient)

Minor criteria
1. Predisposing heart condition or intravenous drug use.
2. Fever: temperature >38°C.
3. Vascular phenomenon-major arterial emboli, Janeway's spots, septic pulmonary infarcts, mycotic aneurysms, intracranial hemorrhage, Janeway's lesions.
4. Immunologic phenomenon: glomeorulonephritis, Osler's nodes, Roth's spots, rheumatoid factor or serologic[14] incidence of active infection with organism coexistent with IE
5. Microbiological evidence: positive blood culture but does not meet a major criterion.
6. Echocardiographic findings – consistent with IE but does not meet a major criterion.

Table 12.5: Modified Duke criteria for diagnosis of infective endocarditis

Definite Infective Endocarditis (IE)
1. Pathologic criteria
   a. Micro-organisms: Demonstrated by culture or histologic examination of a vegetation/embolized vegetation/abscess.
   or
   b. Pathologic lesions: Vegetation or intracardiac abscess.
      - Confirmed by histology showing active endocarditis.
2. Clinical criteria (Table 12.4)
   a. 2 major criteria or
   b. 1 major and three minor criteria
   c. 5 minor criteria

Possible
1. 1 major and 1 minor criterion or
2. 3 minor criteria

Rejected
1. Firm alternate diagnosis for manifestations of endocarditis.
2. Resolution of manifestations of endocarditis with antibiotic therapy in < 4 days or less.
3. No pathologic evidence of infective endocarditis at surgery or autopsy, etc with antibiotic therapy for < 4 days or less
4. Does not merit criteria for possible IE as above.

Complications

Complications are more common in following predisposed conditions:
1. Children < 2 years of age.
2. Cyanotic congenital heart disease
3. Prosthetic cardiac valves
4. IE due to *Staphylococcus aureus* or fungus.
5. Prolonged clinical symptoms > 3 months.
6. Left sided endocarditis
7. Patients with systemic to pulmonary shunts.

Complications arise either due to embolization of vegetation, local extension of infection or rupture or perforation of local structures.

Likely complications include:
1. Congestive heart failure – due to rupture of cusps or chordae.
2. Embolic events – cerebral, renal, coronary, pulmonary.

Flow chart 12.1: Presentation and management of native and prosthetic valve endocarditis

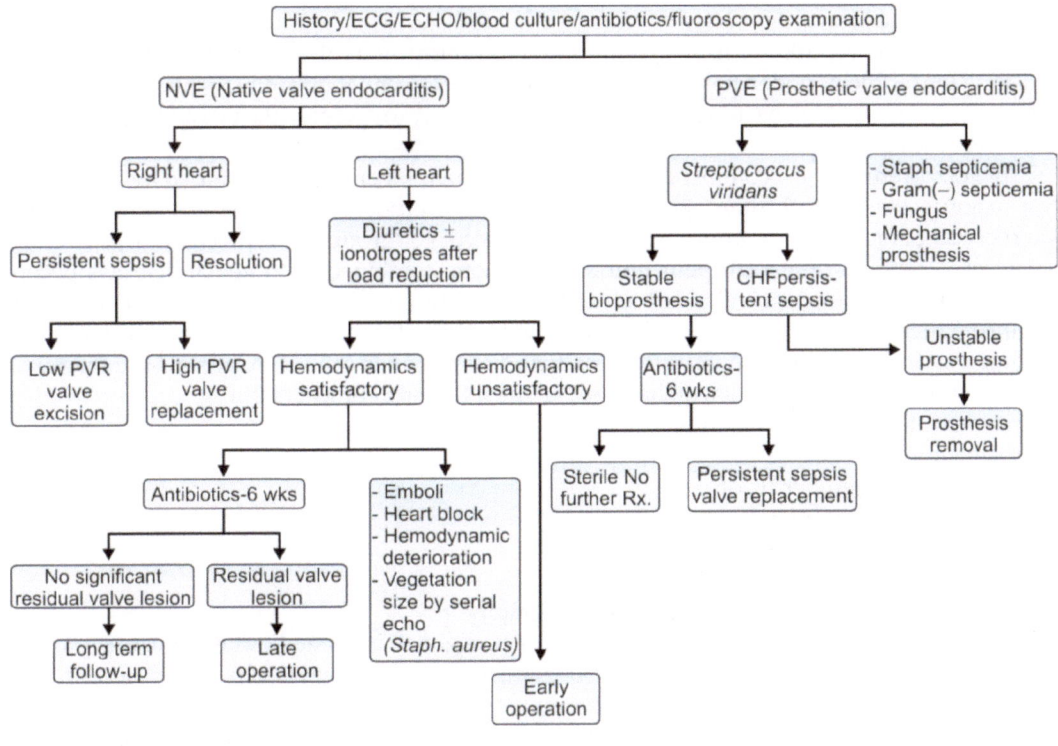

3. Periannular extension of abscess – arrhythmias or new heart block.
4. Prosthetic device dysfunction including valvar dehiscence.
5. Metastatic infection, mycotic aneurysm.
6. Focal diffuse glomerulonephritis leading to chronic renal failure.

Flow chart 12.1 gives the presentation and management of native and prosthetic valve endocarditis.

MANAGEMENT

The principles of management are:
1. Antimicrobial therapy
2. Surgical treatment in some.

Antimicrobial Therapy

In acutely ill case:
1. Three to four blood cultures have to be taken at one hourly interval in the first 24 hours preferably during the febrile period. After the blood culture has been sent, then antibiotics have to be started bactericidal rather than bacteriostatic, given intravenously to decrease the possibility of treatment failure or relapse.

Table 12.6 presents the recommended treatment regimens for endocarditis caused by streptococci, vast majority being of viridians group (α-hemolytic) streptococci, the rest are *S. bovis* (a non-enterococcal penicillin susceptible group D streptococcus) or group A streptococci *(S. pyogenes)*.

A 2 week course therapy with penicillin or ceftriaxone combined with gentamicin has become increasingly popular and results in high cure rates in adults.[15] This regimen is recommended for uncomplicated cases of native valve IE caused by highly penicillin sensitive viridian group streptococci or *S. bovis* in patients at low risk for adverse events caused by gentamicin therapy. It should not be used for patients who have any of the following clinical features:

- Endocarditis > 3 months duration
- Prosthetic valve infection
- Shock or decreased perfusion
- Extracardiac foci of infection
- Mycotic aneurysm or cerebritis
- Renal failure
- Presence of vegetation proved on echocardiography

Relapse rates are low and experience with 2 week regimen is limited but it appears promising. Some of the resistant strains of *S. viridians* or bovis are treated with 4 weeks of penicillin or ceftriaxone combined with 2 weeks of gentamicin.

Individuals allergic to penicillin (or ampicillin) frequently can be desensitized to enable treatment with these agents of choice. An effective alternative can be used safely is intravenous vancomycin. For all streptococci with a high allergy to penicillin, 4 weeks of vancomycin therapy appears adequate. For more resident streptococci treatment for 6 weeks of vancomycin combine with gentamicin is recommended. Patients receiving these regimens should be closely monitored for renal toxicity and ototoxicity.

Staphylococcal Endocarditis

Table 12.7 presents recommended regimens for endocarditis caused by staphylococci. Staphylococci are coagulase positive *(S. aureus)* or coagulate negative *(S. epidermidis)*. Only few strains of *S. aureus* are penicillin sensitive because of production of enzymes called beta lactamases. Therefore antibiotic

Table 12.6: Therapy of native valve endocarditis caused by streptococci

Highly penicillin – susceptible viridian group streptococci and *Streptococcus bovis* (MIC < 0.12 µg/mL)

Regimen	Dosage	Route	Duration, weeks
Aqueous crystalline penicillin G sodium	200,000 Units/kg per day	IV in 4-6 equally divided doses	4
or			
Ceftriaxone sodium	100 mg/kg per 24 h	IV/IM in 1 dose	4
Aqueous crystalline penicillin G sodium	200,000 Units/Kg per 24 h	IV in 4-6 equally divided doses	2b
or			
Ceftriaxone sodium	100 mg/kg per 24h	IV/IM in dose	2
plus			
Gentamicin sulfate	7 mg/kg per 24 h	IV/IM in 3 equally divided doses[1]	2
Vancomycin hydrochloride	40 mg/kg per 24 h	IV in 2-3 equally divided doses	4

Strains of viridians group streptococci and *S. bovis* relatively resistant to penicillin (MIC > 0.12 to < µg/mL)

Regimen	Dosage	Route	Duration, weeks
Aqueous crystalline penicillin G sodium	300,000 U/24 h	IV in 4-6 equally divided doses	4
or			
Ceftriaxone sodium	100 mg/kg per 24 h	IV/IM in 1 dose	4
plus			
Gentamicin sulfate	7 mg/kg per 24 h	IV/IM in 3 equally divided doses	2
Vancomycin hydrochloride	40 mg/kg 24 h	IV in 2 or 3 equally divided doses	4

Streptococci with MIC > 0.5 µg/mL as well as for enterococcal endocarditis caused by strains susceptible to penicillin, gentamicin and vancomycin

Regimen	Dosage	Route	Duration, weeks
Ampicillin sodium	300 mg/kg per 24 h	IV in 4-6 equally divided doses	4-6
or			
Aqueous crystalline penicillin G sodium	300,000 U/Kg per 24 h	IV in 4-6 equally divided doses	4-6
plus			
Gentamicin sulfate	7 mg/kg per 24 h	IV/IM in 3 equally divided doses	4-6
Vancomycin hydrochloride	40 mg/kg 24 h	IV in 2 or 3 equally divided doses	6
plus			
Gentamicin sulfate	7 mg/kg per 24h	IV/IM in 3 equally divided doses	6

Table 12.7: Therapy for endocarditis caused by staphylococci in the absence of prosthetic materials

Staphylococci with MIC > 0.5 µg/mL as well as for enterococcal endocarditis caused by strains susceptible to penicillin, gentamicin and vancomycin

Regimen	Dosage	Route	Duration, weeks
Oxacillin-susceptible strains			
Nafcillin or oxacillin with	200 mg/kg per 24 h	IV in 4-6 equally divided doses	6
Optional addition of gentamicin sulfate	7 mg/kg per 24 h	IV/IM in 3 equally divided doses	3-5 d
For penicillin-allergic (nonanaphylactoid type) patients:			
Cefazolin with			
Optional addition of gentamicin sulfate	7 mg/kg per 24h	IV/IM in 3 equally divided doses	6
Oxacillin resistant strains			
Vancomycin	40 mg/kg per 24 h	IV in 2 or 3 equally divided doses	6 weeks

therapy must involve a penicillinase resistant penicillin (e.g. nafcillin or oxacillin) administered intravenously for 6 weeks. Addition of gentamicin for first 3-5 days helps to rapidly sterilize the blood stream. Cefazolin may be used rather than nafcillin or oxacillin in patients with non-anaphylactoid type penicillin allergy. Oxacillin resistant staphylococci should be treated with vancomycin parenterally for 6 weeks.

Fungal Endocarditis

Fungal endocarditis is a relatively new syndrome and is often a complication of medical and surgical advances. Prognosis is poor with high mortality and morbidity and it can occur in immune compromised patients (preterm infants), injection drug users, in patients on prolonged antibiotic therapy and those with cardiac devices, e.g. prosthetic cardiac valves or central venous catheters. Treatment of fungal endocarditis with antifungal drugs is almost always unsuccessful. Surgical replacement of infected valve and excision of infected tissue is almost always required along with antifungal agents. Surgery is best performed after 2 weeks of medical therapy if the hemodynamic status permits.

Amphotericin B remains the most effective antifungal agent. A test dose of 0.1 mg/kg of amphotericin B (maximum 1 mg) is initially administered. If it is tolerated, it is followed by a dose of 0.5 mg/kg for 1 day and then 1 mg/kg of maintenance dose. Maximum duration of therapy should be 6-8 weeks and renal function and serum potassium levels should be monitored carefully.

Prosthetic Valve Endocarditis

Antibiotic therapy for patients with infected prosthetic heart valves must be appropriate for the specific infective agent. Duration of therapy is usually 6 weeks or longer. Antibiotic therapy depending on the sensitivity is the same as elaborated earlier. Again, for penicillin allergic patients who cannot be desensitized, vancomycin is recommended.

Experience in adults with prosthetic valve endocarditis has emphasized that early surgical replacement of the infected valve may reduce the excessively high mortality rate associated with such infection.

Anticoagulation Therapy

Anticoagulation therapy during treatment of IE remains controversial. Most authorities agree that for prosthetic valve endocarditis and for those who are already on anticoagulation for better reasons, maintenance of anticoagulation is appropriate. This was confirmed as a preferred approach by a consensus by cardiologists and infectious disease specialists.[16]

Surgery

Indications for surgery are:
1. Valvular dysfunction—leading on to resistant congestive heart failure, paravalvular necrosis, aortic dissection or valvular orifice obstruction because of large vegetation.
2. Persistent bacteremia despite adequate antimicrobial therapy for 10-14 days.
3. Fungal endocarditis.
4. Repeated systemic embolization

Less definite indication for surgery
- Single major embolus
- Echocardiographic demonstration of large vegetation.
- Extension of infection to an annular abscess or myocardial abscess.

The infected valve is usually excised and replaced by a homograft valve because of its low predilection to infection. Operative mortality for NVE is 15%. Recurrent endocarditis at 6 years is 20% and at 14 years it is 5%, survival after complete therapy is 40%.

Prognosis

Native valve endocarditis (NVE), complete cure rate varies -for *S. viridans* -it is more than 90%.
- *S faecalis (enterococcus)*—85-90%.
- *Staphylococcus aureus*—60-75%

- Mortality is usually due to resistant CCF, aneurysmal rupture, embolization, renal failure or surgical complications. Prognostic factors are: fungal IE, pseudomonas endocarditis, young age, aortic valve involvement, renal failure, endocardial abscess or large vegetations
- Prognosis of PVE is worse than NVE.

Prophylaxis

Because of the high rates of morbidity and mortality associated with IE, any measure that can prevent the disease is desirable. Theoretically, endocarditis can often be prevented by repairing the underlying cardiac defect or reducing the likelihood of bacteremia. Successful surgical repair of certain cardiac conditions will reduce or eliminate the risk of endocarditis.[17]

Recently, the American Heart Association issued new IE prophylaxis guidelines.[18] It has been concluded that bacteremia resulting from daily activities is much more likely to cause IE than bacteremia associated with dental procedures. Only an extremely small number of cases of IE might be prevented by antibiotic prophylaxis even if prophylaxis were 100% effective, a highly unlikely circumstance. Under these guidelines, prophylaxis is no longer recommended based solely on an increased lifetime risk of acquisition of infective endocarditis. Rather, prophylaxis is suggested only for patients with underlying cardiac condition associated with highest risk of adverse outcomes from IE (Table 12.8). The AHA recommendations state that, for those patients listed in Table 12.8, prophylaxis antibiotics should be given for all dental procedures that involve manipulation of

Table 12.8: Cardiac conditions associated with the highest risk of adverse outcome from endocarditis for which prophylaxis with dental procedures

Prosthetic cardiac valve
Previous IE
Congenital heart disease (CHD)*
- Unrepaired cyanotic CHD, including palliative shunts and conduits.
- Completely repaired congenital heart defect with prosthetic material or device, whether placed by surgery or by catheter intervention, during the first 6 months after the procedure.⁺
- Repaired CHD with residual defects at the site or adjacent to the site of a prosthetic patch or prosthetic device (which inhibit endotheliazation).
- Cardiac transplantation recipients who develop cardiac valvulopathy

* Except for the conditions listed above, antibiotic prophylaxis is no longer recommended for any other form of CHD.
⁺ Prophylaxis is recommended because endothelialization of prosthetic material occurs within 6 months after the procedure.

gingival tissue or the periapical region of teeth or perforation of oral mucosa. Under this framework, postoperative tetralogy of Fallot patients with homografts/conduits would receive antibiotic prophylaxis, same as those with "prosthetic valves" but those with simpler outflow patients would not.

Poor dental hygiene and periodical or periapical infections may produce bacteremia even in the absence of dental or oral procedures. Maintenance of optimal dental care and oral hygiene is important for the prevention of endocarditis in children with underlying cardiac disease. Patients in whom prosthetic valves or other devices are to be placed should undergo needed dental procedure to establish optimal oral hygiene before cardiac surgery.

Antibiotic prophylaxis is also recommended for procedures on respiratory tract or infected skin, skin structures or musculoskeletal tissue (but not GU or GE tract procedures) for those patients with underlying cardiac conditions associated with the highest risk of adverse outcome from IE (Table 12.8). Prophylaxis is most effective when given periprocedurally starting shortly before a procedure. α hemolytic streptococci remain the most common cause of endocarditis following dental, oral or upper respiratory tract procedures. Prophylaxis should be directed specifically against these organisms, which are susceptible to penicillin, ampicillin or amoxicillin (Table 12.9). Children, who are receiving penicillin prophylaxis for prevention of recurrence of rheumatic fever, may have hemolytic streptococci in the oral cavities which are resistant to penicillins. In such case a

Table 12.9: Prophylactic regimens for dental, oral or respiratory tract procedures

	Agent	Regimen (single dose 30-60 min before procedure)
Standard oral prophylaxis	Amoxicillin	50 mg/kg p.o. (maximum 2 g)
Unable to take oral medication	Ampicillin	50 mg/kg i.m. or i.v. (maximum 2 g)
	or	
	Cefazolin or ceftriaxone	50 mg/Kg i.m. or i.v. (maximum 1 g)
Penicillin allergic oral regimen	Clindamycin	20 mg/Kg p.o. (maximum 600 mg)
	or	
	Cephalexin[a]	50 mg/kg p.o. (maximum 2 g)
	or	15 mg/kg p.o. (maximum 500 mg)
Penicillin allergic and unable to take oral medication	Clindamycin	20 mg/kg i.v. (maximum 600 mg)
	or	
	Cefazolin	50 mg/kg i.m. or i.v. (maximum 1 g)

[a] Cephalosporins should not be used in individuals with immediate type hypersensitivity reaction (urticaria, angioedema, or anaphylaxis) to penicillins.

macrolide or a clindamycin should be selected for IE prophylaxis. In addition, prophylaxis should be aimed primarily against *S. aureus* and coagulase – negative staphylococci. A first generation cephalosporin or vancomycin is a reasonable choice and should be used only perioperatively and under most circumstances, for no more than 48 hours.

Finally, new AHA recommendations note the importance of maintenance of good oral health as an important factor in preventing IE in susceptible patients and urge clinicians to educate their patients in this regard.

PERICARDIAL DISEASES

The pericardium is a fibro serous sac which surrounds the heart and roots of great vessels. It consists of outer sac – fibrous pericardium and an inner sac – serous pericardium. The fibrous pericardium is continuous with the pre-tracheal layer of deep cervical fascia.

The serous pericardium is a closed sac that lines the fibrous pericardium. It consists of:
1. The visceral layer – the inner serous layer, which is attached to the outer surface of the myocardium.
2. The parietal layer -outer fibrous layer, which consists of elastic and collagen fibres.

The pericardial space -is a potential space separating the visceral and parietal layers and it is lubricated by lymph, which is less than 50 ml.[19] It is an ultrafiltrate of plasma and contains immune factors.[20]

Blood vessels, lymphatics and nerve fibers are beneath the visceral pericardium and surround the parietal pericardium.

Arterial supply of the pericardium is by the branch of internal mammary artery which originates from the descending aorta.

Nerve supply innervation is via the vagus and phrenic nerves, and by sympathetic nerve fibers.

Conditions Affecting Pericardium

The pericardium helps to reduce the friction resulting from cardiac motion. It acts as a barrier by protecting the heart from any disorders from contiguous structures,[21] and pericardium being a dynamic structure, gets stretched due to accumulation of fluid or cardiac enlargement and will grow to accommodate its contents.
1. Congenital
   - Absent or defects in pericardium
   - Pericardial cysts.

2. Inflammation
   - Acute pericarditis
   - Acute infections
     a. Bacterial – Pericarditis
        – *Staphylococcus aureus*
        – *Haemophilus influenzae* type B
        – Other gram +ve and –ve organisms.
     b. Viral pericarditis
        – Coxsackie A and B
        – Hepatits, HIV, mumps, measles, varicella, etc.
     c. Tubercular pericarditis
     d. Others–Fungal, protozoal rickettsial
     e. Vasculitis and connective tissue diseases
        – Rheumatic arthritis
        – Systemic lupus erythematosus
        – Rheumatic fever
        – Kawasaki disease
     f. Malignancy
     g. Drugs – Anticoagulants, antithrombolytic agents
           Hydralazine, procainamide, phenytoin
           Isoniazide, rifampicin, penicillin,
           Doxorubicin
     h. Miscellaneous – Renal failure, hypothyroidism, trauma.
3. Pericardial effusion (Tamponade)
4. Constructive pericarditis
5. Intrapericardial tumors.

Signs and Symptoms of Pericardial Disease

Clinical Features

1. Chest pain—Sharp pain associated with breathing.
2. Friction rub—It is a grating, scratching sound caused by abrading of inflamed pericardial surfaces with cardiac motion. It is best heard in 2-4th intercostal spaces along the left sternal border or

along the mid clavicular line. It is loudest in the upright position with the patient leaning forward and it is heard both during systole and diastole.
3. Muffled heart sounds in the presence of large pericardial effusion, when rub may not be heard.
4. Ewart's sign—Subscapular dullness on percussion, due to compression of the left lung by massively enlarged heart. There may be associated abnormal breath sounds in that region.
5. Cardiac-tamponade—Features include low cardiac output, elevated central venous pressure, paradoxical pulse, muffled or diminished heart sounds and tachycardia.

Electrocardiography (Fig. 12.4)

Changes in ECG represent the effect of diseased pericardium on the underlying myocardium. Low voltages are seen due to insulating effect of pericardial fluid. Pericarditis is the most common cause of ST elevation, flat or inverted T waves, in children.

Radiographic Findings

In acute pericarditis heart size may be normal.

In pericardial effusion cardiac silhouette is considerably enlarged. Water bottle heart or triangular heart with smooth cut borders is seen in massive pericardial effusion. Associated pulmonary findings may give indication of etiology of pericardial disease, such as bacterial or tubercular pericarditis or in neoplastic disease.

Cystic hygroma with pericardial lymphangiomas may also be detected in chest radiograph of a patient with congenital pericardial defects.

Echocardiography (Figs 12.5A and B)

The detection and quantification of even small volume of pericardial fluid by 2D and M-mode echo-cardiography has simplified the approach to the diagnosis and management of pericardial

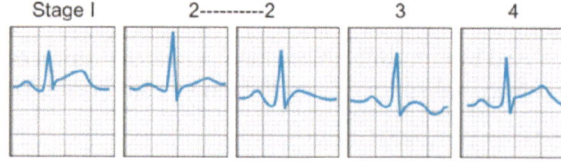

Fig. 12.4: Serial electrocardiograms demonstrating evolution of the stages of pericarditis, which include stage 1: diffuse ST-segment elevation and PR depression; stage 2: normalization of the ST and PR segments; stage 3: widespread T-wave inversion; and stage 4: normalization of the T waves. (From Spodick DH. Electrocardiographic abnormalities in pericardial disease Spodick DH, ed The Pericardium: A Comprehensive Textbook. New York: Marcel Dekker, 1997:42, with permission.)

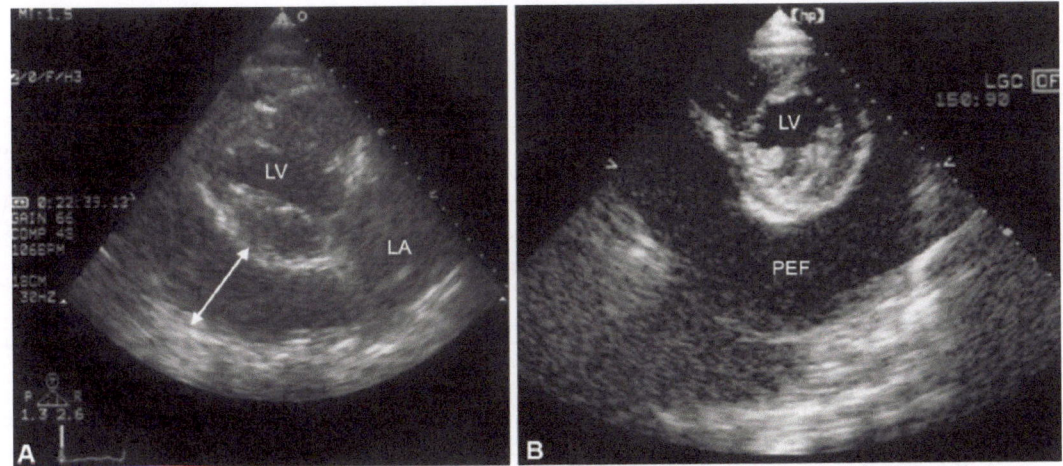

Figs 12.5A and B: Parasternal long and short axis view showing a large pericardial effusion (PE) surrounding the left ventricle

effusion. There might be massive amount of fluid collected in tubercular pericardial effusion which constricts the cardiac shadow, so, in such a situation, a therapeutic pericardiocentesis is indicated (Figs 12.5A and B).

Radionuclide Imaging Technique

Computed tomography and magnetic resonance imaging may be helpful in the assessment of congenital pericardial defects or mediastinal masses involving the percardium.

Drainage of Pericardial Fluid (Pericardiocentesis)

Pericardiocentesis is indicated in patients with pericardial effusion. Ultrasonographic guidance adds to the safety of the procedure but it is not essential when emergent drainage of pericardial effusion is necessary due to hemodynamic compromise.

Complication of Pericardiocentesis

1. Myocardial puncture
2. Coronary artery or vein puncture

3. Hemopericardium and pneumopericardium
4. Pneumothorax.

Acute Pericarditis

Pericarditis is the inflammation of pericardial sac surrounding the heart and the origin of great vessels. It may be acute (< 6 weeks), subacute (6 weeks to 6 months) and chronic (> 6 months). It may occur secondary to infectious agents, collagen vascular disease. cardiac surgery, drug therapy, or in association of renal failure and dialysis. Other systemic diseases leading to pericardial effusion are hypothyroidism, intrapericardial tumors or post-radiation therapy.

INFECTIOUS DISEASES OF THE PERICARDIUM

Purulent Pericarditis

It is a life threatening illness with mortality rates from 25-75%. It may be primary or secondary due to dissemination from another site of infection like pneumonia, septic arthritis, meningitis or osteomyelitis. Incidence of pericarditis due to *Staphylococcus aureus* ranges from 50-80% of reported cases. *Haemophilus influenzae* is the second most common organism. Tamponade is far more likely to occur in children.

N. meningitides, Pseudomonas aeruginosa, Salmonella species, *N. gonorrhea, Campylobacter, E. coli, Brucella, Listeria monocytogenes* are other microorganisms responsible for causing acute pericarditis.

Clinical Features

Pericardial chest pain: It is present in 80% of children with acute pericarditis, excerbated by breathing coughing or movement. Patients are comfortable in upright position.

Respiratory distress: Not a common feature in the absence of pneumonia or cardiac tamponade.

Fever: Present in most cases.

Pericardial rub: It is pathognomonic of acute pericarditis. In the presence of congenital heart disease or valvular rheumatic heart disease, the rub may be obscured by associated murmur. .

Tachycardia: Disproportionate to the degree of fever may indicate pericarditis or myocarditis and may herald impending tamponade.

Diagnosis: Pericarditis must be considered when following features are present:
1. Fever with chest pain.
2. Cardiomegaly on chest X-ray (the absence does not rule out pericarditis).

3. Pericardiocentesis must be performed in suspected cases when diagnosis has not been confirmed by non-invasive methods. Analysis of pericardial fluid should include total and differential cell count, culture for bacteria, viruses and *Mycobacterium tuberculosis* and fungi. Protein specific bacterial antigens may be identified with immunological techniques. In chylopericardium, pericardial fluid triglycerides are elevated and in pericarditis secondary to myxedema pericardial fluid cholesterol levels are high.

Treatment

1. Antibiotic therapy alone may not be sufficient as antibiotic penetration in large abscesses may be insufficient.
2. Pericardiocentesis or placement of pericardial catheter in the pericardial space.
3. Pericardiectomy may be required if the pericardial fluid is viscous.

Broad-spectrum antibiotic coverage should be directed towards the treatment of *Staphylococcus aureus* and *Haemophillus influenzae*. Initial intravenous therapy should include a penicillinase resistant penicillin and a third generation cephalosporin. Once culture reports are known, specific antibiotic should be continued for 3-4 weeks.

Prognosis

Delay in diagnosis, cardiac tamponade with hemodynamic impairment, septicemia due to staphylococcal disease and inadequate drainage of purulent fluid lead to poor outcome. Constrictive pericarditis is a rare but well documented complication of purulent pericarditis.[22]

Viral Pericarditis

It is more frequently seen in children. History of preceding gastrointestinal or respiratory disease is reported in 40-75% of cases.

Viruses, e.g. Adenovirus, echo., coxsackie, mumps, varicella, Ebstein Barr and human immuno deficiency virus are commonly responsible. Fever and chest pain are the main symptoms. Patients are less toxic than those with bacterial pericarditis, unless accompanying myocarditis is present. Pericardial rub is present in 80% of patients with viral pericarditis.

Pericardiocentesis is indicated in patients with cardiac tamponade in immunocompromised patients. Pericardial fluids may be serous or serosanguinous with a predominance of lymphocytes. Peripheral white blood cell count may be normal or lymphocytic.

Diagnosis is confirmed by isolation of virus either from pericardial fluid, oropharyngeal cultures or stool cultures or demonstration of fourfold increase in antibody titer obtained from acute and convalescent serum.

Treatment

It is symptomatic
- Bed rest
- Anti-inflammatory agents—Analgesics and nonsteroidal analgesic agents.
- Steroid therapy—Rarely indicated, should be initiated only when bacterial etiology is ruled out. There is no evidence to prove that steroid therapy reduces the requirement of pericardiocentesis. Pericardial drainage catheter or surgical correction of pericardial window may be needed in refractory cases.
- Relapse may occur in 15% of cases. Constrictive pericarditis is a common complication.

Tubercular Pericarditis

It is more common in underdeveloped countries and it occurs due to direct spread from mediastinal lymph nodes or secondary to hematogenous dissemination even in the absence of pulmonary infiltrates. Tubercular pericarditis accounts for only 4% of cases in developed countries but constitutes about 70% of cases of acute pericarditis in the developing countries.[23] The onset may be insiduous with gradual weight loss, night sweats and dyspnea with chest pain. It may be complicated by pericardial tamponade. Mantoux tuberculin skin test is positive in most patients. The pericardial fluid is serosanguinous with predominance of lymphocytes. Acid fast bacilli are present in fluorescent stained smears of pericardial fluid, or biopsy material. Pericardial biopsy may provide histological confirmation.

Treatment: Because of high prevalence of drug resistant organisms, initial therapy should consist of isoniazid, pyrazinamide, rifampicin, ethambutol and streptomycin, and should be continued for 9-15 months.

Use of steroids is controversial. Although they may have some beneficial effects on morbidity and mortality, there seems to be no beneficial effect on reaccumulation of fluid or prevention of constriction.[24]

Constrictive pericarditis is seen in 35% of patients recovering from tubercular pericarditis due to pericardial thickening, granuloma formation and scarring.

Other Infectious Causes of Pericarditis

These include fungi, protozoa and rickettsia. Immunocompromised patients are at greater risk for the development of pericarditis due to these agents.

Noninfectious causes of acute pericarditis are:

1. *Acute rheumatic fever:* Cardiovascular involvement in acute rheumatic fever is characterized by pancarditis with inflammation of endocardium, myocardium and pericardium. Pericardial involvement is seen in 5 to 10% of patients with acute rheumatic fever. In isolation pericarditis is a rare manifestation of acute rheumatic fever.

    Treatment with anti-inflammatory agents results in rapid reduction of pericardial effusion.

2. *Connective tissue diseases:*
    a. **Rheumatoid arthritis:** Symptomatic pericarditis occurs in 10% of children with juvenile rheumatoid arthritis and may be demonstrated in 50% of patients by echocardiography.

        Pericardiocentesis may be necessary for the treatment and to rule out bacterial etiology in a chronically ill child. Treatment with nonsteroidal anti- inflammatory agents is very effective. Short course of steroid therapy results in rapid resolution of symptoms.
    b. **Systemic lupus erythematosis (SLE):** Cardiovascular manifestations occur in 50-80% of patients with SLE. Apparent pericarditis is the most frequent complication which occurs in 25%.

        Diagnostic pericardiocentesis may be necessary in patients who fail to respond to traditional anti-inflammatory agents.

        Pericardial fluid analysis may show reduced complement levels, positive antinuclear antibodies or positive rheumatoid factor.
    c. **Post-pericardiotomy syndrome:** Post-pericardiotomy syndrome is a relatively benign self limiting condition. Majority of patients respond to bed rest and anti-inflammatory agents. Patients with large or rapidly accumulating pericardial effusion may need pericardiocentesis. Steroids are recommended for severe cases and methotrexate has been used for chronic pericardiotomy syndrome with recurrent pericardial effusion.[25]
    d. **Kawasaki's disease:** One third of patients with Kawasaki's disease in acute phase may develop pericardial effusion but they rarely develop cardiac-tamponade, unless the coronary artery aneurysm ruptures.
    e. **Drug induced pericarditis:** Isoniazid, hydralazine and procainamide may lead to pericarditis and administration of anti-inflammatory agents which controls the drug induced pericarditis.
    f. **Uremic pericarditis:** The association of uremia with pericarditis is considered by nephrologists as a sign of end stage renal disease, though incidence has decreased due to dialysis, from 50-100% of patients with chronic renal failure. Co-existing SLE or previous treatment with hydralazine may contribute to the development of pericarditis in this group of

patients. Pericardiocentesis should be performed in those patients with tamponade or bacterial infection.

In stable patients, dialysis may resolve pericardial effusion. If it fails, pericardial window or pericardiectomy may be necessary.

Constrictive Pericarditis

It is characterized by thickened adherent pericardium that restricts filling of ventricles in the end point of acute or chronic pericardial inflammation.

Etiology

In children, tuberculosis is the commonest cause of constrictive pericarditis as 15-25% of patients with tubercular pericarditis develop constriction. Other causes include trauma, cardiac surgery, irradiation, hemopericardium and others may be termed idiopathic.

Thick, constrictive non-compliant pericarditis produces hemodynamic impairment secondary to restriction of diastolic expansion of the ventricles. Systolic function remains normal initially, but the mid and late diastolic filling is reduced due to incompliant pericardium resulting in elevated central venous pressure and pulmonary capillary wedge pressure and ultimately the features of cardiac tamponade set in.

Pathology

Pathological findings include thickened pericardium with focal areas of inflammation. The underlying myocardium shows atrophic changes due to impaired myocardial perfusion secondary to the effects of an overlying scarred or calcified pericardium.

Clinical Picture

1. Exercise intolerance, easy fatiguability, dyspnea, syncope.
2. Jugular and hepatic congestion.
3. Pedal edema, ascitis
4. Tachycardia—Muffled heart sound signs of low cardiac output.
5. Pericardial knock—A protodiastolic sound, corresponds to abrupt cessation of ventricular filling —is pathognomonic of pericardial constriction.
6. ECG—Low voltage QRS complexes and A-V conduction delay.
7. Heart size is usually normal by chest radiography.

8. 2-D Echo may show pericardial thickening. There are no other specific indicators of constrictive pericarditis. Dilatation of inferior vena cavae and atria and venocaval filling dysfunction may be noted by Doppler echocardiography giving rise to a condition called diastolic dysfunction.

Echocardiography magnetic resonance imaging or CT are sensitive methods for the assessment of pericardial thickening. Clinical and laboratory differentiation of constrictive pericarditis from restrictive cardiomyopathy may be difficult, except by MR or CT. At cardiac catheterization, restrictive cardiomyopathy patients rarely have pulmonary artery pressures greater than 50 mm Hg.

Management

In early stages of constriction, medical management can resolve the constriction by using analgesics, antibiotics and short course of steroids. Resolution of constriction without surgery in pediatric patients has been reported in 60%.[27] Complete or radical pericardiectomy is desirable in advanced cases for improvement in hemodynamics and symptoms but subtotal pericardiectomy may be desirable in some cases. The risk of mortality with pericardiectomy is 15-20%.[28]

MISCELLANEOUS CAUSES OF PERICARDIAL EFFUSION

Hypothyroidism

In hypothyroidism, pericardial effusion may be present. Clinical signs of inflammation are rarely present. The patients with myxoedema have bradycardia in contrast to patients with inflammatory pericarditis.

Treatment with thyroid supplements results in gradual reduction in the size of pericardial effusion. The pericardial fluid in these cases show high cholesterol levels.

Chylopericardium

Chylous or lymphatic pericardial effusion are occasionally seen in children.

Etiology

1. Thoracic cystic hygromas with pericardial imvolvement.
2. Following surgery – for CHD, trauma to thoracic duct.
3. Secondary to obstruction of lymphatic drainage by mediastinal masses.

Diagnosis

Pericardiocentesis to document the type of pericardial fluid. Chylous fluid is serous or milky in appearance with lymphocyte, predominating, triglyceride levels higher than plasma and protein levels more than 3 gm/dl.

Treatment

It should be directed at elimination of the cause of effusion
1. To reduce central venous pressure—diuretics, inotropic agents and drugs to bring about afterload reduction.
2. Mediastinal masses—should be excised to remove obstruction.
3. Palliation—surgical creation of pericardial window or placement of pericardio pleural peritoneal shunt.

Intrapericardial Tumors

Primary malignant neoplasms of pericardium are rare. Congenital, nonmalignant and intrapericardial lesions include:
1. Pericardial celomic cyst
2. Cystic lymphangioma
3. Bronchogenic cyst
4. Pericardial teratoma, mesothelioma, lymphoma and angiosarcoma.

Teratomas are the most common intrapericardial tumors in children.

Echocardiography may show an echogenic lesion within the pericardial space, often associated with pericardial effusion. Congenital pericardial cystic lesions originate at the base of the heart often encircling the great arteries and veins.

Computed tomography and magnetic resonance imaging are useful in diagnosis.

Congenital intrapericardial masses may be associated with hydrops fetalis secondary to compression of fetal venous structures. Pericardiocentesis is the initial life saving measure. Surgical excision is curative.

Radiation Pericarditis

Cardiac side effects of thoracic radiation occur frequently when greater than 4000 rads is delivered to the heart. Pericardial disease is the most common side effect of the radiotherapy to the heart and may present as pericarditis with or without effusion, chronic pericarditis or constrictive pericarditis. Pericardiocentesis should be done to rule out infectious etiology, to assess pericardial cytology and to treat hemodynamic compromise in the presence of pericardial tamponade.

Congenital Pericardial Defects

Partial or total absence of the pericardium is rare and is associated with significant symptoms like syncope, chest pain, arrhythmias and death due to herniation or incarceration of the left atrial appendage through the defect, torsion of the great arteries or constriction of coronary artery at the rim of the defect. Diagnosis of pericardial defects is difficult by echocardiography, chest radiography or ECG. Thoracoscopy or MRI is necessary to confirm the diagnosis.

Treatment

Depends on the size of the defect. Patch closure of the defect or enlargement of the defect to prevent incarceration may be required. Complete absence of pericardium rarely requires treatment, as morbidity and mortality rates are minimal.

Cardiac Tamponade[26]

Cardiac tamponade is a medical emergency. It is life threatening because of slow or rapid compression of the heart due to accumulation of fluid, blood, clots or gas in the pericardial space leading to significant impairment of ventricular filling.[26]

Pathophysiology (Figs 12.6A and B)

Key elements to develop cardiac tamponade include:
1. Rate of fluid accumulation relative to pericardial stretch.
2. Effectiveness of compensatory mechanisms.

The systemic and pulmonary venous pressure rise and as more fluid accumulates, the stroke volume falls. Tachycardia and increase in blood volume compensates this fall in stroke volume. As more fluid accumulates and the initial compensatory mechanism maintains blood pressure and subsequently pulse pressure narrows. Any further increase in fluid accumulation leads to further compromise of the ventricular filling and hypotension. The coronary blood flow is also reduced in tamponade, but there is no ischemic component, as the coronary blood flow remains proportional to the reduced work and requirements of the heart.

Clinical Features

Cardiac tamponade must be suspected in patients with hypotension preceded by purulent pericarditis or other types of pericardial diseases.

Symptoms include:
- Dyspnea on exertion
- Weakness, syncope
- Nonspecific symptoms such as anorexia, dysphagia and cough

Physical signs include:
- Tachycardia, pulsus paradoxus, hypotension.
- Jugular venous distension

- Soft and muffled heart sounds.
- Signs of end organ hypoperfusion

Pulsus paradoxus is the cardinal sign of cardiac tamponade – defined as inspiratory systolic fall in arterial pressure of 10 mm Hg.[26]

Investigations

1. *Electrocardiogram:* Electrical Alternans – especially if it involves both P wave and QRS complexes.
2. Doppler studies–investigation of choice to diagnose tamponade. Marked variation in transvascular flow with respiration is seen. This is the Doppler equivalent of pulsus paradoxus.
3. *Echocardiography:* Evidence of global fluid collection in the pericardial space with evidence of compressed and collapsing chambers with hyperdynamic cardiac function. The inferior vena cava may appear dilated with little change with respiration.

Management

Management of cardiac tamponade consists of drainage of pericardial effusion.

1. *Needle pericardiocentesis:* Should be performed in a controlled setting, e.g. intensive care unit under the guidance of echocardiogram or in the catheterization laboratory under fluoroscopic guidance. The patient is sedated, placed at 30° sitting position. After the subxiphoid area is

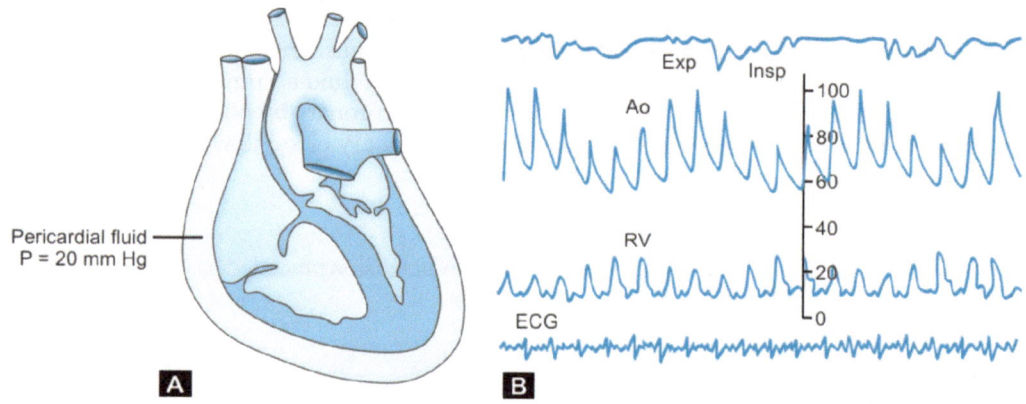

Figs 12.6A and B: Schematic representation of the physiology of cardiac tamponade. Ao, aorta; ECG, electrocardiogram; Exp, expiration; Insp, inspiration; RV, right ventricle. (Adapted from Shabetai R. The Pericardium. New York: Grune and Stratton, 1981:266. In: Braunwald's Heart Disease: A Textbook of Cardiovascular Medicine. 7th ed. Philadelphia: Elsevier, 2005:1764, with permission.)

infiltrated with 1% lidocaine, a 18-22 gauge needle attached to a syringe with sterile saline is inserted and advanced at 45° towards the tip of left scapula, with constant aspiration till the fluid starts coming. Then the needle is attached to an effective drainage system. The catheter is removed when the drainage of fluid is less than 1-2 ml/kg per day.

Complications of pericardiocentesis
   a. Myocardial injury
   b. Laceration of coronary artery
   c. Pneumopericardium
   d. Death
2. Surgical drainage may be necessary when needle pericardiocentesis fails:
   a. Intrapericardial bleeding
   b. Clotted hemopericardium.

REFERENCES

1. The Task force on Infective Endocarditis of European Society of Cardiology: Guidelines on Prevention, Diagnosis and treatment of Infective Endocarditis. Eur. Heart J 2004;25:267-76.
2. Millard DD, Shulman ST. The Changing pattern of neonatal endocarditis. Clin Perinat 1988;15:587-608.
3. Hoen B, Alla F, Selton-Suty C, et al. Changing profile of infective endocarditis: Results of a 1 year survey in France. JAMA 2002;2:75-81.
4. Netzer RO, Zollinger E, Seiler C, Corny A. Infective Endocarditis: Clinical spectrum, presentation and outcome: An analysis of 212 cases. 1980-1995. Heart 2003;83:523-30.
5. Castillo JC, Angnita MP, Ramirez A, et al. Long term outcome of infective endocarditis in patients who were no drug addicts: A 10-year study. Heart 2000;83:523-30.
6. Caviness AC, Cantor SB, Allen CH, Ward MA. A cost effective analysis of bacterial endocarditis prophylaxis for febrile children who have cardiac lesion and undergo urinary catheterization in the emergency department. Pediatrics 2004;113:1291-96.
7. Berkowitz FE. Infective endocarditis in children. St Louis: CV Mosby 1995:961-86.
8. Baddour LM, Wilson WR, Bayer AS, et al. Infective endocarditis, diagnosis and antimicrobial therapy and management of complications. Circulation 2005;111:394-434.
9. Valente AM, Jain R, Scheurer M, Fowler VG, et al. Frequency of infective endocarditis among infants and children with staphylococcus aureus bacteremia. Pediatrics 2005;115:15-19.
10. Tissieres P, Jaeggi ET, Beghetti M, Gerevaix A. Increase in fungal endocarditis in children. Infection 2005; 33:267-72.
11. Tanbort KA, Gewitz M. Infective Endocarditis in Moss and Adam's heart disease in infants, Children and adolescents including fetus and young adults. Ed. Allen HD, Driscoll DJ, Shaddy RE and Feltes TF – 7th Ed: Lippincott Williams and Wilkins, Philadelphia 2008;1299-1311.
12. Kavey RE, Frank DM, Byrum CJ, et al. Two-Dimensional echocardiographic assessment of infective endocarditis in children. Am J Dis Child 1983;137:851-56.

13. Durack DT, Lukes AS, Bright DK. New criteria for diagnosis of infective endocarditis: utilization of specific echocardiographic findings. Am J Med 1994;96:200-9.
14. Li JS Sexton DJ, Miek N, et al. Proposed modifications to the Duke criteria for the diagnosis of infective endocarditis. Clin Infect Dis 2000;30:633-38.
15. Baddour LM, Wilson WR, Bayer AS, Fowler VG Jr. Tanbert KA, et al. (Committee on rheumatic Fever, Endocarditis and Kawasaki Disease; Council on Cardiovascular disease in the young councils on clinical cardiology, stroke and cardiovascular surgery and Anaesthesiology: American Heart Association): Infective Endocarditis, diagnosis, antimicrobial therapy and management of comphealism circulation 2005;111:394-434
16. Kamala Kannan D, Beeai M, Gardin J, Saravolatz L. Anticoagulation in I.E: A Survey of infectious disease specialists and cardiologists. Infect Ds in clinical practice, 2005;13(3):122-26.
17. Morris CD Reller MD, Menashe VD. Thirty year incidence of infective endocarditis after surgery for congenital heart defect. JAMA 1998;279:599-603.
18. Wilson W, Janhert KA, Gewitz M, et al. Prevention of infective endocarditis. Guidelines from the American Heart Association. Circulation 2007;116(15):1736-54.
19. Holt JP. The normal pericardium. Am J Cardiol 1970;26(5):455-65.
20. Gibson AT, Segal MB. A study of composition of pericardial fluid with special reference to the probable mechanisms of fluid formation. J Physio 1978;277:367-77.
21. Ishihara T, Ferrans VJ, Jones M, Boyce SW, Kawanani O, Roberts WC. Histological and ultrastructural features of normal human pericardium. Am J Cardiol 1980;46(5):744-53.
22. Altman CA. Pericarditis and Pericardial Diseases. In: Arthur Garson Jr. TB, David J. Fisher, Steven R. Neish editor. The science and practice of Pediatric Cardiology. Baltimore: Williams and Wilkins 1998:1795-815.
23. Renter H, Burgess LJ, Doubell AF. Epidemiology of pericardial effusions at a large academic hospital in South Africa. Epidemiol Infect 2005;133(3):393-99.
24. Nosekhe M, Wiysonge C, Volmik JA, Commerford PJ, Mayosi BM. Adjuvant corticosterosis for tuberculosis pericarditis. QJM 2003;96(8):593-99.
25. Zuker N, Levitas A, Zalstein E. Methotrexate in recurrent post pericardiotomy syndrome. Cardiol Young 2003; 13(2): 206-8.
26. Shabetai R, Fowler NO. Guntheroth WG. The hemodynamics of cardiac tamponade and constrictive pericarditis. Am J Cardiol 1970;26(5):480-89.
27. Hugo-Hamman CT, Scher H, De Moor MM. Tuberculous pericarditis in children: a review of 44 cases. Pediata Infect Dis J 1994;13(1):13-18.
28. Seifert FC, Miller DC, Oesterle SN, Oyer PE, Stinson EB, Shumway NE. Surgical treatment of constrictive Pericarditis, analysis, outcome and diagnostic error. Circulation 1985;72(3)(2):11,264-73.

CHAPTER 13

Primary Prevention of Atherosclerotic Cardiovascular Disease Beginning in Childhood

Atherosclerotic cardiovascular disease remains the leading cause of both death and disability in the world. Emergence of multiple lines of evidence with regard to the importance of known risk factors for atherosclerotic disease in children and young adults has provided the impetus to develop guidelines for primary prevention in young population.

Atherosclerosis is defined as a disease of large and medium sized muscular and elastic arteries, which is characterized by the presence of atheroma or fibrofatty plaque (Fig. 13.1). Atheroma has a constant distribution which is different from that of a fatty streak. Atheromas occur at the following sites, in descending order:

- Abdominal aorta
- Coronary arteries (in the first 6 cm)
- Popliteal artery
- Internal carotid artery
- Circle of Willis

Atherosclerosis results from deposits of lipid and cholesterol in the intima of arterial wall. The earliest abnormality is thought to be the fatty streak, which is an accumulation of lipid filled macrophages within the intima.[1]

The atherosclerotic process tends to spare the vessels of the upper extremities, the mesenteric and renal arteries, except at their ostia. The other lesions in atherosclerosis are fatty streaks and intimal cushions.

Fatty streaks appear in the aortas of all children older than one year of age, regardless of geography, race, sex and environment. They cover 10% of the aortic intimal surface in the first decade of life and 30-50% in the third decade. In certain locations (e.g., coronary arteries) in predisposed individuals, they may evolve into plaques. It has been noted that smooth muscle fibrous plaques tend to develop at the anatomic sites where fatty streaks are formed in children.[2] Plaques generally tend to develop in the coronary arteries prior to their appearance in the cerebral arteries (Fig. 13.2).

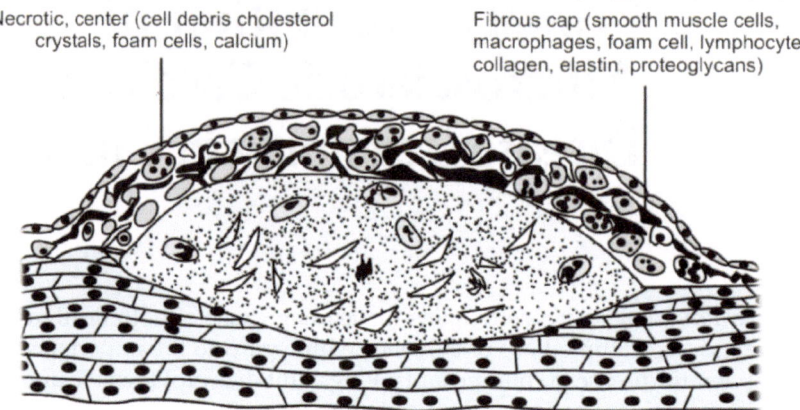

Fig. 13.1: Major components of well developed atheromatous plaque: a cap composed of foam cells, proliferating smooth muscle cells, macrophages, lymphocytes and extracellular matrix. The necrotic core consists of necrotic debris extracellular lipid with cholesterol crystals and foamy macrophages

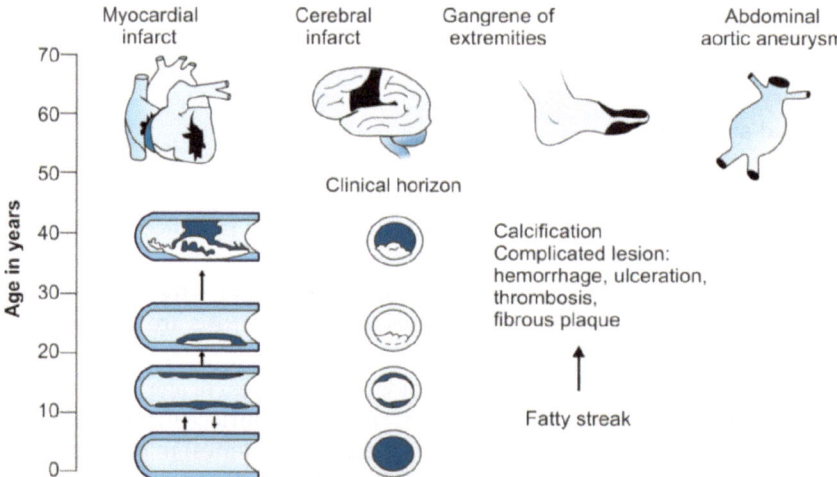

Fig. 13.2:[4] The natural history of atherosclerosis. Plaques usually develop slowly and insidiously over many years, as described in the text, they may progress from a fatty streak to a fibrous plaque and then to a complicated plaque that is likely to lead to clinical events

An intimal cushion or PAD is an additional lesion that may bear a material relationship to atherosclerosis. It is represented by small areas of white thickening at the site of arterial forks or ostia of branch vessels. Microscopically, this thickening is due to accumulation of smooth muscle cells and extracellular matrix in the intima, collagen and virtually no lipid. Intimal cushions occur in young males, at the same sites, that eventually develop plaques, suggesting a casual relationship, but the issue is unsettled.[3]

Epidemiology

Coronary artery disease (CAD) has been described as the greatest epidemic mankind has ever faced and it is responsible for more than 50% deaths, in industrialized countries. The incidence of coronary artery disease is higher in Europe and North America, but is showing a declining trend. On the other hand, the incidence of CAD is showing a risky trend in third world countries including India.[1]

Longitudinal studies as the Framingham study have measured potential risk factors and followed subjects to the development of cardiovascular disease. After decades of research, a group of risk factors often referred to as traditional risk factors has been established (Table 13.1). As can be seen, some of the risk factors are potentially modifiable and others are not. The Bogalusa heart study investigators were able to obtain autopsies in individuals who had participated in a school based risk factor study and were followed longitudinally and died of accidental causes.[4] They found that surface of arteries were covered with fatty streaks and fibrous plaques increased with age and the extent of coverage of arteries (aorta and coronary arteries) was associated with elevation of total cholesterol, low density lipoprotein (LDL-C), triglycerides (HDL-C), decrease in high density cholesterol, blood pressure and body mass index during school age surveys. It was also noticed that prevalence of atherosclerosis increased with an increasing number of risk factors present. This was particularly true for fibrous plaques in coronary arteries where the presence of three or four risk factors were associated with 7% coverage and presence of one or two risk factors were associated with 1 to 2% coverage respectively.[5]

Table 13.1: Established risk factors for coronary artery disease

Non modifiable	
Age	
Sex M > F	
Family history	
Modifiable	
Dyslipidemia	Cigarette smoking
Elevated blood pressure	Obesity metabolic syndrome
Diabetes mellitus	Coagulation factors

Cardinal Features of CAD in Asian Indians

The term "Asian Indians" here refers to all people hailing from the Indian subcontinent, anywhere in the world.[1]

Greater Prematurity

Premature CAD is defined as a cardiac event, occurring before the age of 65 years in women and 55 years in men. "CAD in the young" is defined as CAD occurring in patients less than 40 years of age, representing a more severe form of premature CAD. Of all cases of CAD in the west, only 2 to 5% occur in the young, in contrast to an incidence of CAD in the young of 12 to 16% in India.

Greater Severity

In most populations, young patients with CAD do not have extensive disease, and therefore have a generally favorable prognosis, compared to older patients. However, young Asian Indians with CAD, usually have a poor prognosis, from malignant atherosclerosis and multi-vessel disease, which often resembles the pattern seen in their older counterparts. Three vessel disease is not uncommon even among non-smoking, non-diabetic, premenopausal women in India.
Higher rates of:
- Morbidity, hospitalization and case fatality
- Incidence and prevalence

Insulin Resistance Syndrome or Syndrome X

Clinically evident clustering or coexistence of dyslipidemia, hypertension, hyperinsulinism/insulin resistance and obesity in the same individual is called Syndrome X, and is common in middle aged adults. Recent studies, in a population of young adults aged 18-26 years, revealed remarkable clustering of conditions related to Syndrome X, among those individuals who had very low density lipoprotein (VLDL) cholesterol levels in the top quartile.[3]

Insulin resistance, plays a crucial role in the etiology of syndrome X. This fact, as well as the relationship between total undernutrition and CAD are explained by Figure 13.3.[6]

Lower prevalence of conventional risk factors, i.e.
- Hypertension
- Obesity
- Cigarette smoking
- Serum cholesterol levels (similar to whites, but higher than other Asians)

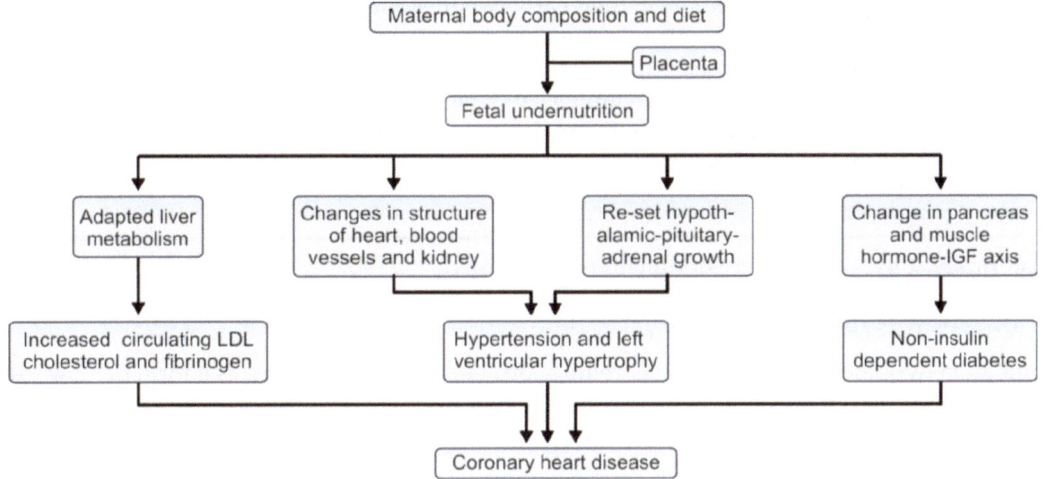

Fig. 13.3: A framework of possible mechanisms linking fetal undernutrition and coronary heart disease

Despite a lower rate of conventional risk factors, Asian Indians have a higher rate of CAD. This paradox is explained by the higher prevalence of new and emerging risk factors like:
- Elevated lipoprotein(a) [Lp(a)]
- Elevated plasminogen activator inhibitor I (PAI-I)
- Elevated triglycerides (TG) level
- Lower high density lipoprotein level (HDL-C)
- Elevated homocysteine levels
- Apple type obesity: (i.e. increased waist to hip ratio).

Therefore, the higher rates of CAD in Asian Indians, are due to combination of nature (genetic predisposition), and nurture (lifestyle factors). The nature is attributed to elevated levels of Lp (a), a common but unrecognized risk factor in Asian Indians, with a prevalence of 25-50%. Given this genetic predisposition, the handful effects of lifestyle factors are magnified exponentially.

Atherosclerosis begins in Childhood, proved by the following facts[6]

The Bogalusa heart study has established that elevated levels of serum low density lipoprotein cholesterol (LDL-C) and decreased levels of serum HDL-C in childhood, persist into adulthood and are important risk factors for CAD.

Autopsies of Korean war soldiers in their early twenties, showed atheromas.

High blood cholesterol, aggregates in families due to both shared environments and genetic factors contribute to the atherosclerotic process. Children with high serum cholesterol, especially LDL cholesterol, frequently come from families in which there is a high incidence of CAD among the adult members (Childhood and youth are defined as the period from birth to 24 years of age– International Youth Year, 1986).

PATHOGENESIS

Historically, 2 hypothesis were dominant until recently.

Imbibation Hypothesis

Imbibation hypothesis by Virchow, i.e. cellular proliferation in the intima is a form of "low grade inflammation", as a reaction to increased filtration of plasma proteins and lipids from the blood. In more recent times, Russell Ross has advocated that atherosclerosis is an inflammatory disease.[8]

Encrustation Theory

Encrustation theory by Rokitansky, i.e. small thrombi composed of platelets, fibrin, and leukocytes, collect over foci of endothelial injury, and that organization of such thrombin and their gradual growth, results in plaque formation.

Current Hypotheses

Reaction to injury hypothesis, i.e. lesions of atherosclerosis are initiated as a response to some form of injury to the arterial endothelium (Fig. 13.4).[4-6]

Monoclonal Hypothesis of Atherogenesis

Monoclonal hypothesis of atherogenesis, i.e. genetic or acquired aberrations of "genetic control" of medial cells, leads to their proliferation. Some human plaques, appear to be the progeny of a single cell (i.e.monoclonal or oligoclonal).[7]

Currently, it is believed that atheroselerosis is a disease of multiple origins (Fig. 13.5).

RISK FACTORS FOR ATHEROSCLEROSIS

Modern disturbances of human culture from early childhood contribute to some risk factors and precipitate the epidemic of atherosclerosis.

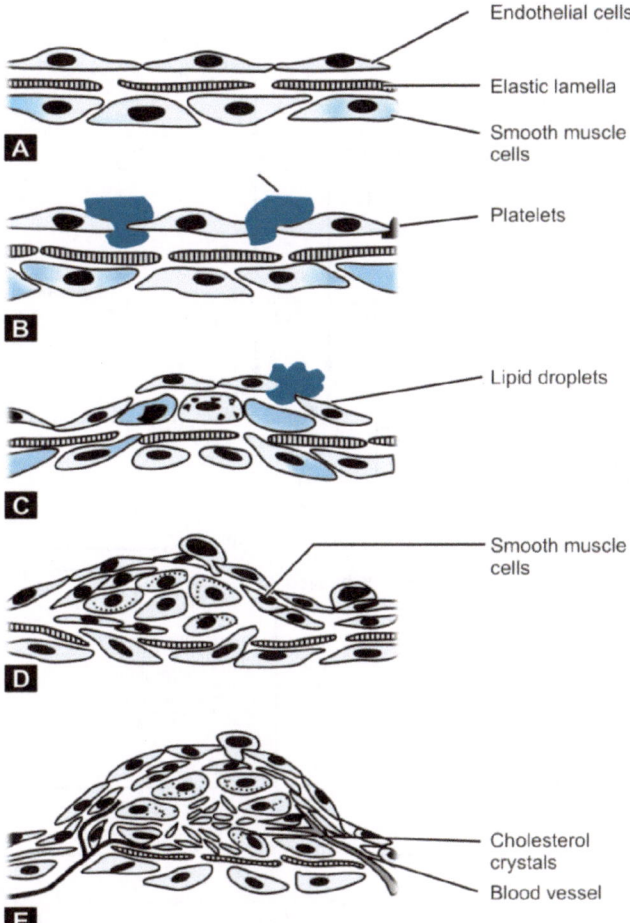

Figs 13.4A to E: Processes in the response to injury hypothesis: A-normal; B-endothelial injury with adhesion of monocytes and platelets (the latter to denuded endothelium); C-migration of monocytes (from lumen) and smooth muscle (from media) into intima; D-smooth muscle proliferation; E-well-developed plaque

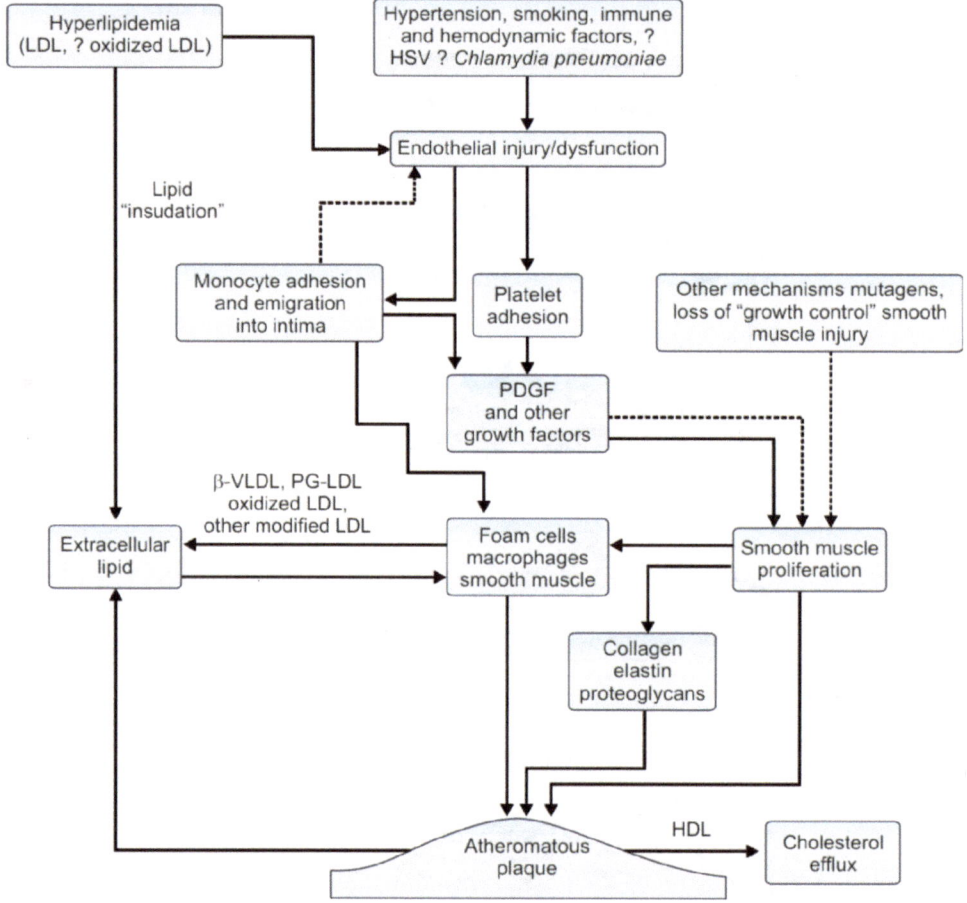

Fig. 13.5:[7] Schematic diagram of a hypothetical sequence of events and cellular interaction in atherosclerosis

The following are risk factors for atherosclerosis:
- *Age:* Clinically overt atherosclerosis, as evidenced by death rates from CAD, rises with each decade of life.
- *Sex:* Death rates due to CAD are higher in male till 55 to 65 years of age, when the incidence in males and females approaches equality. Myocardial infarction is uncommon in premenopausal women.

- *Family history* of premature CAD, cerebrovascular or occlusive peripheral vascular disease (onset <55 years of age in men and <65 years of age in women).
- *Cigarette smoking:* Cigarette smoking is a major independent risk factor for cardiovascular disease. Multiple Risk Factor Intervention Trial (MRFIT) have reported that cessation of smoking will reduce the risk of development of cardiovascular disease. In men who smoke one or more packs of cigarettes per day, the death rate from ischemic heart disease is 70 to 200% higher, than those of non-smokers. In adolescents, atherosclerotic lesions have been seen with increased prevalence in cigarette smokers and HDL-C decreased in adolescent smokers as compared to non-smokers. Chronic cigarette smoking may lead to injury of endothelium which serves as the nidus, for the development of atherosclerosis.
- *Hypertension:* In adults, diastolic BP >105 mm Hg carries a four times higher risk of CAD, than in those with a BP <84 mm Hg.[9]
- *Lipid profile:*
  Decreased HDL-C
  Increased LDL-C
  Increased VLDL-C
  Increased total cholesterol levels
  Increased triglycerides
  This is the kind of unfavorable lipid profile, which is associated with a higher risk of CAD.
- *Diabetes mellitus:* A two-fold increase in the incidence of myocardial infarction is seen in diabetics, as compared to non-diabetics. With the increasing prevalence and severity of obesity in the pediatric population, prevalence of type II diabetes has increased dramatically and risk of cardiovascular disease in the presence of diabetes is increased five folds.[10] However not much is known about the progression of cardiovascular disease in presence of diabetes in the young children and adolescents.

Obesity/Metabolic syndrome (Table 13.2): The prevalence of obesity in children has become more than three fold from 1980 to 2002 and the increase in prevalence of obesity appears to be occurring worldwide. Muscatine and Bogalusa studies have shown that obesity in adolescence is associated with several risk factors for cardiovascular disease including atherogenic dyslipidemia, hypertension, left ventricular hypertrophy and obstructive sleep apnea.

Children and adolescents should be evaluated for being overweight by calculating the Body Mass Index (BMI). This should then be compared with age and sex specific percentiles. Obesity is defined as BMI > 95th percentile, and BMI between 85th-95th percentile is considered at risk of being overweight.

Table 13.2: Metabolic syndrome

• Obesity Atherogenic dyslipidemia ↑ LDL-C, triglycerides ↓ HDL-C Hypertension Hyperinsulinemia Impaired glucose metabolism Inflammation Prothrombotic factors	• Central Obesity

Further research is necessary to determine the optimum definition of the metabolic syndrome. The clustering of risk factors that occur with obesity should be evaluated in the child and they should be treated when the abnormalities are discovered.

- *Physical activity:* A number of cardiovascular health issues have been identified that are related to diminished physical activity. Cardiovascular fitness has been identified as a risk factor for cardiovascular disease in adults and physical fitness probably has both genetic and environmental influences.

  Epidemiological studies in children evaluating the relationship of cardiovascular fitness to lipids and lipoproteins mostly do not show a significant correlation. From the available data, it appears that a minimum of 40 minutes of activity or isometric exercises per day, 5 days per week for 4 months is required to lower triglyceride and increase HDL-C levels. On the other hand, in adolescents with hypertension, aerobic activity programme of 12-32 weeks duration have been shown to have a blood pressure lowering effect. These results suggest that children and adolescents with essential hypertension should be encouraged to engage in aerobic activity to maintain the beneficial effects and it also helps in the management of obesity. Thus it is clear that there are numerous beneficial effects in increasing the level of physical activity in children which may establish better exercise habits into adulthood.
- Increased fibrinogen level has been associated with increased risk of CAD.[11]
- Increased coagulation factor VII is also associated with increased levels of cholesterol and thrombin, both of which predispose to atherosclerosis.[12]
- Decreased fibrinolytic activity.[13]
- Increased plasminogen activator inhibitor (PAI-I).[14]
- *Increased serum homocysteine:* > 16.2 nmol/ml has been associated with an increased risk of atherosclerosis and has been established as an independent risk factor for atherosclerosis.[15]

- *Alcohol:* Moderate consumption of alcohol produces cardioprotection of which 50% is due to increased HDL cholesterol, 18% is due to decreased LDL cholesterol and the remainder is due to decreased thrombogenicity. However, heavy consumption of alcohol over a prolonged period carries an increased risk of CAD.[16]
- *Type A personality and stress:* Type A personalities are highly competitive ambitious and in constant struggle with their environment whereas Type B personalities are passive and less disturbed by environmental stress.
- Type A personality is an independent risk factor for CAD.[17,18]
- Decreased circulating levels of antioxidants,[19] oxidized lipoproteins (Fig. 13.6) which cause
    - Smooth muscle injury
    - Endothelial injury
    - Inhibition of macrophage movement
    - Monocyte chemotaxis
    - Foam cell production

This results in the formation of atheroma.

Increased Lipoprotein (a); Lp(a) > 30 mg/dl is generally considered the threshold at which high risk of premature CAD increases rapidly. Lp(a) is highly thrombogenic and antifibrinolytic by virtue

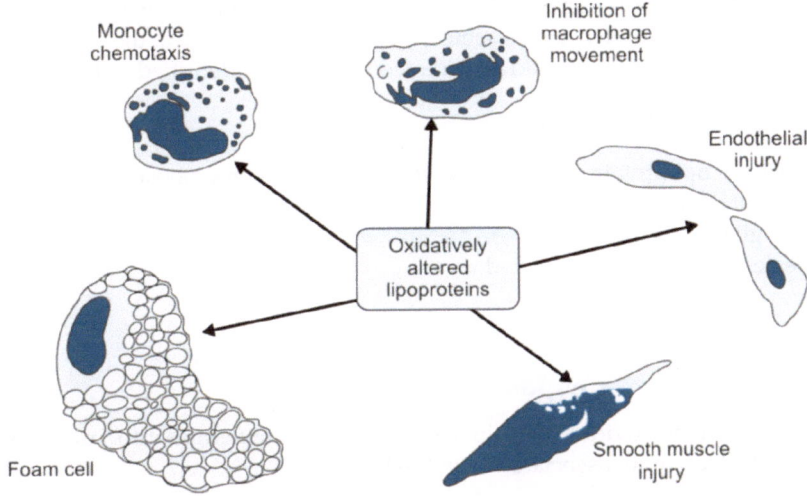

Fig. 13.6: The possible effects of oxidized lipoproteins in atherogenesis

of its structural homology to plasminogen. This genetically determined lipoprotein also promotes early atherosclerosis. Its atherogenecity is 10 fold higher than LDL-C and 15 fold higher than total cholesterol. Therefore, Lp(a) can be called "deadly cholesterol" to distinguish it from HDL-C or the "good cholesterol", LDL-C or the "bad cholesterol" and triglycerides or the "ugly cholesterol". Lp(a) is a strong independent risk factor for premature CAD.[20,21]

Comprehensive Lipid Tetrad Index = Total cholesterol × Triglycerides × Lp(a)/HDL

This index has been proposed as the single best measure of the total burden of dyslipidemia from both nature and nurture. It appears better to explain the markedly different rates of CAD among people of different ethnicity, than any combination of conventional risk factors. Its value varies from approx, 4300 in the Japanese, who have a low incidence of CAD to approx. 24000 in Asian Indians, who have a high incidence of CAD (Table 13.3).
- Possible role of Herpes simplex virus and *Chlamydia pneumoniae*.[8]

These organisms have been identified in atheromatous lesions in coronary arteries and in other organs obtained at autopsy. Increased titres of antibodies to these organisms, have been used as a predictor of further adverse events in patients who have had a myocardial infarction. Nonetheless, there is no direct evidence that these organisms, can cause the lesions of atherosclerosis.

Coronary artery disease is preventable. Death rate due to CAD in Japan is 1/6 in comparison to USA, Australia and European countries. The reason is that their diet is low in saturated fats and rich in omega-3 fatty acids. Prevention can be achieved by breaking the link in the chain of events leading to atherosclerosis. Interventions should be directed against the identified risk factors (Fig. 13.7).

Prevention of Hyperlipidemia

The basic structure of lipoproteins is an outer shell of free cholesterol, phospholipids and apoproteins and an inner core of cholesterol ester and triglycerides. Properties and functions of the major plasma lipoproteins are given in Table 13.4.

Hypercholesterolemia can be classified as:
- Primary
- Secondary

Primary Hyperlipoproteinemias

Fredrickson and Lees have divided the primary hyperlipoproteinemias into 5 phenotypes: Type IV, Types IIa, III, V: The latter are associated with CAD.

Table 13.3: Comprehensive lipid tetrad index by ethnicity and geographic location[1]

	Mean lipid level in mg/dl				
Ethnicity	Index	TC	TG	Lp(a)	HDL
American Whites-men	9342	206	149	14	46
American Whites-women	7318	208	129	15	55
Mexican-Americans-men	6661	202	155	10	47
Mexican-Americans-women	6475	200	142	12	53
Asian Indian in US-Physicians	15024	200	154	20	41
Asian Indian in US-non-Physicians	24035	211	179	21	33
Asian Indian in the UK-men	20629	251	186	19	43
Asian Indian in the UK-women	15615	239	147	20	45
Asian Indian in India-women	10814	196	151	19	52
Asian Indian in India-men	12899	189	182	18	48
Malays in Singapore-men	17349	221	157	15	30
Asian Indians in Singapore-men	22283	218	159	18	28
Asian Indians in Singapore-women	19319	218	131	23	34
Chinese in Singapore-men	11920	215	145	13	34
Chinese In Singapore-women	13211	219	127	19	
Malays in Singapore-women	14266	225	138	17	37
Chinese in Taipei	6471	193	114	15	51
Japanese in Akita	4341	196	106	14	67
American Indian in Arizona	2413	177	160	42	44
Asian Indians CAD patients in UK	37420	236	197	63	41
White CAD patients in UK	18085	233	163	20	42

Adapted from Enas E.A., et al. Indian H J 1996: 49; 25-34. Hughes K.J. Epidemiol Community Health 1997: 51; 394.[1]

Secondary Hypercholesterolemia

All children with LDL levels of atleast 130 mg/dl or more should be evaluated for possible secondary hypercholesterolemia (Fig. 13.8).

Causes of Secondary Hypercholesterolemia

1. *Exogenous factors*
    - Drugs: Steroids, oral contraceptives, beta-blockers, thiazides, anabolic steroids.
        - Alcohol
        - Obesity

2. *Endocrine and metabolic conditions*
   - Hypothyroidism
   - Diabetes mellitus
   - Lipodystrophy
   - Pregnancy
   - Glycogen storage disease
   - Sphingolipidosis
   - Idiopathic hypercalcemia

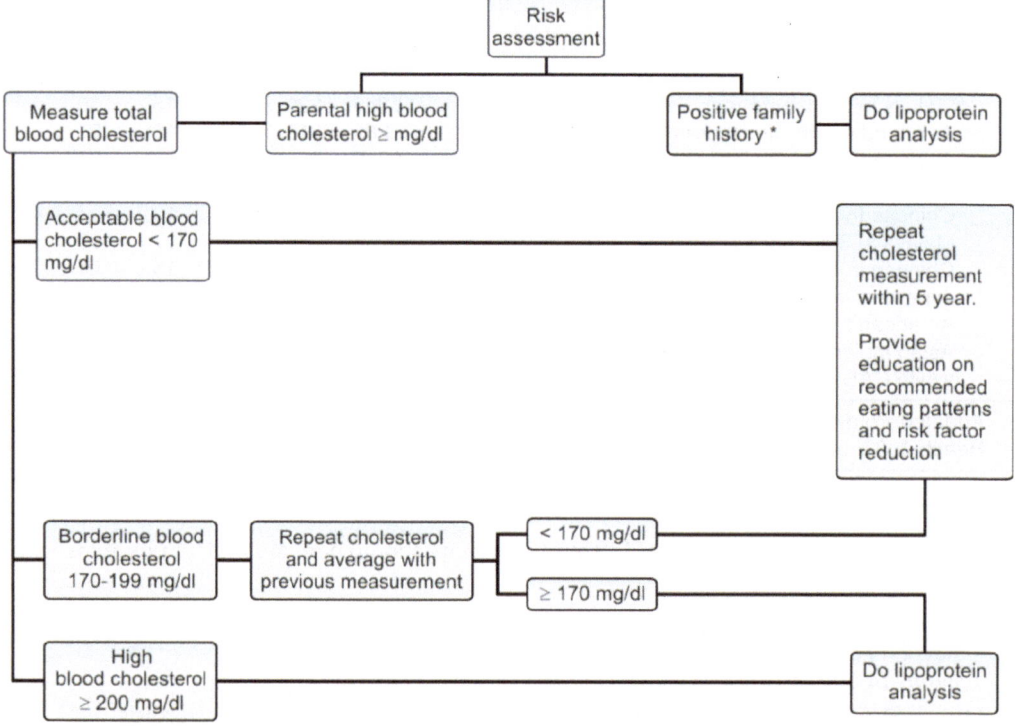

Fig. 13.7: Risk assessment of pediatric atherosclerosis

Table 13.4: Properties and functions of the major plasma lipoproteins

	Chylomicron	VLDC	LDL	HDL
Hydrated density Gm/100 ml)	<0.95	0.95-1.006	1.019-1.063	1.063-1.21
Electrophoresis	Origin	Pre-b	b	a
Major lipid content	Triglycerides (90%) (exogenous)	Triglycerides (55%) Cholesterol (22%) Phospholipid (15%)	Cholesterol (50%) Phospholipid (25%)	Phospholipid (25%) Cholesterol (20%)
Protein content	1%	10%	20%	33%
Apoprotein constituents	B-48 C-I, C-II, C-III A-I, A-II, A-IV E	B-100 C-I, C-II E	B-100	A-I, A-II C-III, C-I, C-II, C-III E
Origin	Intestine Dietary fat	Liver Endogenous Triglycerides	Metabolic product of VLDL catabolism	Liver, intestine catabolism of VLDLs and Chylomicrons
Function	Transports dietary triglycerides	Transports hepatic triglycerides and cholesterol to peripheral tissues to be used as energy or stored as triglycerides	Provides cholesterol to nerve tissue cell membranes, and other tissues for their metabolic needs including steroid hormone synthesis	Participates in reverse cholesterol transport. Provide protection against premature coronary artery disease protection

VLDL – Very low density lipoprotein; LDL – Low density lipoprotein, HDL – High density lipoprotein. Modified from Kwieterovich. PO In: Disorders of lipids and lipoproteind metabolism. In: Rudolph's Pediatrics, Rudolph AM, (ed.), Appleton and Lange, 1991, p 19.

3. *Obstructive liver disease*
   - Biliary atresia
   - Biliary cirrhosis
4. *Nephrotic syndrome*

Cholesterol Lowering Strategies

Expert panel on blood cholesterol levels in children and adolescents:
National Cholesterol Education Panel (NCEP), 1991[22] has recommended two complementary approaches to lower blood cholesterol levels in children and adolescents:

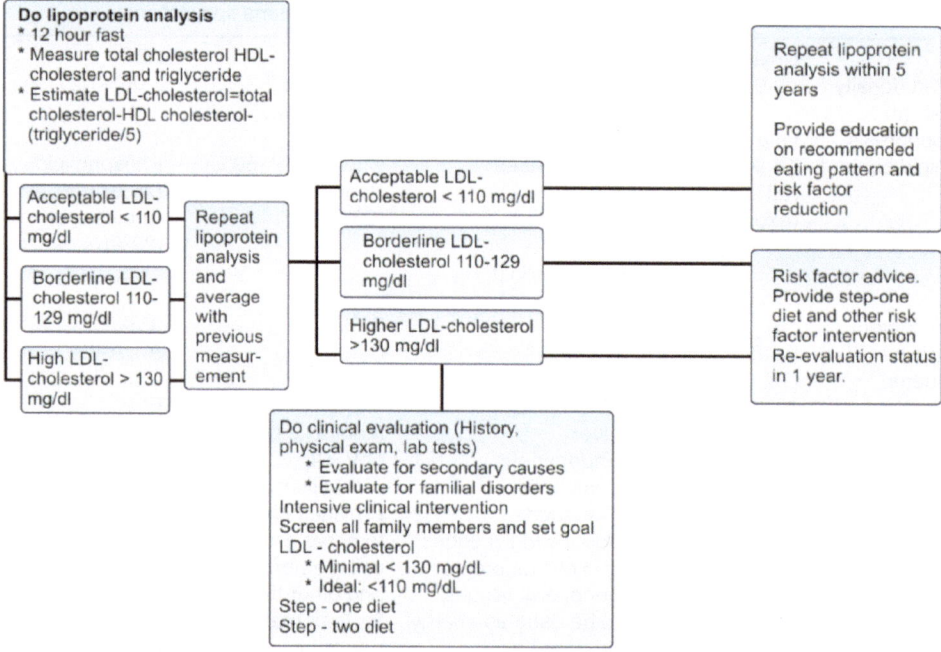

Fig. 13.8: Classification, education and follow-up based on LDL-cholesterol

- Population based approach
- Individualized approach

Population Based Approach

For children > 2 years of age, the following measures are recommended:
1. Nutritional adequacy should be achieved by eating a wide variety of foods.
2. Adequate calories should be provided for normal growth and development.
3. The following pattern of nutrient intake is recommended:
   a. Saturated fatty acids < 10% of total calories.
   b. Total fat not more than 30% of total calories.

c. Dietary cholesterol less than 300 mg per day. Children < 2 years of age, may require a higher percentage of calories from fat.
   d. Limit salt intake < 6 gm/day.

There are three major lipid classes:

Triglycerides

Saturated   65-95%

Monounsaturated
Polyunsaturated
- Arachidonic acid
- Eicosapentanoic acid
- Decosahexapentanoic acid

Phospholipids

Lecithin   1-30%

Sterols

Cholesterol   0-5%
Animal sterols
Plant sterols
Alfalinoleic Acid (ALNA) (18:3, Ω-3) has a double bond on the 3rd carbon atom from the methyl end.

Sources

Chloroplasts of green leaf.
Legumes-linseed, rapeseed, soyabean blackgram, rajmah, lobia-0.5%
Other legumes-0.2%
Fenugreek seeds-(methi)-2%
Linoleic acid (LA) and ALNA yield long chain Ω-3 PUFA (polyunsaturated fatty acids).

Biological Effects of Ω-3 PUFA

- Integral components of structural lipids of membrane bilayers.
- Controls the activity of membrane bound enzymes and transport of various substances hypotriglyceridemic.

- Decreases hepatic synthesis of VLDL
- Doses >3 gm Ω-3 PUFA have a desirable effect on plasma lipid
- Antiplatelet aggregatory-Increases thromboxane A2 (platelet)
    - Decreases prostacyclin PGI2 (endothelial)
    - It is the PGI2/TXA2 balance which maintains vascular homeostasis
    - Antithrombotic activity
    - Decreases insulin secretion therefore, increases the fasting glucose
    - Anti-inflammatory effect
    - Suppresses the immune response.

Linoleic acid (LA) (18:2, Ω-6): LA has a double bond on the 6th carbon atom from the methyl end.

Sources

Oils from plant seeds:
- Groundnut oil (GNO)
- Mustard oil (MO)
- Sunflower oil
- Saffola oil

Except: Coconut oil, cocoa, butter, palm oil

To prevent atherosclerosis, dietary ratio of n-6/n-3 fatty acids should not exceed 10. Oils can be used in combination to achieve the ideal Ω-6/Ω-3 ratio, in the following proportions:[23]

Sesame oil	: MO = 2:1
GNO	: MO = 4:1
Sunflower oil	: MO = 2:1
Saffola oil	: MO = 1:1
Soyabean	: Palmolein = 1:1

In Indian diets, this combination would provide ideal ratios of various fatty acids.

Dietary Advice

Increase PUFA to safe levels.
- Vegetarians can increase ALNA by eating ALNA rich diet.
- Non-vegetarians-100-200 gms fish-twice a week or 30 gms fish/day.[24]

Individualized Approach

This approach identifies and creates children and adolescents at risk of having high cholesterol levels. The "Expert Panel" NCEP recommends selective screening of the following:[22]

1. Children with a positive family history of premature CAD as defined by cardiovascular disease in men < 55 years and women < 65 years of age.
2. Children and adolescents whose parents/grandparents at < 55 years of age had documented:
   - Myocardial infarction
   - Angina
   - Peripheral vascular disease
   - Cerebrovascular disease
   - Sudden cardiac death
3. The offspring of a parent who had total cholesterol level of >240 mg/dl.
4. Children and adolescents whose family history is not available, but other risk factors are present.

TREATMENT

Diet therapy

This is prescribed in two steps that progressively decrease the intake of saturated fatty acids and cholesterol (Table 13.5).

Step-one diet $\xrightarrow{\text{fails}}$ Step-two diet

Drug Therapy

Recommended for children >10 years, if after diet therapy for 6 months-1 year:
1. LDL > 190 mg/dl.
2. Positive family history of premature cardiovascular disease (< 55 years-men, < 65 years-women).

Table 13.5:[22] Nutrient composition of step-one and step-two diets

Nutrient	Step-one diet	Step-two diet
Total fat (% total calories)	< 30%	< 30%
Saturated fatty acids	<10%	<7%
Polyunsaturated fatty acids	Up to 10%	Up to 15%
Monounsaturated fatty acids	10-15%	10-15%
Carbohydrates (% total calories)	50-60%	50-60%
Protein (% total calories)	10-20%	10-20%
Cholesterol (per day)	< 300 mg	< 200 mg
Total calories	To achieve and maintain desirable weight	To achieve and maintain desirable weight

3. Other lipids and lipoproteins
    a. Fasting triglycerides–more than 200 mg/dl.
    b. HDLC–less than 30 mg/dl[24]
4. More than 2 risk factors are present.

Drugs used

1. Bile acid sequestrants (Table 13.6)
    - Cholestyramine
    - Colestipol

    These are the only drugs routinely used in children.
2. Nicotinic acid
3. HMGCoA reductase inhibitors
    - Lovastatin
    - Pravastatin
4. Probucol
5. Fibric acid derivatives
    - Clofibrate
    - Gemfibrozil

Table 13.6: Suggested initial dosage of a bile acid sequestrant for treatment of children and adolescents with family history of hypercholesterolemia

Daily doses	TC and LDL levels after diet (mg/100 ml)	
	TC	LDL
1	<245	<195
2	245-300	195-235
3	301-345	236-280

* One dose is the equivalent of a 9 g packet of cholestyramine (containing 4 g of cholestyramine and 5 g of filler), one bar of cholestyramine or 5 g of Colestipol. FH: Familial hypercholesterolemia; TC: Total cholesterol.

Hypertension: Roots of essential hypertension extend back to childhood, control of blood pressure can significantly decrease the risk for future development of CAD.

Obesity: Screening of obese school children especially from affluent families should be done.

Promotion of physical activity: In the form of drills, PT, yoga, aerobic exercises and walking is beneficial. The physical activity recommended is for 60 minutes/day.

Smoking should be stopped for the children: The prevalence of smoking is increasing between 13-19 years of age. Smoking is today, the commonest risk factor for CAD. Even passive smoking free environment should be created.

Follow-up and evaluation of risk factor intervention: Two year trial should be given to see if interventions have succeeded.

REFERENCES

1. Enas A Enas. Why is there an epidemic of malignant CAD in young Indians? Asian J Clin Cardiol 1999;1:43-55.
2. Barker DJP. The undernourished baby. In: Mothers, Babies and Health in Later Life, 2nd Ed. Churchill Livingstone 1998;129-45.
3. Stary HC, Chandler AB, Dinsmore RE, et al. A definition of advanced types of atherosclerotic lesions and histological classification of atherscelerosis. A report from the committee on vascular lesions of the council on Arterioscler Thromb. Vasc. Biol 1995;15:1512-31.
4. Ross R. The pathogenesis of atherosclerosis. An update. New Engl J Med 1986;314:488-500.
5. Newman WP, Freedman DS, Voors AW, et al. Relation of serum lipoprotein levels and systolic blood pressure to early atherosclerosis. The Bogalusa Heart Study. New Engl J Med 1986;3:24:132-44.
6. Berenson GS, Srinivasan SR, Bao W, et al. Association between multiple cardiovascular risk factors and atherosclerosis in children and young adults. The Bogalusa Heart Study. New Engl J Med 1998;338:1650-56.
7. Benditt EP, Benditt JM. Evidence for a monoclonal origin of human atherosclerotive plaque. Proc Natl Alad. Sci-USA 1973;70:1753-56.
8. Ross R. Atherosclerosis–An inflammatory disease. New Engl J Med 1999;340(2):115-26.
9. Macmohan S, Peto R, Cutler J. Blood pressure, Stroke and coronary heart disease, Part A, prolonged differences in blood pressure; Prospective observational studies corrected for the regression dilution bias. Lancet 1990;335:765-68.
10. Kannel WB, McGee DL. Diabetes and cardiovascular disease: The Framingham study. JAMA 1979;241:2035-38.
11. Heinrich J, Ballerisen L. Schulte H, et al. Fibrinogen and factor VII in the prediction of coronary risk. Results from PROCAM study in healthy men. Arteriosclerosis Thromb 1994;14(1):54-59.
12. Miller GJ. Hemostasis and cardiovascular risk. The British and European Experience. Arch Path Sub Med 1992;116(12):1318-21.
13. Meade TW, Ruddock, Stirling Y, et al. Fibrinolytic activity clotting factor and long term incidence of isochemic heart disease in Northwich Park Heart Study. Lancet 1993;342(8879):1076-79.
14. Jahan-Vague I, Alessi MC. Plasminogen activator inhibitor and atherothrombosis. Thromb. Haemostat 1993;70(1):138-43.

15. Glueck CJ, Shaw P, Lang JE. Evidence that homocysteine is an independent risk factor for atherosclerosis in hyperlipidemic patients. Am J Cardiol 1995;75(2):132-36.
16. Langer RD, Criqui MH, Reed OM. Lipoproteins and blood pressure as biological pathways for effect of moderate alcohol consumption on coronary heart disease. Circulation 1992;85(3):910-15.
17. Lachar BL. Coronary prone behavior: Type A behavior revisited. Texas. Heart Inst J 1993;20(3):143-51.
18. Littman AB. Review of psychosomatic aspects of cardiovascular disease. Psychother Psychosom. 1993; 60(3-4):148-67.
19. Hoffman RM, Garewal HS. Antioxidants and prevention of coronary heart diseases. Arch Int Med 1995; 155:241-45.
20. Scam AM. Lipoprotein (a), a genetic risk factor for premature coronary artery disease. JAMA 1992; 267:3326-29.
21. Enas A Enas. Rapid angiographic progression of coronary artery disease in patients with elevated lipoprotein (a). Circulation 1995;92(8):2353-54.
22. Kromhout D, Bosschieter EB, Conlauder CD. The inverse relation between fish consumption and 20 year mortality from coronary heart disease. N Engl J Med 1985;312(19):1205-09.
23. National Cholesterol Education Program, expert panel on detection, evaluation and treatment of high blood cholesterol in adults (Adult Treatment Panel-II). JAMA 1993;269:3015-28.
24. Kavey RE, Daniels SR, Lauer RM. American Heart Association guidelines for primary prevention of atherosclerotic cardiovascular disease beginning in childhood–Circulation 2003;107(11):1562-66.

Index

A

Abnormal
   blood pressure 110
   chest
      roentgenogram 109
      X-ray 232
   ECG 230
   heart with SVT 69
Accessory pathway re-entry
      tachycardia 51
Acquired heart diseases 3
Acute
   management principles 258
   pericarditis 378
Acyanotic
   pressure overload 145
   volume overload L-R shunt 124
American College of Cardiology 74
American Heart Association 74
Amiodarone 62
Anatomic sites of obstruction to
      pulmonary venous drainage 178
Anatomy and physiology of
      conduction system 42
Anemia 4
Angiotensin
   converting enzyme inhibitors 16
   II receptor blockers 16
Anomalies of aorta 93
Anticoagulation therapy 371
Antimicrobial therapy 368

Anti-rheumatic therapy 276
Aortic
   regurgitation 297
   stenosis 149
   valve disease 297
Arrhythmias 4, 42, 259
Arthritis 269
Associated cardiac
      anomalies 178, 191
Asymptomatic WPW 69
Atrial
   fibrillation 57
   flutter 56
   hypertrophy 230
   septal defect 124
   septostomy 118
Atrioventricular
   block disturbance 65
   re-entrant tachycardia 50
Augmenting myocardial
contractility 10
AV nodal re-entry tachycardia 52

B

Bacterial endocarditis
      prophylaxis 279
Balloon
   angioplasty 119
   valvuloplasty 119, 290
Benefits of fetal echocardiography 238
Beta adrenergic antagonists 17

Blood
   flow 191
   pressure correlation with
      height and weight 24
   pressure measurements 228
Bradyarrhythmias 62
Brock's procedure 196
Bundle branch blocks 69

C

Calcium 29, 33
   channel blockers 16
Cardiac
   arrhythmias 42
   catheterization and
      angiocardiography 136
   functional assessment 97
   imaging 77
   infections 357
   tamponade 385
Cardiomyopathy 330
Cardiovascular sequelae of
      prematurity 243
Carditis 270
Catheter device closure 129
Catheteric intervention procedure 118
Causes of secondary
      hypercholesterolemia 401
Central cyanosis 250
Chagas disease 319
Changes in circulation after birth 112

Chest roentgenography 232
Cholesterol lowering strategies 403
Chorea 273
Chronic
    management 258
    treatment 62
Chylopericardium 383
Classification of
    hypertension 24
    tricuspid atresia 197
Clinical cardiac MR spectroscope 98
Closure of ductus arteriosus 223
Coarctation of aorta 157
Collagen diseases 322
Collete and Edwards
    classification 186
Complete heart block 261
Complication of pericardiocentesis 377
Conditions affecting pericardium 374
Congenital
    heart disease 3, 101, 105, 122
    pericardial defects 384
Congestive cardiac failure 1
Constrictive pericarditis 382
Course of fetal circulation 221
Currective surgery 196
Current hypotheses 394
Cyanosis in newborn 250
Cyanotic
    congenital heart disease 252
    TOF 193
Cytomegalovirus 320

D

Definition of hypertension 24
Device
    closure techniques 119
    therapy 17
Diagnosis and noninvasive
    testing 312
Dilated congestive
    cardiomyopathy 330
Dimensions of cardiac chambers 111

Direct blood pressure
    measurements 228
Disorders of cardiac rhythm and
    conduction 42
Disturbances of atrioventricular
    conduction 260
Diuretics 13
Doxorubicin cardiomyopathy 349
Drainage of pericardial fluid 377

E

Ebstein's anomaly 203
ECG characteristic of SVT 53
Echocardiogram 286
Echocardiographic techniques 89
Eisenmenger syndrome 117
Ejection fraction 86
Electrocardiogram 286
Embryology of heart 214
Encrustation theory 394
Endocardial fibroelastosis 339
Endocarditis 271
Erythema marginatum 273
Evaluation
    in specific cardiovascular
        disorders 93
    of congenital heart disease 93
Evidence of cardiac abnormalitiy in
    newborn 226

F

Factors determining MRI images 97
Fate of subdivisions of heart tubes 215
Features of chronic MR 292
Fertilization to primitive heart
    tube 214
Fetal
    and perinatal circulation 110, 221
    cardiac output 111
    circulation 110, 221
    echocardiography 89, 238
First degree atrioventricular block 66

Formation of external part of heart 217
Full term newborns 259
Fungal endocarditis 370

G

Genetics 340
Giant cell myocarditis 321
Greater
    prematurity 392
    severity 392

H

Hallmark finding 160
Hazards and contraindications of
    MRI 99
Heart 268
    Heart disease 105
    failure
        in the newborn 256
        syndromes 1
    murmurs 249
HIV infection 321
Hyperoxia test 250
Hypertension 4, 408
    in children 22
Hypertensive
    children 29
    emergencies 39
Hypertrophic cardiomyopathy 340
Hypothyroidism 383

I

Ibuprofen 117
Imbibation hypothesis 394
Infants 7
Infectious diseases of pericardium 378
Infective endocarditis 357
Infracardiac type-features 182
Innocent murmurs 249
Inotropic drugs 10
Insulin resistance syndrome 392
Intrapericardial tumors 384

Intrauterine interventions 241
Intravascular echocardiography 90

K

Kawasaki disease 323

L

Large PDA 142
Left
   bundle branch block 70
   ventricular
      hypertrophy 230
      outflow obstruction 167
Lifestyle modifications 33
Long QT interval syndrome 60
Low birth weight newborns 259
Lyme disease 321

M

Magnetic resonance
      imaging 92, 93, 135, 161
Management of
   SVT 53
   ventricular fibrillation 60
   blood pressure in children 25
Mechanisms of postnatal closure 139
Mexiletine 62
Miscellaneous causes of pericardial
      effusion 383
Mitral
   regurgitation 290
   stenosis 283
   valve
      disease 283
      prolapse 294
Mobitz type II atrioventricular
      block 67
Monoclonal hypothesis of
      atherogenesis 394
MRI angiography 98
Mucocutaneous lymph node
      syndrome 323

Myocardial disorders 303
Myocarditis 304, 321

N

Neonatal hypertension 37
Neonates 6
Newborn 23
   cardiac assessment 224
Nitrogen washout test 250
Non-infectious inflammatory
      myocarditis 322
Non-pharmacologic therapy of
      hypertension 32
Normal
   cardiac findings in newborn 214
   ECG 229
   heart with SVT 69

O

Obesity 33, 408
Optimal timing of screening 239

P

Pacemaker
   implantation 74, 75
   in children 73
   types 75
Palliative
   procedure 187
   shunt procedures 196
Parasternal windows 78
Patent ductus arteriosus 138, 243
Pathologic heart murmurs 249
Pathophysiology of ductus
      arteriosus patency 244
Pediatric cardiac MRI
      spectroscopy 99
Pericardial diseases 374, 375
Pericardiocentesis 377
Perinatal
   cardiology 214
   echocardiography 236

Peripheral cyanosis 250
Persistent
   pulmonary hypertension of
      newborn 253
   truncus arteriosus 185
Pharmacological treatment of
      hypertension 34
Phenytoin 62
Phosphodiesterase inhibitors 12
Phospholipids 405
Polyarteritis nodosa 322
Population based approach 404
Potassium 28,
Pre-excitation syndromes 50, 53
Premature
   infant 144
   ventricular contraction 58
Pressure overload R-L-shunt 189
Preterm neonate 242
Prevention of
   hyperlipidemia 400
   sudden cardiac death 348
Primary
   hyperlipoproteinemias 400
   prevention 119
      of atherosclerotic
         cardiovascular disease 389
   prophylaxis 277
Procainamide 62
Prophylaxis 372
Prosthetic valve endocarditis 371
Pulmonary venous obstruction 180
Pulmonic stenosis 145
Purulent pericarditis 378

Q

QRS axis 230
Quinidine 62

R

Radiation pericarditis 384
Radiofrequency energy catheter
      ablation of SVT 69

Radionuclide imaging technique 377
Recognition of
  cardiac
    abnormality 240
    disorders in fetus and
    newborn period 239
  tachyarrhythmias 48
Reducing heart size 13
Relationship of pericardial cavity to heart tubes 216
Restrictive cardiomyopathy 350
Rheumatic
  fever 4, 263
  heart disease 4, 383
Right
  bundle branch block 69
  ventricular hypertrophy 230
Risk factors for atherosclerosis 394
Role of cytokines in myocarditis and dilated cardiomyopathy 311
Ross classification 257

S

Salt 33
Second degree atrioventricular block 67
Secondary
  hypercholesterolemia 401
  prevention 278
Sedation protocol 83
Severity of LV dysfunction 248
Shunt procedures 196

Sinus
  arrhythmia 49
  bradycardia 63
  node dysfunction 64
  rhythm 45
  tachycardia 49
Small PDA 142
Sodium intake 28
Sotalol 62
Specific causes of myocarditis 319
Staphylococcal endocarditis 368
Sterols 405
Subcutaneous nodules 274
Supraventricular tachycardia 50
Sydenham's chorea 273
Sympathomimetic agents 12

T

Tachyarrhythmias 48
Tachycardia 378
Target organ effects 23
Tetralogy of Fallot 189
Third degree A-V block 68, 261
Total anomalous pulmonary venous connection 177
Toxoplasmosis 320
Transient myocardial ischemia 248
Transposition of great arteries 167
Treatment of
  chorea 277
  hypertension 32
  infective endocarditis 118
  intercurrent infection 118
  severe hypertension 38

Tricuspid
  atresia 197
  regurgitation 302
Triglycerides 405
Tubercular pericarditis 380
Two-dimensional echo examinations 238

U

Use of
  indomethacin 117
  indomethacin 247

V

Vaccination 319
Valvular defects 383
Ventricular
  arrhythmia 58
  conduction disturbances 231
  fibrillation 60
  septal defect 130, 167
  tachycardia 58
Viral pericarditis 379
Volume overload R-L shunt 167
VSD classification 130

W

Wolff-Parkinson-White syndrome 53
X-ray
  chest 159, 292, 300
  studies 133, 153, 181, 193, 285, 339